DIPG

ETERNAL HOPE

VERSUS

TERMINAL CORRUPTION

DEAN FACHON

DIPG: Eternal Hope Versus Terminal Corruption

Visit our website at **www.StillwaterPress.com** for more information.

First Stillwater River Publications Edition.

ISBN: 978-1-963296-57-0

Library of Congress Control Number: 2024911769

1 2 3 4 5 6 7 8 9 10
Written by Dean Fachon.
Published by Stillwater River Publications, West Warwick, RI, USA.

Names: Fachon, Dean, author.
Title: DIPG : eternal hope versus terminal corruption / Dean Fachon.
Description: First Stillwater River Publications edition. | West Warwick, RI, USA : Stillwater River Publications, [2024]
Identifiers: ISBN: 978-1-963296-57-0 (paperback) | LCCN: 2024911769
Subjects: LCSH: Fachon, Neil. | Brain—Cancer—Patients—Biography. | Brain—Tumors. | Diagnostic errors. | Medical care—United States. | LCGFT: Biographies.
Classification: LCC: RC280.B7 F33 2024 | DDC: 362.196994810092—dc23

This book is dedicated to everyone who feels abandoned by the very institutions we believed were established to safeguard our Rights.

To Eric,
Let's keep pushing!
Yours,
Dean Jackson

CONTENTS

Freedom. What is it? We view it as the ability to make choices of and for ourselves, so we may live our lives as individuals with free will. Yet, it would seem that humanity's freedom has led it to the brink of chaos. I think freedom is the right to live a natural life unimposed upon by others. But to true freedom, there is more than one's own freedom. To grasp true freedom, one must understand the freedom of others, and in so doing, respect all others with their freedom as deeply and dearly as we hold our own. This includes protecting the balance of our world because if we do not, we eliminate the freedom of all Earth's occupants. I wish I could understand and interpret this more deeply, but it gets confusing. Maybe what I mean by freedom comes back to yin and yang. There is a balance to everything, even freedom.*

— **NEIL FACHON**

* Quotes and phrases from Neil are interlaced throughout his story.

NOTE TO READERS:

While excerpts of Neil's medical reports are included chronologically throughout this text, they were not available to us in real time. It was months later when we finally cut through the red tape to gain access. I include these records to offer insight into Neil's frame of mind and experience.

If the middle of this book seems a chaos of emails, that's reflective of the struggle we were in. Every effort has been made to document the facts of Neil's story. The opinions expressed are those of his parents. This book is not intended as medical advice for any specific condition or treatment.

PROLOGUE

"All of a suddenly" NF

MARCH 3, 2016

It was late afternoon on a sunny day in March. Wendy and I were in our home office, each typing on our respective computers. Wendy is a writer for *Natural Awakenings*, a magazine that promotes healthy living and a healthy planet. I was working on a book about the nature of money and how it has influenced our culture.

In addition to writing, we were spending more time thinking about what comes next in our lives. Both of our children were off to college. We were "empty nesters" and getting used to life after kids. It was time for some changes; it was time to simplify and decongest our lives. Several friends had moved to South Carolina and urged us to come check it out, and a few weeks before, that's exactly what we had done! We liked it so much we were planning our next trip. Of course, a parent never stops being a parent, and our children were never far from our minds. Neil in particular seemed to be caught in a struggle. These were the thoughts occupying our minds on the last day of life as we knew it, then the phone rang:

I picked up the receiver. "Hello?"

"Hey Dad," Neil answered.

"Hi Neil," I said brightly, and Wendy picked up her extension when she heard it was Neil.

"Hi Honey," she said.

"Hi Mom, Dad," he spoke haltingly, subdued. "It turns out you were right to be worried about me. I have a brain tumor."

1

AN INFORMAL INTRODUCTION

"Never underestimate the power you have to touch another person's life." NF

SEPTEMBER 2015

The late summer sun shone on another day at Northeastern University, a metropolitan campus full of life at all hours, everyone energized, motivated, and on the move. For one young man, though, it had been a "really bad day." We'll call him "Glum," and by late afternoon, he just padded back to his dorm and sat hunched on the steps, gently weeping. Other students walked by, most averting their gaze with studied indifference, then a young man approached. Instead of looking away, he looked Glum straight in the eyes, like maybe he cared, but then he strode past and up the steps into the dorm. "Gee thanks," Glum muttered to himself, his head drooping. A moment later, however, the young man returned and sat down next to Glum, handed him a box of tissues, and said, "Hi, I'm Neil. Wanna talk about it?"

Besides having an empathetic character and a dry sense of humor, Neil was a "high honors" student in Northeastern's school of engineering, president of his dorm council, a skilled chess player, a budding philosopher, and a gifted athlete. These qualities had drawn him into a group of like-minded friends, knit together in the academic and social rigors of freshman year. Now a sophomore, Neil was happy to be back on campus. His older sister Evie was a Northeastern student too, but she was in New Zealand on a work-internship — a semester-long "co-op." There was no one to look over Neil's shoulder. He was on his own, and he seized every opportunity: He was thinking hard about pledging the Eta Zeta Chapter of Beta Theta Pi, a fraternity well-known on campus for its academic excellence and civic commitment. Neil also planned to try out once again for Northeastern's club tennis team, a dream sustained through diligent practice after a disappointing tryout freshman year. Then, there was the "slackline" in Centennial Park. From the first moment he saw it during a campus visit two summers before, the slackline tugged at Neil like a magnet. He loved testing his balance and making friends with other kids doing likewise.

Most things were right with Neil's personal world. If something wasn't, he would come up with a strategic plan to help make it better. This was a skill honed by long hours playing chess: at the age of twelve, Neil was ranked among the top fifty players his age in the US. He eased back from the game when he entered high school, but he still ranked as an "expert," and he was eager to play the chess game of life. He was thirsty for experience and knowledge — a sponge for profound thoughts and teachings, which he used to help analyze events. In notes for a piece he was writing, he juxtaposed the following:

> "All the world is a stage, and all the men and women merely players. They have their exits and their entrances, and one man in his time plays many parts." —*William Shakespeare*

> "Every day is a journey, and the journey itself is home."
> —*Matsuo Basho*

Upon these coupled quotes, Neil elaborated:

> *"Throughout our lives, we all go through countless challenges. Sometimes, these challenges can overwhelm us — work overload, health difficulties, relationship troubles. We ourselves swivel and swerve as these challenges confront us, and with*

them, we change as people. Our worlds change along with the settings of our lives and the people of our company.

We go through stages in life, playing all sorts of roles — son/daughter, grandson/granddaughter, neighbor, student, friend, teammate, acquaintance, observer, counselor, counseled, employee, boss, lover, caretaker, father/mother, grandfather/grandmother, problem solver, problem creator, follower, leader. And through these roles, we interact with others. Every person you observe, every friend you hug, every smile you share defines a piece of you.

As we go through life, there are innumerable hellos and goodbyes, some marking mere moments or single interactions, and others marking entire chapters. But no matter what, these events make up who we are in life. Life isn't a destination or a goal. Life is a journey."

Neil tried to anticipate life's twists and turns and make intentional adjustments to help bring about positive outcomes. He tried to be logical and pragmatic, but of course — as with most college students — "making the world a better place" was his principal goal.

2

CONCUSSIONS

"Don't bulldoze through time.
Let time flow through you." NF

LOW BRANCH

One moment, Neil was running like a gazelle, six feet tall and one hundred fifty-five pounds of agility. The next, he was stopped — dead in his tracks. He was playing "capture the flag" with friends at one of Northeastern's spiritual centers. Plunging through some bushes to evade an opponent, he did not see the tree branch at head level as he popped out from the bushes. The impact nearly threw him off his feet, and he stood dazed, hands on knees.

Everyone froze. "Are you okay?"

"Yeh," Neil nodded gingerly, panting. "Didn't see that coming!" He rubbed his forehead and could feel a lump forming. "Maybe I'll guard home base for a while."

"Maybe you should go get some ice," a teammate suggested.

"And a dubbie!" another joked.

Neil shook his head gingerly. "I guess you're right." Waving goodbye, he started back toward his apartment.

The next day, his head was still aching. It didn't help much that a month earlier, before school had even begun, he and his best friend from home, Andrew, had been horsing around, and Neil ended up getting punched in the head. He wasn't knocked out then, but it hurt, and now this. He decided to visit the school's infirmary.

Northeastern Clinic, September 10, 2015 excerpts:

Chief complaint: ?concussion.
This well appearing 19 year old man was punched in the head one month ago with no loss of consciousness and then hit his head on a tree branch while running yesterday, again with no loss of consciousness or fall.

Plan:
Head Injury NOS (Neurological Outcome Scale) - 959.01 (head injury, unspecified).
Notes: Pt was reassured his recent head injuries were <u>mild concussions at worst</u> and that sufficient recovery time passed between episodes to avoid hit on hit situation.

After his visit, Neil breathed a sigh of relief, perhaps even recalling the "headgear" we made him wear when he first started playing soccer — to protect his "chess-head." The headgear had singled him out for some ribbing from his teammates, but as his skills became evident, the jibes

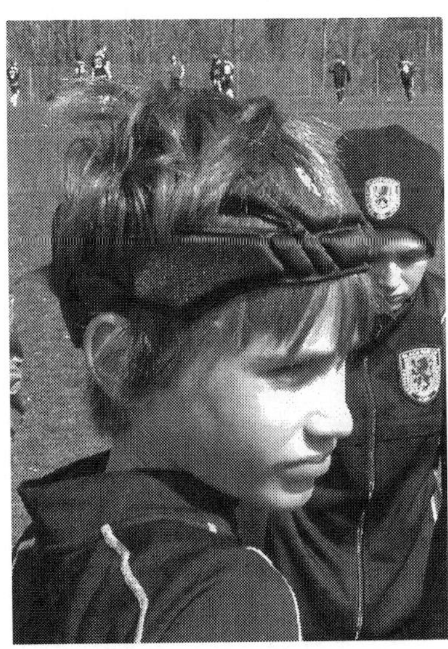

stopped, and the headgear helped earn him the nickname of "Ninja" on his middle school soccer team. Such recollections might have put a smile on his face as he digested the doctor's report. Thankfully, it was nothing to tell us about. He just stowed the episode in his mental footlocker and resumed his normal routine. His school year was going well; he liked his professors; his classes were challenging; he loved his friends; the fraternity continued to encourage his interest; and he continued playing tennis.

Tennis: Neil loved the game, but unlike his chess career, which began very early, he was a late bloomer at tennis. His high school tennis coach had been reluctant to bring Neil on board — a sophomore with almost no experience — but she liked his will to improve, his relentlessly positive attitude, and his work ethic She hoped these traits would rub off on the team, so she brought him on board as a backup. From there, Neil worked his way up to playing third doubles at the start of his junior year. By the end of his senior year, he was playing third singles, and his wins helped the team take second place in their state division. Neil brought this momentum to tryouts for Northeastern's club team. He did not make the cut freshman year, but he kept his head in the game and practiced as much as he could — whenever he could. He even started a tennis-partnering club to help students find someone to hit with. His effort was paying off, and Neil felt good about his chances of making the club team this time around — as a sophomore again.

EARLY WARNINGS
OCTOBER 2015

While school life was rewarding, its demands took their toll, so Neil looked forward to taking a break at our upcoming family reunion at Migis Lodge in Maine. Wendy and I had made plans to pick him up on our way north, and he was packed and ready to go when we pulled up to his dorm. During the ride, he filled us in with great gusto on his latest activities, briefly mentioning his capture the flag incident.

"It was a mild concussion at worst," he assured us. "I've got it covered."

This pricked our parental concern, but he was nineteen and taking charge of his life, so we held our tongues.

With Evie off-campus on co-op, Neil planned to spend lots of Migis-time with his cousin Christopher, especially playing tennis. Chris is an advanced player, and throughout the weekend, the boys traded some aggressive volleys, with Chris often getting the upper hand. This frustrated Neil. He was having some trouble with his "ground strokes." Nonetheless, their competition was great entertainment. When they weren't hitting tennis balls, they were playing Frisbee golf, shuffleboard, or ping-pong; kicking around a soccer ball; kayaking; or "banging heads" over a chess board, where Neil was indomitable.

At the close of the weekend, Migis held a dinner party with a band and dancing. Neil and Chris were particularly full of mirth, and for much of the time, Neil wore a Cheshire grin, which drew smiles from all those around him. When the dance music took over, he swayed like a willow in swirling winds, so loose as to be almost comical, and he was quick to laugh. We chalked it up to "high" spirits (he was in college, after all) and enjoyed the evening with everyone else. The next morning, we left early enough to return Neil to school for his classes, then Wendy and I headed home.

Life resumed its normal course at home and at school, and soon thereafter, Neil was invited to join the tennis team. Hooray! He was thriving, or so we believed. Unfortunately, Neil took a backwards fall off the slackline. Perhaps it happened while he was celebrating his new status as a club tennis player. We'll never know. But the jolt was sufficient to send him back to the campus clinic:

Northeastern Clinic, October 27, 2015 excerpts:

Chief Complaints: Concussion
19 year old male seen 1 month ago for 2 head injuries felt to be mild post traumatic head aches or mild concussions. Now had another injury where he fell off a slackline and hit back of head. No loss of consciousness. This was three

> weeks ago. Now still having mostly visual symptoms where increased exertion in tennis will cause him to have some difficulty tracking ball, and he is inaccurate with hits and "seeing double" when trying to track ball. Intermittent mild headaches, but denies other symptoms, no nausea/emisis, no dizziness, no cognitive slowing/decline noted.
>
> **Assessment:**
> Unspecified injury of head, initial encounter - S09,90XA (Primary) possible delayed/persistent vestibular and convergence problems s/p head previous head injuries. Appears to have little to no other symptom domain problems and normal neuro exam.
>
> **Plan:**
> Recommend seeking vestibular PT with Dr. H of MGH Sport PT/ RTC for any other concerns or with persistent/worsening symptoms.

Translation: Neil was having trouble with his peripheral vision — with seeing objects off to the side unless he turned his head. He was also having trouble tracking objects that were moving across his field of vision — things like tennis balls. This made it difficult to practice with the team. After his visit to the clinic, Neil felt compelled to make an admission.

> **To: Dean & Wendy Fachon**
> **From: Neil Fachon**
> **Subject: Concussion**
> **Date: Tue, 27 Oct 2015 20:26:11 -0400**
>
> Hey Mom and Dad,
>
> I am sorry to say it, but I do in fact have a concussion... back to back concussions actually. In the past 2 and a

half months I have had 3 head traumas. The first one was at the beginning of August, and I honestly didn't want to tell you guys because I didn't want to say how it happened, I didn't want you to worry, and I wasn't really feeling any symptoms so I didn't want to make a mountain out of a mole hill. I kind of figured it would just go away and wouldn't really matter.

The second trauma was a month after in the first week of the semester when I was playing a game similar to capture the flag with friends at the catholic center. Running back with the flag I went through some brush and hit my head on a tree branch. After this one, I went to health services and based on their diagnostic they told me it was no worse then a mild concussion and that I could continue with my life pretty much normally just making sure to get plenty of sleep, not to over exert myself, or to eat to much sweets. They even said I was fine to try out for the tennis team. Also, despite being after a previous concussion they said that there was enough elapsed time between the two concussions that the second should not have been impacted by the first. So once again, I realize I should've told you guys, but I didn't want to make a big deal out of it.

The third one happened about 3 weeks ago, or another month after the previous one. I was slack lining and trying to learn a new trick when I flipped off and hit my head on the ground. Happening a month after the previous concussion, having hit a different part of my head, and not thinking the blow was that hard (I braced my fall with my arms a little and it was from a sitting position not a standing one) I figured once again that it was just a mild concussion and that the doctor wouldn't tell me anything he hadn't told me the last time I saw him. So... I didn't visit the doctor again until tonight.

For the past 3 weeks I have been having difficulty with my vision. I'd had a little bit of difficulty after the first 2, but it wasn't too bad and I figured it would get better. On a day to day basis I am relatively fine, but when doing physical activities I get double vision. The more strenuous the activity the worse my focus. So immediately after the impact I cut out all athletics except working out and slowly but surely I brought the physical activities back on. My first really physical activity after that fact was playing tennis with Chris at Migis. I was having a little difficulty with my vision then, but I was able to play through it alright. The following week, I tried to play dodge ball with my intramural team however and that was pretty bad, so I quit that altogether. The same week I played tennis with Marcus though and I once again was able to play fairly well without too significant a trouble.

Fast forward to yesterday at my first practice with the tennis team, 3 weeks after the last concussion. I figured after this point I should be fine, however the combination of the bright indoors lights and the fast paced drilling nature of practice, and I had a very tough time handling it. After this weekend I was already planning to see the doctor again, but that confirmed that I needed to. I saw the doctor today, about an hour ago now and he said most of the same things as the last doctor said. You look fine, you're performing well enough on the little tests I gave, but clearly strenuous physical activity clouds your vision. He says I am in no danger and that performing physical activity is fine for me, but that I just need to avoid overdoing it and take breaks when necessary. He did however refer me to a physical therapist to get some possible therapies for my vision. I am going to call her tomorrow and set up an appointment. There will be a copay for it. I will pay out of pocket for it.

I thought it was about time I let you know, and I'm sorry I didn't tell you guys sooner. I imagine that you're probably angry that I didn't, and I know that I really should've. Having never had a concussion before I definitely underestimated its severity and seriousness.

School work is going fine, and I'm handling the stress of life without too much difficulty. It's really just my vision and physical activities which are giving me a lot of trouble. I'll keep you posted on the physical therapy, in the meantime I am going to continue trying to practice with the team because I clearly can't just stop after a first day. I'll just plan to take it easy and to go at my own pace. Regarding other activities I'm sure you might be worried about, no I am not doing physical activities other than tennis, working, and intramural soccer every other week for half an hour. No, I am not slack lining at all, and yes I am staying away from alcohol.

I'll talk to you guys soon.

Lots of Love,
Neil

GET AN MRI!

Huh? We wondered if something might have been wrong at the family reunion. Neil had struggled with tennis, and at times, he'd seemed a little too giddy, as if he were trying to compensate for something. He had been trying to handle his own affairs, but this condition was too much to keep from his parents. We called him immediately.

"Hey," he picked up. "You got my email."

"Oh yes," Wendy answered. "Quite a surprise."

"I know," he said quietly. "Not a good one."

"I'll say," I agreed. "After all those years wearing headgear, too."

"Okay, okay," he pushed back gently. "I'm doing okay."

"You should go see a neurologist," Wendy coached him. "Don't mess around."

"I'm not messing around," he said. "But I hear you."

"Seriously," I added. "And get an MRI."

"Okay," he answered. "I will."

"What else is going on?" Wendy asked to lighten the mood.

"The Husky Hunt is coming up," he said, his animation returning. "I'm pulling together a team."

"First things first," I said, doubtless rolling my eyes. "Your health is number one."

"Agreed," he acknowledged. "But it's not like I'm going to just drop everything."

"No one is saying that," Wendy added. "But you need to take more care of yourself."

"I hear you," he said. "We may not even make the cut," he explained. "Just to be in the Husky Hunt, teams have to qualify."

"Cross that bridge when you get to it," I suggested. "Get checked out."

The conversation wrapped up with his promise to get an appointment, and Wendy followed up later that evening to emphasize our concerns.

To: Neil Fachon
From: Wendy Fachon
Subject: Re: Concussion
Date: Tue, 27 Oct 2015 20:57

Take a deep breath, and go see a neurologist, ASAP. Bring

along the documentation you have typed in the email. Ask about getting an MRI. You have health insurance for a reason.

Was the first concussion the pole in Josh's basement? I'd say "no" on the Husky Hunt, Honey.

Love,
Mom

* * *

To: Wendy Fachon, Dean Fachon
From: Eugene (Neil) Fachon
Subject: Re: Concussion
Date: Tue, 27 Oct 2015 21:31:11 -0400

As far as the husky hunt goes, if we do make it, I am planning to be one of the brains of the operation making sure everything is organized and people are working well together. Last year we had poor organization which led to a lot of people becoming disenchanted and stop trying. Also people didn't know what exactly to do or when to do it, so I was already planning to be more of an organizer than a biker this year. At this point I would probably give my bike and my helmet to someone else because we still need as many bikes as we can get. Although, this is all if we do in fact make it.

"If we do in fact make it." Leave it to Neil to be thinking game strategy just in case. I could not help but smile, and the next morning, I sent him a hug:

To: "Eugene (Neil) Fachon"
From: Dean Fachon

Subject: How are you doing today?
Date: Wed, 28 Oct 2015 10:04

Just thinking of you.
Hug,
Dad

* * *

To: Dean Fachon
From: "Eugene (Neil) Fachon"
Subject: Re: How are you doing today?
Date: Wed, 28 Oct 2015 14:34

Heya, I'm doing fine. I've been living with whatever brain problems I have for awhile, so I don't really notice anything out of the ordinary other than my vision and I haven't been doing much since Monday so that hasn't been much of a problem either. I have my math midterm tomorrow, so I am studying up for that today. Found out earlier that we made the Husky Hunt, which is great! So now we have some planning to do for that. I'll probably just be an organizer from a main base so I shouldn't be doing too much running around. Though it would still be good to get my bike and helmet here at some point, so I can give them to someone else to use. Also have my first tennis team party coming up this Friday which should be sweet! I've wanted to go to one for awhile but obviously, this is the first one I can attend.

* * *

To: "Eugene (Neil) Fachon"
From: Dean Fachon
Subject: Re: How are you doing today?
Date: Wed, 28 Oct 2015 15:30

Did you get an appointment with a neurologist? That's more important than hunting or partying.

* * *

To: Dean Fachon
From: "Eugene (Neil) Fachon"
Subject: Re: How are you doing today?
Date: Wed, 28 Oct 2015 18:28:57 -0400

I went to the clinic but I have to go back tomorrow morning because the doctor who writes referrals wasn't there.

* * *

To: "Eugene (Neil) Fachon"
From: Dean Fachon
Subject: Re: How are you doing today?
Date: Wed, Oct 28, 2015 at 6:50 PM

This is priority one. Everything else distant 2nd. Keep us posted.

* * *

To: Dean Fachon
From: "Eugene (Neil) Fachon"
Subject: Re: How are you doing today?
Date: Wed, 28 Oct 2015 21:28

I realize. I'll be going to NUHS *(Northeastern University Health Services)* right after my math test tomorrow.

Upon his return to NUHS, Neil was told he could not get a referral until the following week. We cannot recall what the exact reason was, but now our parental instincts were on full alert, so we told him we'd start looking for other resources he could contact directly.

To: "Eugene (Neil) Fachon"
From: Dean Fachon
Subject: Neurology department, Mass General
Date: Thu, Oct 29, 2015 at 2:07 PM

Neil,

Here is a link to the neurology dept at Mass General.

http://www.massgeneral.org/neurology

To set up an appointment:

If you are a new patient to MGH, the first step to making an appointment with MGH Neurology is to register as an MGH patient and get a medical ID number by calling 1-866-211-6588. The next step is to call the Neurology department at 855-644-6387, and a patient care coordinator will assist you in finding the most appropriate neurologist for your condition. Business Hours: 8:00 am to 4:30 pm.

It would be worth calling to create an ID if you can. You will no doubt have to hold for a few minutes. Have your insurance info available. If they throw up road blocks about waiting for Northeastern, explain that you've had three concussions in three months and Northeastern is making you wait until next week just to get a referral. Hopefully that will clear a path. Then call the department to set up an appointment. Be sure to explain the complete history for this situation. That should open the door to a prompt appointment.

We have other feelers out too. Whatever comes through first. Call when you can.

Oh, are you taking any aspirin or other pain killers?

Talk soon,
Dad

* * *

To: Dean Fachon
From: "Eugene (Neil) Fachon"
Subject: Re: Neurology department, Mass General
Date: Thu, 29 Oct 2015 17:42:14 -0400

No, I rarely ever take anything. Elderberry juice and vitamin C pretty much the only things I use. I have an account number at MGH now that I set up to get an appointment for physical therapy next Thursday, so I'll try calling tomorrow and asking about the neurologist – letting them know about the wait on the referral.

By the way, did a little research myself. The part of the brain associated with vision the most is the Occipital Lobe which is in the back of my head where the last hit I received occurred. Also, I figured out that I have kind of a "blind spot", so to speak. At the corner of my right eye is where I have the worst focus, so thats roughly where the center of my left eye is looking and further left. This would also explain why tennis was so tough because I hit mostly forehands and you turn that side of your body towards the ball to hit a forehand. Also I was worse at volleys cross court from the Deuce side as opposed to when I was on the Ad side. Not sure what exactly this means for my brain and what's damaged, but it does give me a way to try and work around my weakness and to tell the doctors when they are trying to figure out what's wrong.

Oh yeah, pretty sure I aced my math test today btw, so I'm doing well right now. : ^) I'll call MGH again tomorrow.

Lots of love,
Neil

* * *

To: "Eugene (Neil) Fachon"
From: Dean Fachon
Subject: Re: Neurology department, Mass General
Date: 10-29-15, 6:12 PM

Yes, call the neurology department first thing - 8AM sharp. Explain EVERYTHING. Hopefully they will find a way to see you tomorrow. A cab might be the fastest way to get there. If you take one, just be sure to get in and out carefully. As for PT, not worth much until you have a thorough work-up, including MRI or CAT scan, to know what is going on and the best way to approach it. Hopefully any "damage" will heal, but could take a long time. Need to be extra careful. Seriously. Must say, the medical folks at NE are not earning any points in East Greenwich. Very disappointed with their nonchalance. Glad to hear the test went well. Keep us posted. If we don't talk to you before, go easy on the late nights and parties this weekend. No drinking, obviously, but no antics, and try to get a solid 8+ hours of sleep every night.

Love,
Dad and Mom

By this time, we were also reaching out to friends and family in the medical field, looking for any advice that might be useful for Neil's situation. One such contact came through Wendy's brother Jeff, who is good friends with Dr. Drew Breen, a family physician. As luck would have it, Dr. Breen's wife also happened to be a neurologist.

To: "Eugene (Neil) Fachon"
From: Dean Fachon
Subject: Re: Concussion
Date: On Thu, Oct 29, 2015 at 7:20 PM

From Uncle Jeff's friend. Pay attention to this:

> ***On Oct 29, 2015, at 11:28 AM, Dr. Drew Breen wrote:***
>
> Hi Jeff--Sorry to hear your nephew has been concussed. General common sense advice includes: no sports, concerts, nor high-stimulation activities; limiting close-up screen time; lots of rest; and staying well-hydrated. I would also suggest Neil discuss his situation with his advisor at school - so his teachers are aware of his struggles. Academic stress can interfere with mood and sleep and make things worse.
>
> Good Luck, Drew

* * *

To: Dean Fachon
From: "Eugene (Neil) Fachon"
Subject: Re: Concussion
Date: Fri, 30 Oct 2015 00:27:29 -0400

I'm keeping my stuff to a minimum, and I'm going easy at tennis. I can't cut it out though, not unless I have no choice. And I have been pretty low key with everything though I also can't miss my first tennis get-together. I'll just stay aware of myself and know if I need to step out.

> Screen time is tough to cut out but I can try. I've been staying well hydrated and rested, and I have a meeting with my adviser tomorrow regarding class registration, but I'm not really feeling stressed and [school] work hasn't been a struggle. My biggest stress is simply not being able to see well when I might want to.

Which would be pretty much when your eyes were open, I wanted to shout. While Neil was doing his best to advance the situation, a part of him seemed a bit too cavalier — the "invincible youth" — so we kept up a steady drumbeat.

> **To: "Eugene (Neil) Fachon"**
> **From: Dean Fachon**
> **Subject: Re: Concussion**
> **Date: Fri, 30 Oct 2015 8:14AM**
>
> That's why it's so important to see a neurologist and get an MRI. Seeing well all the time would pretty much be the goal... We'd like to visit on Sunday – for brunch maybe – if you have time. Have some things to bring. Let us know what transpires with your MGH conversation.
>
> Big hug,
> Dad

* * *

> **To: Dean Fachon**
> **From: "Eugene (Neil) Fachon"**
> **Subject: Re: Concussion**
> **Date: Fri, 30 Oct 2015 13:47**
>
> God damn this medical system needs some industrial

> engineers to fix it's problems – holy crap! Just got off the phone with a woman in the neurology department telling me I couldn't get an appointment until December and that if I wanted to get my head checked out sooner I'd need to go to the emergency room. What a load of bull crap. I am currently emailing with a neurologist at MGH, and I fully explained my situation and he says he'd be willing to see me so I'm really hoping I can set some sort of appointment up there. This sh*t is taking way too much time though to figure out.

No kidding! His frustration was ours. It shouldn't be taking this long to schedule a test that seemed critical! Of course, hindsight is always twenty-twenty, and we should have insisted he go to the emergency room. But we didn't.

> **To: "Eugene (Neil) Fachon"**
> **From: Dean Fachon**
> **Subject: Re: Concussion**
> **Date: Fri, 30 Oct 2015**
>
> Okay. Frustrating, but sounds like some progress. Fingers crossed here. Good luck and talk later, if possible.
> Dad

Fortunately, Halloween presented a great opportunity to offset our growing chagrin with a bit of distraction. We sent Neil a photo of him and his sister from ten years before. He was dressed as a pile of leaves — literally. It was a costume Wendy made. She stitched autumn-colored plastic leaves to a cape she made using a leaf-patterned fabric. Coupled with camouflage paint on his face, Neil could crouch low to the ground, gather the cape over himself, and look just like a small pile of leaves.

NOVEMBER 2015

To: Dean Fachon
From: "Eugene (Neil) Fachon"
Subject: Re: Happy Halloween!
Date: Sun, 1 Nov 2015 01:27

Oh my god, I remember that, loved that costume! I think that was honestly my favorite costume!

To celebrate Halloween at Northeastern, Neil had dressed up as Link, the hero in Nintendo's game, *Zelda*. Of his time out and about with his friends, Neil told us people driving by would shout, "LINK!" and wave. Even if it was just for a few hours, he was glad to set his worries aside and submerge in his universe, and we were glad for him.

Otherwise, Neil's difficulty getting a timely appointment with a neurologist continued. We later learned that he'd managed to reach one doctor (or the doctor's receptionist), but something about the conversation just didn't feel right to Neil, so his anxiety led him down the one available path he knew.

Northeastern Clinic, November 3, 2015 excerpts:

Chief Complaints:
19 year old male presents for referral - see previous notes from concussions.
Patient discussed with his parents who felt he needed to see a neurologist and get an MRI. Still doing well except for visual symptoms with tennis.

Assessment:
Concussion without loss of consciousness, initial encounter - S06.0X0A (Primary)

> discussed with patient that I am a concussion specialist and [there is] lack of need for MRI. He would still like to get second opinion.

Of course, we never saw this report until months later. The "Health Insurance Portability and Accountability Act" (HIPAA) forbade us from seeing any of Neil's medical reports, but in our next phone conversation, Neil adopted the confidence of this particular doctor.

"I saw a concussion specialist at the clinic who said MRIs don't tell anything about concussions," his voice held a note of finality. Some push-back again.

"Okay," we demurred, but after the call, Wendy had to comment.

"It reminds me of when Neil was a toddler," she started. "You remember this story? He and I were playing in the basement. [It had barn-board walls and a plush padded carpet — an ideal "romper room."] I was chasing Neil around the play gym [a Little Tikes gem that was his castle], the evil dragon in pursuit of the brave knight." Her eyes smiled. "I'll never forget when he suddenly stopped, turned around, and brandished his toy sword. He spoke his first complete sentence: 'You have no power here!' Game over."

Yes, I remembered that precious story. Now, Neil was telling us once again that we had no power. He had the situation under control, so we shouldn't try to make it our business. Of course, he was technically correct. As parents of a nineteen-year-old, we were prohibited from seeing his medical records or contacting his doctors without Neil's explicit written permission, all in accordance with HIPAA. Heck, even his school records were off-limits unless he gave us explicit permission to see them. Neil told us what he wanted to tell us — and he was generally open — but when it got down to brass tacks, we had no power.

3

SPORTS THERAPY

"Find something to be passionate about and jump on board." NF

For his next doctor's appointment, Neil went to Mass General to have a "neurologic evaluation" with Dr. Lenore Herget. The appointment was under the aegis of sports therapy:

> ***MGH Sports Physical Therapy, November 5, 2015 excerpts:***
>
> Physical Therapy Neurologic Evaluation - Post Concussion Syndrome
>
> **Patient Profile:**
> Patient is right-handed male, referred to PT by NUHS with a diagnosis of post concussion syndrome, and chief complaint of headaches and dizziness.
>
> **History of present illness/condition:**
> Patient has sustained 3 concussions over the past few months in August (punched in the face during a fight). September (playing capture the flag and front of head hit tree) and October (was on a slack/tightrope line and fell backward and hit back of his head).

Dizziness initially with all three. Did not recover fully from either of the first 2 concussions (sleep schedule off, blurred vision when running, etc.) After the 3rd concussion, this got worse. Started club tennis at NEU and it was too difficult to track the ball.

Saw HUHS last week.
Next week sees a Neurologist at Children's [Hospital].

Imaging: none.

Home Exercise Program:
Head Turns: Vestibular Ocular Reflex, (VOR) exercise 1. Target must remain clear and stable throughout exercise.

Place "X" card at arms-length distance from you. With eyes focused on "X," move your head side to side at rate of 50-beats per minute. Make sure "X" remains clear the entire time. If there is even the slightest blur to X, slow the speed down (as blurriness not beneficial). Repeat the entire cycle 10 times total side to side.

Then do the same, but moving your head up and down at rate of 80-beats per minute. Again, slow down if any blurriness. Repeat this 10 times total up and down.

As long as your symptoms do not increase, do this routine multiple times (at least 3) throughout the day.

Neil commenced physical therapy for his eyes with determination and positivity, the hallmarks of his personality. He just knew if he worked hard enough, he'd get better. And why not? He was living his "immortal" years. As instructed, he performed these exercises at least three times per day, but otherwise, he was glad to just plunge back into the life of a Northeastern student-athlete.

Classes went well (he consistently made the "Dean's List"); his connection with the brothers at Beta Theta Pi grew increasingly rewarding; and his participation in the tennis team's practice sessions and social events seemed destined to be the highlight of his year. His biggest complaint was the trouble he had with tracking the tennis ball, but he was devising strategies to help compensate for the handicap. In short, he was putting his worries behind him.

Neil's confidence was bolstered even more by his next medical appointment — the long-awaited neurological assessment.

> ***Boston Children's Hospital, Sports Therapy, November 10, 2015 excerpts:***
>
> **History of Present Illness:** Eugene is a 19-year-old male tennis player, who presents for evaluation of 3 concussions sustained consecutively over the past 3 months. The 1st one he sustained in August 2015 when he was in a fight. He got hit in the head, did not lose consciousness, and thinks that his symptoms, which were primarily vestibular symptoms and headaches, lasted about a week. He was not clinically evaluated for this. Then in September 2015, he was playing capture the flag and ran into a tree, sustaining his second concussion. He did see a doctor at MGH, who recommended vestibular physical therapy. Then in October 2015, he fell off a slack-line and hit his head, sustaining his 3rd lifetime concussion. He also saw a doctor at Mass General Hospital for this...
>
> **Plan:** At this time, we cannot clear him for contact sports, and we recommend no soccer. All non-contact activity is fine for him to participate in, provided that he is not having

> worsening symptoms. We will hold off on an MRI right now, as he is continuing to improve, per his report. We will refer him to an ophthalmologist here at Children's for further assessment of the visual disturbances... We will see him back in 4-6 weeks for another clinical re-evaluation...

With this reinforcement of his November 5 appointment, Neil's optimism grew. Between his dedication to physical therapy for his eyes and the power of positive thinking, he convinced himself he was slowly improving. He was master of his universe once again, and having felt the pangs of stepping back for a while, it was a universe he loved all the more, especially with the Husky Hunt close at hand!

THE HUSKY HUNT NOVEMBER 13

The Husky Hunt, a city-wide scavenger hunt lasting twenty-four hours, has become a Boston tradition. Only fifty teams make the cut, and in 2015, Neil's was one of them.

"I'll mostly coordinate the team from 'HQ' in Snell Library," he assured us.

"Okay," we nodded reluctantly, as if there was really a choice. "Please just take it easy."

"I will," he said, barely containing his glee.

Though "taking it easy" may have been his intention, the event's excitement was overpowering. When we spoke to Neil afterwards, he admitted to doing "some running around." So much for his good intentions. But it was hard to blame him. Participating in the Husky Hunt must have been akin to playing a city-sized, neon-lit pinball machine with a soundtrack mix from Imagine Dragons, Linkin Park, Coldplay, and fun."

While you might think a twenty-four-hour game marathon would have exhausted him completely, rather than "crashing," Neil kept right on motoring the following day. His personal calendar showed he attended his classes, did some lab work for one of them, and held a Husky Hunt debriefing session with his friends — among other things. In an interview published in a school newspaper long after the Husky Hunt, we learned even more.

> "John Lambert, a junior who met Neil as a freshman, recalled Neil inviting him to be part of his Husky Hunt team during the Fall of Neil's sophomore year. John said Neil was one of the few members on the team who stayed awake for the whole 24 hours. He did anything that needed to be done, whether it was going out into the city to fulfill one of the challenges or staying where the team was set up in Snell Library in order to organize their next move."

"That's our Game Boy," I shook my head and smiled when we finally saw the article.

CONSEQUENCES
DECEMBER 2015

Unfortunately, there was a price to be paid for his exploits. The progress he'd been making with his physical therapy was largely erased, and his difficulty playing tennis increased so much that he later had to admit he'd put himself "on the bench."

"I'm still going to practice," he told us. "Working things through. But I would be a liability if I tried to compete."

On December 3, he went to MGH Sports Therapy:

> ***MGH Sports Therapy, December 3, 2015 excerpts:***
>
> Patient states his symptoms have remained fairly consistent. He experienced an initial improvement and had returned to practicing tennis, but then did the "Husky Hunt" (a 24-

> hour scavenger hunt where he was awake for 24 hours and did some running) after which he experienced a decline.. His vision became worse and he subsequently stopped practicing tennis. Classes have continued to go well and he had not had any difficulty concentrating. He states his vision symptoms are worse after longer days and increased walking, especially in a busy area. Of note, he states he is currently feeling worse due to the T ride and the walk from Bowdoin, which was crowded...
>
> He went to Children's to be seen by Neurology, but cannot recall who he saw. He states they were supposed to follow up with a referral...but he cannot recall what type of appointment and he never heard back from them.

It was uncharacteristic of Neil to forget things like this, and hearing it secondhand seemed negligent on Neil's part, and unfortunate. When we spoke with him on the phone, he was his usual confident self.

"I'm getting better at compensating," he assured us. "I'm doing okay. Don't worry about me."

Right, I thought wistfully. "Okay Pal."

Before coming home for winter break, Neil had a meeting called "Mindful Meditation" scheduled in his calendar. Interesting. He also had two separate reminders to call his new neuro-optometrist. These entries were doubtless related to the appointment he had at New England College of Optometry on the tenth:

> ***New England College of Optometry, December 10, 2015 excerpts:***
>
> Patient had a series of 3 concussions in Aug/Sept/Oct and is now having difficulty tracking, is seeing double. Symp-

toms are exacerbated by physical activity. Patient plays tennis and is seeing two balls when tracking.

Diplopia in leftward gaze since last concussion 2 months ago. EDMS: L on 6 palsy? (last injury was posterior head on left side.)

Monocular Saccadic Workbook #2: OD easier than OS. Good posture, accuracy and speed.

Monocular Circling: Patient reports OD=OS in terms of difficulty. Good accuracy, but had to remind patient about posture and to avoid using finger or pen to track.

Monocular flippers: Patient reports +0.50/+1.00 [lens] is a little more difficult. Switched to +0.75/+1.25: No blur lenses, similar difficulty.

Brock String: 2 beads, 8" and 16." Patient has no trouble fusing bead at either distance.

Mild left CN VI palsy.

Neil also had what was becoming a routine visit with MGH Sports Therapy:

MGH Sports Therapy, December 17, 2015 excerpts:

Current Condition: Reports exercises have been going well overall and feels he has progressed most with five finger accommodation exercise. Is able to visually focus after walking longer distances, but still has difficulty biking. He has been consistently biking and maintaining his HR between

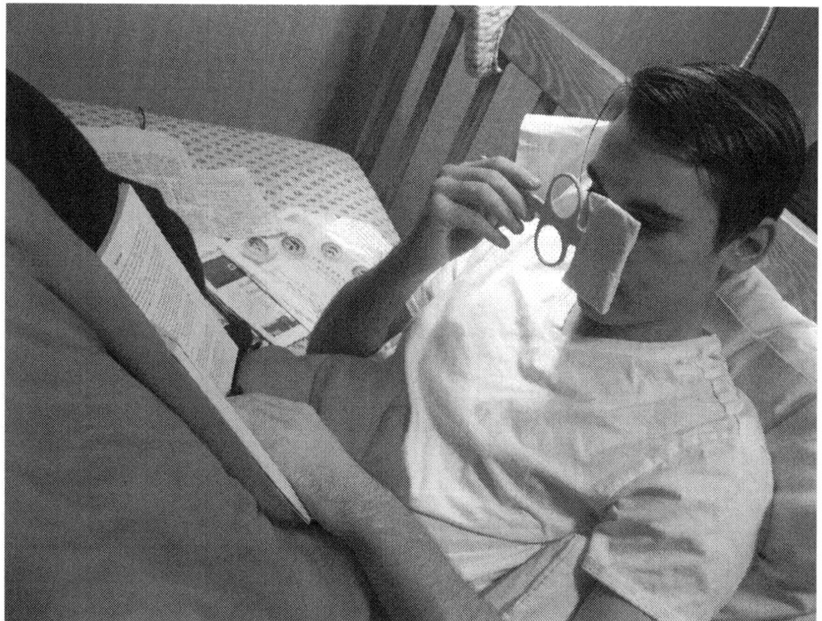

> 130 and 135. He experiences no exacerbation of symptoms except for an occasional mild headache. He has been doing yoga with minimal difficulty. He had follow-up at the New England Eye Center for exercise prescription...
>
> Assessment/Plan: Patient to continue with gradual increase in exertion and cardiovascular challenge without contact. He will progress his vestibular exercises as well to include more complex backgrounds. He is demonstrating good progress overall. He will continue visual exercises until his next appointment at the NE College of Optometry, at which point he will discontinue [current exercises] and replace with exercises from neuro-optometery.

Anxious inklings aside, Neil had things under control as far as we knew, and his doctors seemed to think so too. If fitfully, he was making progress with his physical therapy — to which new exercises had been added, and for which he had been prescribed a variety of new therapeutic tools. He referred to terms like "physiological diplopia" and "vestibular vision," both of which he was working on by doing exercises with a suite of new tools: a "Brock string," a "saccadic workbook," and a "visual tracing workbook" to name just a few. He added these new exercises into his routine with the same diligence and enthusiasm he applied to his coursework or tennis practice.

WINTER BREAK

When he came home for his holiday/winter break, Neil would sit at the breakfast table every morning to do eye exercises, a regimen that had become considerably more complex since his last visit home at Thanksgiving. On his first morning home, he demonstrated his "focusing flipper" with side-by-side lenses of different magnifications and tints and the "Slayer 3D Variable Tranaglyph" composed of overlapping transparencies. We watched in fascination and, quite honestly, with growing unease at this collection of gadgets. It seemed obvious, despite assurances to the contrary, that Neil was coping with significant issues. This was further underscored when he calmly announced he would avoid driving his car while he was home.

Wait... What?!

What kid home from college doesn't want to use his car to get around to see friends? Nevertheless, Neil assured us he was doing well — that he had been eating well, taking time to relax, and doing his daily eye exercises. Making progress. On a particularly warm, sunny day before Christmas, Neil even asked me to play tennis.

"Do you want to hit some balls," he asked after doing his exercises.

"Sure," I nodded, "if you're up for it!"

"I need to work on my ground strokes," he nodded.

Among the things he brought home was his tennis bag. It contained a pair of Babolat tennis rackets and some reasonably firm tennis balls.

"Shall we take the punch-buggie?" I asked, referring to his green '03

Volkswagen Beetle with a stick shift. It had belonged to his Grandma Carolyn, who had given it to his cousin Elise, who left it in New Hampshire when she moved to California. The car had been sitting neglected when Neil's Grandpa Gene — Grumpa — offered to buy it back and give it to Neil. It wasn't a masculine car, but being fans of the *Need for Speed* video games, Neil and I planned to make a few tasteful mods to give it some snap.

"Absolutely," Neil grinned. "Let's give the old girl some exercise too."

We went to the high school to hit on the courts he once played on with his old team — the "good old days," when tennis became his favorite sport:

> Neil hadn't played much tennis before sophomore year in high school, but something about his determination convinced the coach to squeak him onto the roster, and she never looked back. Neil gave everything he had to improving his game. He approached tennis, like everything else, with his mind. He hadn't yet learned how to hit the ball with much power, so he became a master of "dinks," lobs that looked more like dainty badminton shots than tennis. Even after his game skills improved enough to play singles, Neil still liked to lob, especially when he was outmatched. There was one match in particular when he had to "play up" because one of his teammates was sick. Neil had to play a much stronger player who was favored to "crush" him. His attitude? "Let's do it!"
>
> The boy hit rockets, and Neil had to hustle like a scared rabbit just to get within reach of these shots, then he'd stretch out and somehow manage to "dink" the ball back. Taking a page from his Grandpa Ferd's playbook, Neil would do this over and over, stretching nearly into splits just to put his racket on the ball and dink a return. After a while, this began to infuriate Neil's opponent, making him try even harder to mash the ball past Neil's stubborn

> defense. Instead of winning points, however, his opponent began drilling the ball into the net or sending it sailing past the back line. And Neil ended up winning the match...
>
> By the end of his senior year, Neil was hitting some rockets himself, and he had advanced enough to play third singles, but he still enjoyed mixing in dink shots just to throw his opponents off stride.

As we loosened up and began playing that warm day in December, I could see Neil struggle with some of his shots, shifting his body to get a better read on the ball's approach so he could make a return.

"I'm not seeing the ball clearly on my forehand side," he said. "It's double sometimes, and my tracking is off. Keep hitting to my forehand."

That's what I tried to do, and he adjusted his stance and cocked his head at different angles as he swung through gently. As he found a groove, he increased his power until he could blow the ball by me at will. That wasn't the point, though. We were playing to volley, and several times, we sent the ball back and forth a few dozen times each, running each other around just enough to test skills and endurance without being brutal. It was a great hour of play, reminding me of the father/son tournament we had played the previous summer. How I looked forward to playing again!

During the extended holiday break, Neil also suggested we play a game of blindfold chess. The last time we did that he was about ten years old:

> We were moored on our boat in Dutch Harbor, one of our favorite weekend get-aways, located at the mouth of Narragansett Bay. Another delicious dinner was history, and we were settling into the evening, a time when our snug little foursome often liked to play games — usually together, but not always.
>
> "I'd like to try playing a game of blindfold chess," Neil announced.
>
> "What's that?" I asked.

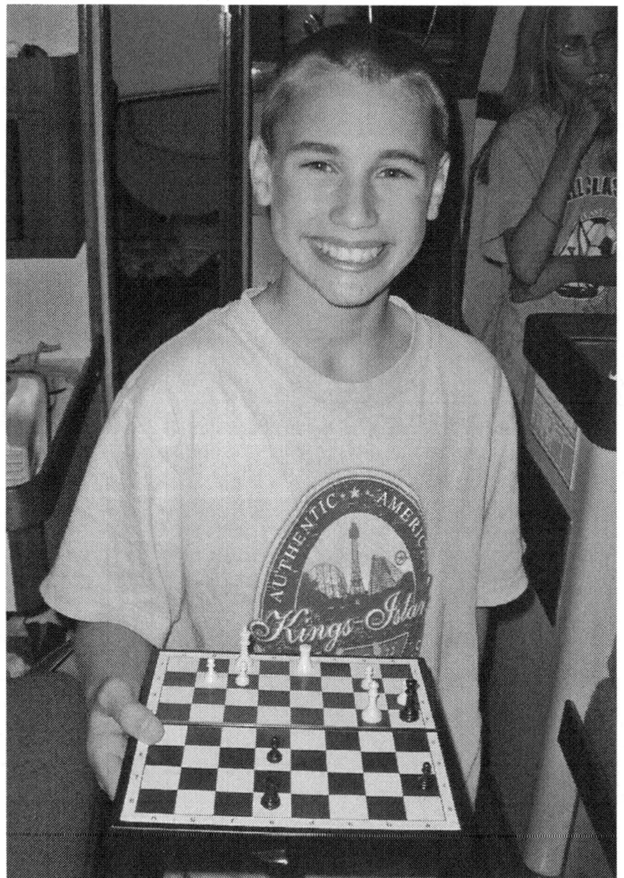

"That's when I play a game without ever looking at the board," he explained.

"Are you kidding?"

"C'mon Dad. All you have to do is tell me your moves, and I'll tell you mine, and you move my pieces how I tell you so you can keep track."

"And you won't look at the board," I was doubtful.

"Nope," he crossed his heart.

"But I get to look at the board?"

"Yup," he smiled. "Just be sure to make my moves like I tell you and tell me your moves correctly."

I still looked incredulous.

"That's why the board's ranks and files are marked," he explained. "You know that."

Right. Looking at the board from white's side, the squares from left to right, called the "files," are labeled A through H, and the squares from bottom to top, called "ranks," are numbered one through eight. I knew that. I wasn't fluent with chess nomenclature, but I knew that much. "Okay," I agreed.

While some might think playing blindfold chess is impossible, by that time, Neil was ranked in the top fifty players his age in the US. He had played in many large tournaments and had even once beaten a "master," a player with a rating of over 2200. A "Grandmaster" rating is 2400. Neil's rating was getting close to 2000, and it had been years since I'd taken a game off him. This might be my big chance.

We set up our little magnetic chessboard. Thankfully, the board's ranks and files were indeed labeled. Otherwise, I would have struggled, and roughly thirty minutes and two dozen moves later, I was in checkmate. Neil never once looked at the board. Scout's honor. It was an intellectual feat far beyond my capacity. To say I was proud would be a gross understatement. Truth be known, I was more than a little bit awed, and a bit jealous too.

Neil just smiled his big grin, proud of himself but not smug. "GG, Dad!"

We never did play blindfold chess that December. I dodged his request, not because I feared he would beat me — that was a forgone conclusion — but because I feared he could no longer hold the moves in his head, and I was afraid of what that might mean.

Neil had one appointment with his local optometrist while he was home. He was due for a new prescription for glasses. We all hoped that would help with some of his vision issues, and doubtless a bit more clarity was a benefit, but it made no difference to his underlying complaints.

Still, all in all, it was a wonderful break. Neil always looked on the bright side, and his positive attitude had a way of rubbing off. He even seemed to discover more humor in life, laughing easily and sometimes for reasons that were apparent only to him. To cap off the vacation, Evie returned home from her co-op in New Zealand, so we had everyone together for New Year's. Then, all too soon, it was time for the next semester to start.

4

SOMETHING ISN'T ADDING UP

"We'll leave that as a hanging note to come back to later." NF

JANUARY 2016

We drove the kids back to campus and unloaded their gear around 1:00 p.m.. We were lucky enough to find a parking place near Neil's apartment, so I asked about going out for a bite.

"Yes, let's do that," Wendy quickly agreed. Anything to extend our time all together. And what better way than appealing to appetite.

"Boston Burger is just a short walk," Evie said.

"Sounds like a plan," Neil agreed.

Boston Burger concocts some of the best and most outrageous hamburgers one is likely to find, so we walked over and were lucky enough to get a table in less than five minutes. We exchanged small talk until the food arrived, then we laughed at the mess we were making. It was a great way to wrap up our vacation, then, all too soon, we were saying goodbyes, the kids heading off to meet friends and the "rents" heading home to our "empty nest" with an ill-defined sense of concern.

Communications with both kids resumed their normal tenor — emailing links to events in the news and quick "check-ins" to see how things were going. Neil resumed his routine, including his regular visits to MGH Sports Therapy:

> ***MGH Sports Therapy, January 12, 2016 excerpts:***
>
> [Patient] tried some weights in the gym (light weights) - had HA (head ache) the next few days. Didn't do too much over break, but was doing stationary bike at home getting HR up a little higher without problem. Did play tennis with his father for 1 hour without too much issue....
>
> Back to school 1/10, classes started 1/11. Has had more headaches...
>
> Plan: Continue with assessment and progression. Continue increasing cardiovascular demand tennis moves.

Again, this report was not one we would see until months after the fact, but it still sets me on edge when I read it. It validates the ill-defined sense of concern that was creeping around in my nightmares. What were "more headaches" if not a red flag? But we were not "privy." As far as we knew, everything with Neil was status quo, and we started thinking again about our next trip to South Carolina.

At mid-month, both Neil and Evie "trained" home for a weekend to celebrate my birthday and collect a few more things they needed at school. We drove them back Sunday afternoon, thinking how terrific it was for their school to be close enough we could do that, yet Boston provided them with a "whole other world" of experience — as good as being a thousand miles away, but right at our doorstep. Not a bad combination. Then, too, because Boston is a "hub" of medical excellence, we took solace in believing Neil was where he needed to be to get the best possible care.

After tennis practice one day, Neil was feeling dizzy, so he trekked to the clinic again.

Northeastern Clinic, January 28, 2016 excerpts:

Chief complaint: Dizzy

Consult: General student presents with c/o lightheadedness and dizzy x 1 day. He states he had 3 concussions in the past year in August, September and October of 2015 playing soccer. He also plays club tennis. He has a vision issue that he is seen for to exercise his eye muscles due to damage with one of his concussions.

Assessment: Dizziness and giddiness - R42 (Primary)

Plan: LAB: Complete CBC with Differential...

This report contained no references to his previous clinic visits or his regular appointments with MGH Sports Therapy. Instead, the report reads as if this was Neil's first visit to the clinic. Had all of his records been put into context — "lightheadedness," "more headaches," "dizziness," and "giddiness" — it might have provided a clue that something more was going on. Instead, Neil was initially diagnosed with "mild concussions at worst," but then over time, this diagnosis had morphed. "Concussions" were taken as a given, and no one was inclined to look for anything else, even when Neil's symptoms failed to improve and were in some ways getting worse. It was a similar story with this follow-up visit to New England College of Optometry at the end of the month:

Dr. Laudon, New England College of Optometry, January 30, 2016 excerpts:

Patient reports good compliance with visual training. SIP 3 concussions.

- Double vision in far leftward gaze remains stable.

- HA's are variable but overall improving.
- Dizziness for a few days with lying back. Went to doctor and awaiting results of blood work.

To the best of our recollection, Neil made no special mention of these two visits except to say he was he was keeping up with his appointments and "making good progress."

FEBRUARY 2016

Valentine's month found Neil much as he had been the last several weeks. Although it was doubtless a hassle to incorporate off-campus appointments with doctors and physical therapists — some occurring as early as 8:00 a.m. and halfway across town — he did so without fuss. He met with the tennis team and tried to play when he could; classes were going very well; and time with his friends was his manna from Heaven.

> ***MGH Sports Therapy Appointment, February 2, 2016 excerpts:***
>
> Playing tennis with the team again; notices that total body coordination is difficult. Had a dizzy spell after doing sit-ups and then for a few days afterwards every time he put his head backwards (wasn't getting good sleep that week)...
>
> Sports Psych referral? (<u>If he gets to a point where he can no longer talk himself out of stress headache</u>)..."

Despite continued "dizziness" and "headaches," now the focus seemed to be on the possibility Neil was just stressing out...

While Neil tried to think positively and take things in stride, an objective assessment of his collective records clearly suggests a lack of significant improvement. In some cases, his symptoms worsened, and he even began to exhibit new symptoms. Unfortunately, it seems no one ever looked at his collective records, and changes that were noted in isolation were chalked up to stress. Through it all — as far as we knew — Neil was "making progress." Then, this came out of the blue:

Social media post, February 8, 2016:

Recovering from three concussions while going through some other serious life traumas has made the past four months of my life some of the toughest I can remember. Each day has provided its own struggle, and some days, I have just plain felt like quitting. I'd say to my resigned self, "That's it, let me just hibernate for the winter and wake up a new man in May. I'm done." It is on these depressed days that I would pull out my bookmark from "Walk in Their Shoes," dive a couple pages deeper into Jim Ziolkowski's life story, and find myself moved, in many cases, to the point of tears. Every page is filled with so much heart, compassion, and inspiration that saying I was/am inspired is almost an understatement.

As one of the most moving stories I have ever had the pleasure of hearing, "Walk in Their Shoes" has given me more than just the motivation to keep plugging away at life. It's given me the inspiration and the aspiration to make more of it. In his awe-inspiring story, Jim takes you on a journey away from the comfortable recesses of your home, out into the streets of Harlem, and off through the wastelands of some of the poorest countries in the world on one of the most touching and meaningful journeys that life has to offer. From the most forsaken corners of Haiti to the deep recesses of Nepal, he has traveled forming bonds, building schools, and spreading light. His story represents a beacon of hope, in what often seems a dark and desolate landscape.

For anyone out there having a rough time with life right now and looking for motivation to get back to making a difference in the world, I highly recommend picking up a copy of this book for yourself. Each and everyone of us has such an incredible potential to make a difference, all it takes is the right key to unlock this potential.

So for all of you out there having a bad day or a rough time with life right now, I have a short poem from the book to share:

"Never Give up
No matter what is going on
Never give up
Develop the heart
Too much energy in your country
Is spent developing the mind
Instead of the heart
Develop the heart
Be compassionate
Not just to your friends
But to everyone
Be compassionate
Work for peace
In your heart and in the world
Work for peace
And I say again
Never give up.
No matter what is happening
No matter what is going on around you
Never give up."
~Dalai Lama~

Was this a cry for help, a cry that was not being answered by his routine appointments? Neil was having more trouble — balancing his recovery efforts with his desire to participate in tennis, fraternity gatherings, hall council meetings, relationships, and just about everything related to being a college student — than he told us. His post shook us up.

MORE SYMPTOMS

On February 11, 2016, Neil had another appointment at MGH Sports Therapy:

> ***MGH Sports Therapy Appointment, February 11, 2016 excerpt:***
>
> "Playing tennis with the team again; notices that total body coordination is difficult. Had a dizzy spell after doing sit-ups and then for a few days afterwards every time he put his head backwards (wasn't getting good sleep that week)."

Oddly, this report was a near duplicate of his report from February 2, and sometime after this appointment, Neil called Wendy. He told her he was having difficulty swallowing, and he was experiencing coordination issues with his handwriting. He also admitted to having slipped on some ice, but he assured her he had not hit his head. As always, Neil said he was fine, but he wondered if Mom had any suggestions.

These new issues just turned up the volume on alarm bells that had never stopped ringing, but Wendy kept her cool. Immediately after their conversation, Wendy did some research and sent Neil the following note:

> **To: Eugene (Neil) Fachon**
> **From: Wendy Fachon**
> **Subject: Swallowing...**
> **Date: Sun, 21 Feb 2016**

Hi Hon!

Looking on the Internet with regards to swallowing I found...

"Brain injury frequently affects the skilled coordination of the nerves and 26 different muscles in the neck and esophagus that are used during the normal swallowing process."

This may also explain the challenges with writing.

Have you called your neuro-opthamologist to discuss these new symptoms... and your loss of balance on Monday?

These issues are not about the eyes. If I were you, I would ask him to refer you to another neuro-specialist ASAP. You may need some additional diagnosis and therapy.

Call his office tomorrow and express a degree of nervousness and anxiety.

We're here for you!
Love, Mom

It felt like the situation was beginning to spin out of control, and our hands were effectively tied. Our efforts to get more involved had been mostly rebuffed, thanks largely to privacy laws that may have gone to Neil's head, laws that blocked any recourse we might have had to discussing his condition with his doctors.

To: Wendy Fachon
From: Dean Fachon
Subject: health-care debacle
Date: Sun, 21 Feb 2016

Write an article about how health-care rules have put a barrier between us and helping our son through the biggest health-care challenge of his life, seriously jeopardizing the chances of a full recovery.

* * *

To: "Eugene (Neil) Fachon"
From: Dean Fachon
Subject: Your current health
Date: On Sun, Feb 21, 2016 at 6 PM

Neil,

When did you first notice you were having new symptoms? What might have triggered them? Did you stay up late a few nights in a row? Have a beer? Take a really hot shower? Work out really hard? Think and write anything down. And while you did not hit your head when you fell, the blow rattled your already delicate brain. You need to start taking the seriousness of your situation up a few notches. Your quality of life, for the rest of your life, may hang in the balance. Make it clear to your doctor that your family is that concerned. A physical therapist is not a neurologist. I would also not rule out that you may even need to drop out of school for a year. You need to be in a situation that minimizes risk of further aggravation as much as possible. I'm not kidding, nor am I overreacting. I do not want you to panic, but this needs to become your first and foremost priority. Get your advisor in the loop, but not for advise, just to keep him/her advised. There is nothing more important! We love you and are thinking of you and sending our positive thoughts and prayers.

Love,
Dad and Mom

* * *

To: Dean Fachon
From: "Eugene (Neil) Fachon"
Subject: Re: Your current health
Date: Feb 21, 2016

I'm going to be honest here, you're scaring me with this. And no these are things that I've noticed kind of develop over time aka the past few weeks. But please stop telling me to take the seriousness of my situation up a few notches, it's already on the highest pedestal possible, and I'm not about to make a new pedestal (that would require wrapping me in bubble wrap). That fall is a hazard of winter, I can be as careful as you like, ice is a hazard of living in the Northeast and that was an especially slippery day. As soon as I had the opportunity I took the underground route back to my dorm. I will go back to health services and talk to them again this week. Really I'm fine. You guys are worrying about me way too much. Your concern honestly makes me feel worse than I know I actually am. And please don't tell me I'm not taking this seriously enough because I have taken it very seriously for a very long time, and I am continuing to take it just as seriously. Please don't lose sleep over it. I'll get checked out, and I am going to be fine.

Love you guys,
Neil

I was very sorry to upset my son, but I wonder if he hadn't been harboring larger fears of his own. Could he feel his world slipping from his grasp? If so, I had poked him where it hurt. That's a regret. Thankfully, he set aside any resentment — if indeed he felt any — because he reached out immediately to his medical team.

To: Dr. Herget and Dr. Laudon
From: Eugene (Neil) Fachon
Subject: Update + what should I do?
Date: Feb 21, 2016, at 6:09 PM
CC: Wendy and Dean

Hi Dr. Herget and Dr. Laudon

I've been noticing some different symptoms lately with my condition, including poor balance, an inability to swallow water, and loss of fine motor dexterity aka writing. At first I didn't think much of these symptoms as they kind of came on slowly, but they've been persisting for the past few weeks, so I thought they were worth noting. Furthermore, I slipped on ice and landed on my back this past Monday, and though I didn't hit my head luckily, I did get a bit jostled. I have talked things over with my parents (who I have CCed on this email, so they can stay in the loop), and was wondering what I should do as they believe I should seek further help. Should I look into other specialists, and if so could I get a referral or are these symptoms that should go away quickly?

I will see you this Wednesday, Lenore, so you will be able to take a peak at me again then, but I won't be seeing you, Dr Laudon, until March 6. Recommendations are appreciated, and I looked forward to hearing from you both soon.

Cheers,
Neil Fachon

* * *

To: Eugene Fachon
From: Dr. Herget, P.T.,D.P.T.,SCS,M.Ed.,CSCS
Subject: Re: Update + what should I do?
Date: Feb 21, 2016

Hello Neil,

These newly experienced symptoms are not consistent with a typical concussion, nor are they found with BPPV (your most recent positional vertigo). I would contact your PCP. Who are you seeing in the concussion clinic? I would contact that physician as well. I am happy to refer you to a concussion specialist: neurologist or psychiatrist if needed.

Best
Dr. Herget

Neil forwarded this response to Wendy, and she promptly replied.

To: Dr. Herget, P.T.,D.P.T.,SCS,M.Ed.,CSCS, Eugene (Neil) Fachon
From: Wendy Fachon
Subject: Re: Update + What should I do?
Date: Mon, 22 Feb 2016
CC: Dr. L, Dean Fachon

Hi Neil!

Do you have a Primary Care Physician (PCP) at the University clinic? Your PCP at home is Dr. John Slattery, however, he is more likely to refer doctors in Rhode Island. Who provides your referrals at the University? In November you reported you met with a neurologist in Boston, who you said was not helpful. Get a recommendation for a good neurologist. Drs. Herget and Laudon are on your team, and, if I were you, I would start with doctors they respect, have worked well with, and would recommend.

Mom and Dad

On the heels of sending this note to Neil, we immediately wrote and hand-delivered a letter to Neil's pediatrician/physician at home.

February 22, 2016

Dear Dr. Slattery:

We're writing with regards to Eugene Fachon, a sophomore at Northeastern University. Beginning last August, he suffered a series of three head traumas over three months. After the third incident he began suffering symptoms of concussion: Dizziness, blurred double vision, and headaches. He went to the Northeastern infirmary and was ultimately referred to a neuro-optometrist and a physical therapist. He followed a regimen of special eye exercises and cut back on physical activity and was making good progress. In the last three weeks, however, he has begun having issues with balance, fine motor skills and swallowing. (He also slipped and fell on the ice last Monday, although these symptoms were cropping up before then.)

Upon Eugene notifying his care providers, they suggested he speak with his PCP for a referral to a concussion specialist/neurologist. In all this time, Eugene has not had an MRI, even so it was requested. The push back has always been that in cases like this an MRI would not be that useful. With these new symptoms, we wonder if that was being a little too lax.

Water under the dam at this point. We wanted to let you know what is happening in case you might care to offer any suggestions or refer Eugene to someone in Boston to work with.

Thank you for you time. We hope to hear from you, or hear that you have contacted Eugene, at your earliest convenience.

Regards,
Dean and Wendy Fachon
East Greenwich, RI

In the meantime, because he did not have a primary care physician at school, Neil went back to the only place that came close, the university clinic.

Northeastern Clinic, February 23, 2016 excerpts:

Chief Complaints: Possible re-occurring concussion.

HPI:
Follow Up: **19 year old male here with concern about progressive post-concussion symptoms.** See previous notes. Reports he sustained three concussions last semester, no recent head injuries since but slipped on ice and "jarred" himself. Reports that initially symptoms were all visual in nature, saw a neurologist at CBH and has been following up with neuro-ophthalmologist and ophtho PT. **Now reports that for several weeks has felt more dizzy, having some balance issues, difficulty initiating urination and defecation and posterior headache with laughing.** Denies worsening vision, incontinence, weakness, difficulty sleeping or trouble with school work. Has not followed up with his neurologist with these concerns.

Assessment:

1) Concussion without loss of consciousness, initial encounter - S05-0X0A
2) Encounter for screening for other disorder - Z13.89

Plan:

Concussion without loss of consciousness, initial encounter. Notes: Advised student to follow-up with neurologist given new neuro changes. **Student says he didn't like the neurologist he saw**, given 3 additional contacts. Discussed need to go to ER if he develops acute change, pain, gait disturbance or any other concerns.

Note: When we finally saw Neil's medical reports, the lack of continuity was distressing. For instance, the above report states, "See previous notes," yet the subsequent words belie the suggestion: "Now reports that for several weeks has felt more dizzy..." Now reports?! Dizziness had been a constant refrain in his official reports dating back to October of 2015! It seemed like each time Neil had a medical visit, it was as if he was being seen for the first time. "See previous notes" (as in "connect the dots") wasn't happening.

INCREASING ANXIETY

Neil had no PCP, and he had no neurologist, and finding either had proven problematic, beginning with the delay in getting a referral from Northeastern's clinic. This had led Neil to try as best he could to find one on his own, and that hadn't worked out. Now, he had three referrals, and he immediately tried to make an appointment with any one of them. He later called to tell us the soonest he could get a follow-up with a specialist was March 10. Knowing we were scheduled to leave on a "spring break" vacation to Florida on March 6, Wendy took the initiative to contact Dr. Herget directly.

To: Dr. Herget
From: Wendy Fachon
Subject: Regarding Eugene Fachon concussion
Date: Fri, Feb 26, 2016 at 9:57 AM
CC: Neil Fachon

Dr. Herget,

Just spoke with Neil and learned the first appointment he is able to get with the neurologist is March 10. We have a couple of questions...

We are scheduled to fly to Florida, as a family, March 6-11. Is it okay for Neil to travel by air with changes in air pressure?

Is it fine for Neil to wait until the following week for an appointment? Or should he see someone as soon as possible?

Is there physical therapy Neil can do in the meantime to help with his swallowing or his fine motor skills?

Wendy and Dean Fachon

There's little doubt Neil's frustration had pushed him out of character. He was not happy when he saw Wendy's note to his doctor.

To: Hey Mom and Dad
From: Eugene (Neil) Fachon
Subject: Re: Eugene Fachon Concussion
Date: 2/26/2016

You can let me handle this. I have been working with her for awhile so it really would've been better to just let me handle communication. Remember, I'm not a little kid any more, I can handle setting up appointments and communicating with my doctors. I appreciate the concern, but I think it would be more appropriate for me to take care of this as I have been keeping up with Dr. Laudon in a separate email chain.

Love you guys,
Neil

This made Wendy feel guilty, so she quickly replied:

To: Eugene (Neil) Fachon
From: Wendy Fachon
Subject: Re: Eugene Fachon Concussion
Date: Fri, 26 Feb 2016

I'm sorry.
Forgive me.
Thank you.
We love you.

Which, of course, made Neil feel terrible, so he called to apologize and voice his eagerness to get away on spring break.

"I can't wait to get to Florida and put this aside for awhile," he lamented.

Unfortunately, Florida was the furthest thing from our minds.

To: Eugene (Neil) Fachon
From: Dean Fachon
Subject: Need to get to the bottom of this...
Date: Sun, 28 Feb 2016
CC: Evie Fachon, Wendy Fachon

Neil,

Evie is worried about you too. If these new symptoms are caused by a physical trauma, could rapid changes of cabin pressure cause further trouble? You think you are well enough to fly, but please forgive us if we're not as confident. Recall that you thought it was ok to use the slack line after you'd had two concussions; that it was okay to go running in the Husky Hunt when you felt you were doing better; that you have been ramping up activity and now these new symptoms have cropped up.

No, neither of us is a doctor and we cannot diagnose you telepathically. No one can tell you what's going on in your head without a complete work-up, but you must think in terms of risk/rewards. Is today's enjoyment worth chancing another downturn? Maybe the stress-relief would be worth it, if the risk is truly minimal, but who is best to assess that?

If you can't see a neurologist right away, what are the opinions of your doctor/therapist team, including Dr. Slattery? If any of them thinks it would be wiser to avoid flying until you get a complete work-up, then do you think Florida should wait for another time? We hope you can see the wisdom in this caution. If you want to discuss further, we would be happy to come see you. We will be bringing Evie back to Boston later today. Call if you want to get together later. Otherwise, please communicate with your team ASAP, and let us know what they say.

All our Love,
Dad and Mom

Thankfully, Neil's communications with Dr. Herget led to a referral with Dr. Walter Panis, a neurologist affiliated with Harvard and Mass General. Neil was able to schedule an appointment to see Dr. Panis on March 2, 2016.

5

REAL ANSWERS AT LAST

"Tell me about an instance where you failed or did something you are ashamed of." NF

MARCH 2016

It was a relief to know Neil would finally be seeing a neurologist, but we could not help worrying about what might be revealed. Neil, too, was wrestling with this, but as always, he tried to put things in a positive light:

Social media post by Neil, March 2, 2016:

"An arrow can only be shot by pulling it backward. So when life is dragging you back with difficulties, it means that its going to launch you into something great. So just focus, and keep aiming." —*Anonymous*

From the moment he met Dr. Panis, Neil liked him. Dr. Panis seemed affable and attentive, and he gave Neil a thorough neurological exam. Dr. Panis also wanted to order an MRI for the following day. Some more answers would be forthcoming, at last.

Doctor Panis Office Visit, March 2, 2016 excerpt:

Eugene is a 19-year-old, right handed young man who is

> a sophomore at Northeastern. He is studying industrial engineering. He begins by telling me that he has had 3 concussions in August, September and October. In August he had been punched in the face. He had a headache. He made a quick recovery. In September while playing a game, he ran into a tree. He made another quick recovery. In October he fell 3 or 4 feet while he was playing on a slack line; that is like a tightrope. He fell and hit his head. He developed double vision. He saw someone who told him he had a palsy in the left eye. He was told to see a neuro-optometrist. He was in physical therapy. However, for the 1-1/2 months, things have been worsening. He has difficulty with his writing. He has developed difficulty swallowing water. He chokes. He has lost coordination. He has tripped. He has developed difficulty with initiating both bowel and bladder. He notes he has a change in his behavior as well. He will start to laugh out of control. He had an episode when he walked like he was drunk and he was not. When it is very cold, he has difficulty with his speech. He could not be understood. He can get intermittent vertigo with movement. He gets a headache in the back or his head with neck extension. He feels his memory is impaired. He continues to have double vision...
>
> He has a very abnormal neurologic examination. I do not think it is related to the concussions. I am concerned about him enough that I am going to try get an MRI with gadolinium as quickly as possible.

Of course, Neil did not see this report. He was just relieved to feel he was on track at last and called later that evening to tell us the good news.

"Hi Mom. It's me."

"How was your appointment?" Wendy asked as soon as we both picked up the phone.

"It was a good," Neil told us with a smile in his voice. "I really like Dr. Panis. He's my kind of guy. And he's ordered an MRI for tomorrow."

"Wow," Wendy exclaimed. "Tomorrow. That's great Honey!"

"Truly," I joined in. "Maybe now we'll get some better answers."

"I'm sure," Neil agreed.

"How are you feeling?" Wendy asked him.

"I'm okay," Neil bluffed a little. "But really, I'm fine. I've got some lab work to do so I really can't talk much right now."

"Well, we love you," Wendy answered.

"Keep us posted," I said.

"I will," he promised and hung up.

We don't know how Neil slept that night. Was he relieved to be getting the long-awaited MRI, or was he nervous? As his parents, we were both.

MARCH 3, 2016

The day began like so many recent days when Neil had had to work doctor's appointments into his routine. The MRI must have loomed a bit more in the forefront of his mind, but he would take it in stride.

To: Eugene (Neil) Fachon
From: Wendy Fachon
Subject: Thinking of you
Date: Thu, 3 Mar 2016

Hi Neil!

Good luck with the MRI today. This test is meant to give us the piece of mind that comes with knowledge and information.

With your interest in learning more about the brain, ask questions today! Learn all you can.

Sorry, if it seems we have been a pain with all of this. It's because we love you so much! Your Taurian stubbornness will frustrate me at times, but I admire the resilience at the core of your soul.

May we all grow in strength and wisdom.

Smiles and hugs,
Mom

* * *

To: "Eugene (Neil) Fachon"
From: Dean
Subject: Good luck today!
Date: March 3, 2016 8AM

Big HUG!
Dad

THE LONG-AWAITED MRI

Prior to getting the MRI, Neil had an appointment with his physical therapist, Dr. Hergot.

Excerpt from MGH Sports Therapy Appointment, March 3, 2016:

Patient has experienced many new symptoms since our last visit including difficulty with speech, swallowing' ataxia, dis-coordination; bowel/bladder problems, etc. I referred him to neurology. Saw Dr. Panis yesterday. Ordering MRI as he had a very abnormal neurologic exam...

I would encourage the patient to go to Florida (for planned family vacation) for some relaxation and positive visualization, as well as working on some total body coordination in the pool.

After this meeting, Neil reported to Mass General's radiology department. Getting there and back from Northeastern was no doubt a hassle, but Neil managed, and after the MRI, he went on with the rest of his day. Meanwhile, reports flew through the ether:

> ***MRI at Mass General, March 3, 2016 excerpts:***
>
> **History:**
> Abnormal gait (Ataxia) - Concussion mild or acute, no neurological deficit - Coordination changes, new or progressive...
>
> **IMPRESSION:**
> 3.6 x 5.7 x 5.1 cm T@/FLAIR hyperintense, T1 dark, expansile and exophytic nonehancing ill-defined lesion centered in the pons concerning for neoplasm, specifically diffuse infiltrative with exphytic component brainstem glioma.

Upon receiving this report from Mass General, Dr. Panis called Neil. In his own words — written months later about that day's events — Neil said:

> That same day, sometime in the early afternoon, I received a call from my neurologist:
>
> "Your MRI results came back, and they are abnormal. I am sorry to inform you that you have a brain tumor."
>
> Completely taken aback and stunned, I asked him, "How scared should I be?"
>
> He replied, "It's safe to say you should probably cancel your vacation plans and be seen up at MGH neuro-oncology as soon as possible. I'm setting up an appointment for tomorrow."

> After a few parting words, he hung up, and I proceeded to quake. I walked slowly from the common area of my apartment to my bedroom, turned to my roommate Steve, and announced in a shaky cry, "It turns out...I have a brain tumor."
>
> I proceeded to sit on my bed and quake for the next hour and a half as I tried to gather my composure to call my parents with the news.
>
> Steve [Neil's college roommate], in just as much shock, had no idea what to do other than to put his arm over my shoulder and tell me, "Dude, I'm so sorry! You're gonna figure this out."
>
> Once I gathered some semblance of composure and could speak without stammering, I began to spread the news to those closest to me.

"ALL OF A SUDDENLY..."

The phone rang. Wendy and I anticipated the call and picked up together, then we heard Neil deliver those fateful words.

"It turns out you were right to be worried about me. I have a brain tumor."

Life as we knew it was over. Neil seemed to be falling in over his head. In the space between heartbeats, another fall came to mind:

> Neil was three, and we were on our sailboat, tied up at a dock in Block Island — an old-fashioned pier with pilings and a platform bolted to them well above the high-water mark. At a dock like this, the boat rides up and down with the tide while the platform remains stationary. It was early evening, and the sun cast long shadows. The tide was low, too, so the platform was three or four feet above the boat's deck. We were planning a "shore party." The kids were eager

> to go, but we told them to sit on the cabin top while we closed up the boat. Neil, being a monkey who climbed effortlessly up and down his bunk bed at home, decided he'd waited long enough. I looked just in time to see him reaching up and out towards the platform, and then he was gone. He fell down between the dock and the boat with a splash and vanished under water. What happened next is a blur. Wendy says I did not want to risk jumping in on top of him, so I hooked my left foot on the boat's toe rail and gripped a lifeline stanchion with my left hand, draping my body over the side of the boat with my head just touching the water. Neil was nowhere to be seen — just bubbles rising to the surface. All I really recall is how deep and dark the water looked in the shadows under the dock and how easily a small boy could be swallowed. I thrust my arm down into the water, reaching as far as I could, and like a miracle, he was there. I grabbed hold of an arm and pulled him to the surface. Then, reaching around his waist, I hoisted him up into Wendy's outstretched hands. He was hardly phased by the incident, but we were in a mild state of shock.

Wendy inhaled sharply. "I'm so sorry Honey! We'll beat this!"

"Do you want us to come up?" I asked. "We can be there in less than two hours."

"No, that's okay," he said, being stoic. "I'll be fine. I have an appointment tomorrow at Mass General Oncology. Come for that."

"Of course," we answered together.

Saying goodbye was unbearable.

"Call for any reason," Wendy said. "We love you!"

"I will," Neil promised.

"We'll be there to take you to the oncologist," we promised and hung up.

As soon as the receiver was down, I was seething. "Holy sh*t! Five months! He should have had an MRI five months ago!"

Wendy stared blankly into space. "I don't believe this."

We held each other for a while, trying as best we could to process this impossible news. In between bouts of anger and tears, we began calling family members and close friends. There was a lot of stunned silence, punctuated with, "Oh my God!" Then, we began casting a net for resources and potential solutions. I'm not sure we ever went to bed that night.

To: "Eugene (Neil) Fachon"
From: Dean and Wendy
Subject: BIG HUG
Date: March 3, 2016, 11:30 PM

We hope you are sleeping by now, and that you do not see this until you wake up. But if you are still up, then go to bed! And sweet dreams, son. We'll see you soon.
Love,
Dad & Mom

In hindsight, "Sweet dreams!" was a moronic thing to say. Chalk it up to traumatic stress.

LIFELINES

The next day, I wrote another hand-delivered note to Neil's pediatrician:

To: Dr. John Slattery
Date: March 4, 2016
From: Dean

Dear Dr. Slattery:

We're writing again with regards to Eugene (Neil). Since last communicating with you, he managed to be seen by a neurologist at Mass General and get an MRI. The results were not good. His concussion symptoms were masking a brain tumor. We are meeting with a neuro-oncologist at Mass general later today to learn details, but in the meantime we're trying to assemble a list of the top neuro-surgeons and care-centers in the US, so we hopefully have options for reaching out for a second opinion. Your input on this matter would be greatly appreciated! Obviously time is critical.

Thank you,
Dean and Wendy Fachon

Dr. Slattery replied by email within hours:

From: Dr. John Slattery
To: Dean Fachon
Date: March 4, 2015

I am sorry to hear of the mass found in the brain during the MRI. I hope that it does follow the odds of being a benign tumor. If needed there is a very good doctor in RI that deals with malignant brain tumors named Dr. Heinrich Elinzano:

I wish you all the best in this time.

Dr. S

Wendy immediately reached out to Dr. Elinzano's office. I also reached out to Susie and Tom, dear friends in Switzerland whose family ties go back the better part of a century. We had just taken the kids to visit with them a couple of years before in the summer after Neil's junior year of high school — Evie's first year at Northeastern. One recollection in particular still haunts me:

> With a perfect day forecast, Susie and Tom invited us to join them and their hiking friends for an alpine excursion. We would walk from the Madulain railway station to the "Es-cha hut," a cabin-stübli at the end of a trail about six miles long and ascending three thousand five hundred feet into the alps. Surrounded by snowcapped peaks, the lower slopes were strewn with scattered outcroppings of rock, lush with tall grass and prolific wildflowers — including edelweiss. It was perfect grazing for the cows dotting the slopes, their legendary cowbells clanking musically. Postcard perfect.
>
> We walked a well-trodden cow path that zig-zagged back and forth up steep inclines, in some places so vertical it provoked an instinctive lean toward the slope to offset the vertigo. There was one comical moment when we looked up to see a cow gazing down at us as it chewed. The skies were so deep we could wish to dive into them, and when we reached a plateau, we found pools of water that were teaming with tadpoles. Rocks poked up haphazardly from the pool's surface, close together like steppingstones. Neil hopped from rock to rock until he was right in the middle of the pool. We took a photo, and by a trick of the light and the reflections in the pool, it looked as if he were hovering a few feet above the pool — an apparition.

Apparitions aside, I contacted Susie and Tom because their daughter, Chantal, is a doctor, and so is her husband, Raffaele — a pediatric oncologist. He and his colleagues are among the "top doctors" in this field, and this family connection would prove a blessing.

> **To: Susie and Tom**
> **From: Dean and Wendy Fachon**
> **Subject: Urgent request**
> **Date: March 4, 2016**

Dear Susie and Tom,

We have just learned that Neil has a brain tumor. We are meeting with a neuro-oncologist this afternoon at Mass General to get details, but we want to find the best possible care/second-opinion as quickly as possible. Who would you or Chantal and Raffaele say is the best neuro-surgical specialist and/or center in the US? Or the world for that matter? Would you have any personal connections that might expedite contact? We're trying to assemble a list of alternatives as quickly as possible. I'm very sorry to be the bearer of this bad news. We are still in shock. We had been planning a family trip to Florida for his upcoming break, and it was by luck that he managed to get an MRI before we left...

Love,
Dean and Wendy

* * *

To: Raffaele
From: Dean Fachon
Subject: Urgent request
Date: March 4, 2016

Dear Chantal and Raffaele,

I just sent the [appended] note to your folks and decided I should just contact you directly. If you have any thoughts or suggestions, we would welcome them! We hope you are well and hear little Hadrien is thriving. Enjoy these precious years as much as you can!

Love,
Dean

* * *

To: Dean Fachon
From: Raffaele
Subject: Re: Urgent request
Date: Fri, 04 Mar 2016

Dear Dean,

Just read your email with great sadness. Yes, it's always better to get in touch with us directly. Never hesitate, please.

We would be very happy to assist in finding the best team for Neil. Let me just say upfront that I think you are already in an outstanding institution. Neurosurgery and Neuro-Oncology at MGH is phenomenal, and I think you are in very good hands. Boston in general, I think, is a city where both fields are among the best in the world. People travel from everywhere to be treated there.

To help you effectively, I think the conversation with the Neuro-Oncologist today will be the guiding element. In fact, brain tumours are many and different. Depending specifically on what the Neuro-Oncologist thinks Neil suffers from will determine the advice we can give you, and influence its quality. In short, to really personalize our opinion, we need to know more information.

To help you have the best conversation with the Neuro-Oncologist today, here some questions I would personally ask:

- What is the most likely nature (type) of the brain tumor seen on the MRI?
- Has a Neurosurgeon seen the MRI, and if yes, can the tumor be removed surgically?
- Can it be removed completely or only in part?
- If there is to be a surgery, what are the risks? Will Neil loose any of his functions?
- If the tumor cannot be removed, what are the recommendations for the Neuro-Oncologist? Chemotherapy? Radiotherapy?
- If the tumor can be removed, is the Neuro-Oncologist recommending other treatments before or after the surgery? Chemotherapy? Radiotherapy?

Again, I think the most important information for you is that you are in a great place (MGH has been US Best Hospital for many years in a row) and in Boston you have the world's best people around the corner. If you can get the information to the above suggested questions, you'll have a good understanding of what this disease is, what it means for Neil and you will be able to make the best decisions. If you send us more information after the conversation today, we'll be able to give you some more thoughts and recommendations, if needed.

Please give Neil a very big hug from us. You are in our thoughts at all times. If we need to talk on the phone at a later time, we are available.

Warmest wishes,
Raffaele

THE MOMENT OF TRUTH
FRIDAY AFTERNOON, MARCH 4, 2016

As we drove to Boston to pick up Neil and take him to his appointment, the idea that he had a brain tumor was still almost impossible to grasp. We gave him a call as we parked, and he came out to meet us. The difference in his gait and demeanor since the last time we saw him was startling. Gone was the athletic spring in his step, replaced by a slow flat-footed step, as if he was drunk and trying to hide it. He greeted us with big hugs and spoke clearly enough, but he had an odd tendency to giggle for no apparent reason. We were early, so we walked to his apartment to use the facilities and freshen up. It was a mild day and spring break had begun. Neil's roommate Steve had already gone home. He and Neil had roomed together freshman year and formed a tight bond. We were sorry to miss him but thankful Neil shared his apartment with such a close friend.

About an hour before the appointment, we drove to Mass General and parked in the patient lot. Mass General is a sprawling metropolitan hospital with several big buildings. Neil was supposed to report the Stephen E. & Catherine Pappas Center for Neuro-Oncology on the ninth floor of the Yawkey Center for Outpatient Care. It was as difficult to get to as it is a mouthful to say, but finding our way through the labyrinth offered a bit of distraction. Once on the ninth floor, we exited the elevator onto a long hallway lined from floor to ceiling in glass overlooking Boston. We looked down on the miniaturized street, tiny cars moving slowly through sluggish traffic and even tinier people — like ants — weaving around each other on the crammed sidewalks, each person with a life we would never know. It was impossible to avoid feeling a pang of jealousy for their apparent freedom, while Neil was being shunted down a narrow and frightening path.

The neuro-oncology waiting area was just off the hallway. Neil checked in and did not have to wait long before he was greeted by a neuro-oncology fellow, Dr. Ina Ly, a young woman with fine features and precise movements. She asked if he wanted us to be with him for the meeting, and he nodded. So began our full participation, after nearly six months, in Neil's health crisis.

Dr. Ly escorted us to a room with an exam chair, some padded chairs for family members, and a desk with a workstation. She directed Neil to the exam chair and began by asking him a few questions about how he was doing. Once up to speed on his current symptoms, she sat at a computer and pulled up Neil's MRI. She windowed through horizontal slices of Neil's brain, working down from the top, almost like a flip-book animation.

If you've never seen an MRI of a brain, it looks somewhat like a cauliflower divided in roughly symmetrical halves and colored all shades of gray. The halves of Neil's brain grew larger as she moved downwards until she arrived at one image in particular with a lighter area, almost white in comparison to the surrounding tissue, located right in the middle, and about the size of a golf ball. Dr. Ly told us the lighter area was the tumor, but she added no context for understanding the meaning of what we were looking at.

Neil stared at the screen, mouth agape.

My thought was, *Okay, that's the bastard that needs to come out.*

Wendy recalls thinking, *My God, how is it even possible he's still walking around!*

Dr. Ly made no comment, as if we understood the implications of the image just by seeing it, then she excused herself. A few moments later, we were joined by the attending neuro-oncologist, Dr. Isabel Arrillaga. Active in appearance and exuding compassion, she was apparently the doctor who would be calling the shots. Her kind demeanor took the room's tension down a notch as she gave Neil a physical examination.

Among her many questions, she asked him, "When was last time you had a bowel movement?"

It seemed a bizarre thing to ask.

"At least a week," he told her.

At least a week! (This might have been another unnoticed clue. Was the part of Neil's brain in control of involuntary movement under siege?)

Dr. Arrillaga took notes as she quizzed him, then she began to explain the type of brain tumor that was ensconced in Neil's head. "It's called DIPG," she said. "It stands for diffuse intrinsic pontine glioma."

We had no idea what that meant in terms of severity, but she cleared things up quickly.

"Left untreated," she said with empathy, "you have roughly three months to live."

"What?!" Neil sat bolt upright.

Our hearts stopped, and we just looked at Neil, our field of vision narrowing in shock, like a movie moment when the camera zooms in and pans back at the same time. Neil's eyes were riveted on Dr. Arrillaga, registering his first hint of panic and telegraphing the obvious question.

"What's the treatment?!"

"We can extend that to six months," she nodded soberly, "but we have to start radiation right away."

He was stricken. How could this moment possibly be real? In the vacuum left by her pronouncement, Dr. Arrillaga tried to breathe some hope.

"There's a slim chance your tumor could be something less malignant than DIPG," she said. "Or possibly even something that could cause similar inflammation, like MS."

"What are the chances?" Neil pleaded.

She admitted the odds were probably less than 1 percent, but if that were the case, Neil's prognosis could be completely different.

"To help know for sure," she explained, "we'll need an MRI of your spine. If the tumor has spread to your spine, it could be something different than DIPG."

"Of course," Neil nodded mechanically, just beginning to process his shortened horizon.

"And you should start radiation," she gently reiterated. "Now I'll leave for a few minutes to give you some private time."

THE MONSTER OF DESPAIR

After she closed the door, Neil gave an agonized groan. "I'm f*cked," he said in a rare moment of despair, dropping his head into his hands with a sob.

There was a monster in the house, a monster that did not even have the decency to hide under Neil's bed. It was inside his head! All Wendy and I could do was huddle close and hug him. Six months? How could this possibly be?!

"Let's pray it turns out to be less malignant," I said quietly. "We'd gain some time to figure things out," and my voice trailed off. No matter what, we would have to reach deeper and pull harder than we had ever dreamed of before.

"A one percent chance is better than none," Wendy held back her despair.

Dr. Arrillaga returned a few minutes later, looking rather shaken herself. Delivering mortal news must take a terrible toll, but she soldiered on. She professed genuine hope that some of the newer treatments might hold more promise, and she discussed one in particular that could be done at Mass General.

"If we could take a small biopsy," she explained, "it's possible we can isolate the genetic flaws and search for a match among the chemotherapies known to impact those mutations."

From this, we inferred that DIPG varies genetically from patient to patient. (If a good chemo-match can be found, the trick is to deliver it effectively into the brain. No small detail, as we would learn soon enough.)

"The prognosis for this strategy is unlikely to be much better than radiation," Dr. Arrillaga admitted, "but there is always a chance. Research is ongoing. Clinical trials are happening all the time. Something could be right around the corner that will change everything," she smiled hopefully. "If nothing else, a tissue sample would aid ongoing research to develop better treatments for DIPG patients in the future."

In a way, she was "singing Neil's song" — positivity and altruism. "I'd like to learn more about the biopsy procedure," he told her. "But I'm not ready to start radiation. I need to think more about it."

"Of course," she nodded. "Take a few days, but if that's the direction you decide to take, the sooner we start, the better. It could buy you more time to find a suitable clinical trial."

"I'll think about that too," Neil sighed heavily.

"I'll schedule an appointment with the neurosurgeon who does the biopsy procedure," Dr. Arrillaga continued. "It will most likely be first thing next week; the nurse will call to confirm. And I'll take a look for clinical trials."

"Thank you," Neil smiled.

"In the meantime, I'd like you to start taking three milligrams a day of dexamethasone. It's a steroid that should help to alleviate symptoms."

Neil nodded as Dr. Arrillaga wrote him a script. "Call anytime with questions," she handed him her card to wrap up the appointment.

After some commiserating hugs, we departed.

6

REGROUP

*"All things are relative,
even advice." NF*

Wendy and I huddled around Neil in silence as we navigated the busy hallways and sidewalks back to the car, but I imagine the lyrics from Bastille's "Pompeii" were looping through his mind: *"How am I gonna be an optimist about this."* They sure crossed my mind.

"We'll find a better solution," I tried to reassure him — reassure all of us — as we buckled in. "We won't just accept this."

"No," Neil agreed, perhaps indulging a little in the innocent notion his parents could make things better. "Radiation, just to buy a few months? That makes no sense. Maybe the biopsy and chemo-matching. At least that's pushing the envelope."

"We'll find out more about that," Wendy nodded, "but you need to get that spinal MRI, and we need to get a second opinion as quickly as possible."

"In the meantime, we'll research everything we can find," I said. "We have a lot of friends who can help. We'll get their suggestions and ask them to put out feelers as well."

As we were driving back to Neil's apartment on Huntington Avenue, he called Evie and told her the details of the meeting with Dr. Arrillaga. Evie seemed to absorb it all quietly, her heart aching more with each word, and she promised to come right over to his apartment. Amazingly, when we arrived at Neil's building, a parking space was open within fifty feet of the door.

"Thank you parking angels," Wendy said, putting a smile on Neil's face.

We "checked in" at the building's security desk and trundled inside.

WHAT HAVE YOU BEEN EATING?

"First things first," Wendy said as Neil unlocked his door. "Let's get your digestive tract moving. How can you not have pooped in more than a week?!"

"Do you eat anything besides pizza," I joked lamely.

"C'mon, Dad," Neil scowled. "I do a good job with my cooking! Ask Steve."

As part of graduating from a "dorm" to an apartment after freshman year, Neil had dropped the meal plan and started cooking his own meals. Contrary to my pizza quip, sitting on the kitchen counter was a box of fresh produce from a local "CSA" (Community-Supported Agriculture program). The box was full of fresh vegetables, and the frying pan on the stove showed every indication of regular use in creating stir-fries. Neil was eating as well as we could have hoped, and the kitchen sink proved it. Full of dishes.

"Sorry about that," Neil apologized. "Steve and I have a deal. I do the cooking, and he does the cleaning," Neil explained. "He took-off for break, and I've let it lapse."

"Not like you had anything else on your mind," I commiserated.

"This won't take five minutes," Wendy rolled up her sleeves.

Neil offered to help when the door buzzer sounded, announcing Evie's arrival. She gave everyone a hug and clung to Neil. She and he were always close. No sibling rivalries to speak of, just two peas in a pod.

"Oh Buddy," she held him tight, but held back any tears. "We'll beat this!"

"Now that you're here," Neil smiled. "I'm sure of it!"

We all pitched in with the cleanup, getting lost in small talk, then Wendy and Evie began chopping veggies and heating the skillet.

"Where's the olive oil?" Wendy asked.

"On that shelf," Neil pointed, "alongside the hot sauces and sesame oil."

"Good stuff," Wendy nodded in approval.

"See Dad," Neil gave me smirk.

The smell of stir-fry filled the apartment, and we opened a couple of windows, exchanging some aroma wafting out for the sounds of the city wafting in.

"This is great," Neil exclaimed when he took his first bite.

"We just threw in everything you had," Wendy smiled. "Good ingredients."

Neil looked at me and chuckled once more. I just raised my palms. QED.

After dinner — and another cleanup — we "hung out" while those of Neil's friends still on campus stopped by to commiserate. The talk was all positive, and there were some very big hugs! After a couple of hours, we began to think about leaving. I assumed Neil would come with us, but as soon as I mentioned it, he protested.

"I'd like to stay here."

Wendy cringed. "Are you sure you're okay?"

Neil opened his arms in a gesture to take in Evie and his friends. "I'll be fine."

"Okay," we hesitated, but we knew Evie would be close. "Call if you need us for anything! We'll come back late tomorrow morning to help you pack-up and come home."

One more night in his dorm. Neil wanted to bask in his college life and friends for as long as he could. We shared a group hug, then Wendy and I departed, struggling to reorient ourselves to this new "surreality." We learned later that Evie had offered to stay overnight, but with his friends all around him, Neil had also told her he'd be fine.

"I don't like leaving him," I said when we settled into the car for the ride home.

"He can't stand the thought he might never come back," Wendy nodded, barely containing a sob.

"We'll make sure he does," I reassured her. "Thank God Evie is home!"

"Yup."

The first tears began to roll down our cheeks as we wended our way out of Boston and began plotting a strategy: We would scour the Internet for more information about DIPG; send out urgent email requests to family and friends with medical connections; start learning everything we could about clinical trials; and get connected as quickly as possible with the very best doctor we could find for a second opinion.

It was way past our normal bedtime when we got home, but despite our emotional exhaustion, sleep was obviously the last thing on our minds. Still moving through a fog of disbelief, we sat at our respective computers and began regrouping for a long marathon.

DEXAMETHASONE?

The first thing Wendy did was look up dexamethasone to learn more about its benefits and side effects: She discovered that dexamethasone is a "corticosteroid" that interacts with the hypothalamic-pituitary-adrenocortical (HPA) axis. The hypothalamus secretes corticotropin- releasing factor (CRF), which causes the pituitary gland to secrete adrenocorticotropin (ACTH). In turn, this stimulates the adrenal glands to release about twenty milligrams of cortisol per day, with peak levels occurring in the morning. Through a negative feedback mechanism instigated by dexamethasone, an increase in circulating cortisol results in the inhibition of this cycle and suppression of its activity. Suppression of the HPA axis affects a patient's ability to respond to an acute stressful event, and chronic dexamethasone-use causes the axis to atrophy. The patient's face and extremities also begin to swell noticeably. While dexamethasone might help to reduce inflammation of the tumor, the drug's side effects sounded daunting. A day later, when Wendy told Neil what she had learned about dexamethasone, he elected to refrain from its use unless and until it was absolutely necessary.

ALTERNATIVES?

When the best mainstream medicine has to offer is a three-month reprieve on a death sentence, you either accept it as fate or you look outside the box — clinical trials and alternative therapies. Dr Arrillaga promised to get a head start on the clinical trials, so I began the search for alternative cancer treatments from both the past and present. Over the following days, some of the people and treatments we discovered include:

- Dr. Otto Warburg
- Dr. Max Gerson
- Royal Raymon Rife
- Rene Caisse Essiac
- Dr. Nicholas Gonzalez
- Dr. Stanislaw Burzynski

Some of the alternative cancer therapies espoused include:

- Laetrile
- Medical Marijuana
- IV Vitamin-C
- Resveratrol
- Antineoplastons
- Nutritional modification
- Fasting

While these doctors and their therapies are generally dismissed by mainstream medicine as outdated or quackery, the theories and science behind much of their work is ingenious. In particular, Dr. Burzynski had taken the brunt of ridicule in recent years. However, real-world evidence — "anecdotal evidence" — suggests there have been many patients for whom these outside-the-box therapies — including Burzynski's — have been very effective. Way too effective to dismiss out of hand.

After taking some initial bearings on these possibilities, Wendy and I sent off a few urgent emails, especially this one to Raffaele:

To: Raffaele
From: Dean Fachon
Subject: Re: Urgent request
Date: March 4, 2015

Raffaelle,

The doctor we met with is Isabel Arrillaga. She seems exceptionally knowledgeable and sympathetic. Unfortunately, she had no good news. Neil's tumor is, she and her colleagues are almost certain, a DIPG (defuse intrinsic pontine glioma). "Aggressive." About 300 cases occur each year, and generally they are pediatric. We looked at the MRI. Neil's brain stem is heavily compromised and there is no chance of surgery. The option she proposes is doing a biopsy – not without risk – to ID the tumor for sure and do a molecular scan to determine if there are any drugs that might knock it back. She is also looking to see if there are any promising clinical trials within the US. She thinks radiation should be done regardless of whether we elect to do the biopsy, and she said a clinical trial would not be possible if we do not do the biopsy. She did not give us any time frame for what to expect except to gently imply that the long-term prognosis is poor. Our heads are in a fog. I'm not sure I got all of this exactly right, but pretty much that's the gist. Your thoughts and input are more than welcome. We are not giving up! If you know of anything happening outside the US that we should investigate, we would not hesitate to bring Neil anywhere that offered an honest chance of hope. We are thinking outside the box. All for now.

Thank you and thank you!
Dean and Wendy

By then, it was well after midnight, and we headed for bed, but sleep came fitfully, if at all. Meanwhile, we knew our friends would be strapping on their "thinking caps." Besides our correspondence with Raffaele, one of the first suggestions we received was from Charles, also a doctor. After an initial review of what's happening regarding DIPG, he sent this:

To: Fachon Wendy
From: Charles
Subject: Mark Souweidane, Neurological Surgery, Weill Cornell Medicine
Date: Fri, 4 Mar 2016

Mark Souweidane, MD and neurosurgeon. He seems the closest to a treatment for DIPG if that is what Neil truly has. It tends to occur in younger kids under 10. He has completed "Phase I" trials at Memorial Sloan Kettering, and he is determined to find a treatment.

https://weillcornell.org/mmsouweidane

There is a foundation to support families of children who are diagnosed with DIPG.

Charles

This would not be the last time we would hear of Dr. Souweidane and Sloan Kettering.

March 4, 2016, excerpts from MGH Neuro-oncology report:

HISTORY OF PRESENTING ILLNESS:
Two months ago patient developed new symptoms. He had difficulties with initiating urination and defecation. He has had a lack of coordination, e.g. when getting out of bed, affecting both arms and legs. He has had problems with penmanship. He has had difficulty swallowing thin liquids, resulting in choking. He noted symptoms (except swallowing) have been worsening progressively... He has had headaches that began 2-3 weeks after the 3rd concussion. They were originally over the left side and more recently over the back of the neck and top of the right side. He has had episodes of laughing inappropriately since the 3rd concussion. His parents also feel that his mannerisms have been a little bit "off" recently. He saw Dr. Walter Panis from PM&R on 3/2/16 who ordered and MRI brain...

RADIOGRAPHS:
I personally reviewed the patient's MRI brain dated 3/3/16. This reveals an expansile, exophytic, nono-enhancing T2/FLAIR-hyperintense lesion in the pons with extension into medulla and midbrain, most consistent with a suspected diffuse intrinsic pontine glioma.

WHAT IS "DIFFUSE INTRINSIC PONTINE GLIOMA?"

It's "diffuse" because the cancer spreads in and around healthy tissue; "intrinsic" because the cancer is so intertwined it's impossible to tease it apart from healthy tissue; "pontine" because the cancer specifically takes up residence in the pons, the base of the brain (brainstem), which controls many crucial bodily functions (many autonomic); and "glioma" because the cancer invades "glial" cells, the cells which, as irony would have it, form the protective cushion which surrounds healthy neurons. As "diffuse intrinsic pontine glioma" grows, it stretches synaptic connections and squeezes neurons, slowly degrading their ability to relay signals until those signals are completely cut off. DIPG for short.

DIPG is quick, and it's stealthy. At first, its symptoms are so imperceptible they could easily be ignored, all the more so because DIPG's victims are often very small children who can't articulate what they're feeling. Even then, a pediatrician might chalk symptoms up to sleep loss or fighting a low-grade infection: "Fill this prescription and make sure she gets enough rest."

Until one day, the victim's eyes cross, or her movements become fumbled. Then, the alarm bells go off, and tests are ordered. By then, the prognosis is bleak. In the latter stages of disease, symptoms range from increasing difficulty with swallowing to being unable to take a deep breath. The progressive loss of autonomic functions and motor control is akin to beheading the victim one nerve strand at a time. Death by any combination of critical system failures usually occurs within less than a year of diagnosis.

HOW MAINSTREAM ONCOLOGY TREATS DIPG

Fortunately, DIPG is quite rare, afflicting less than three hundred children per year in the United States. Of those, patients Neil's age number less than 1 percent. Unfortunately, this scarcity makes it less attractive to pharmaceutical research — no obvious monetary incentive. Thus, mainstream oncology's "standard of care" is the same trio of cancer treatments that have been employed for the last fifty years:

- Surgery: Surgical options for DIPG are almost nonexistent. The tumor is so intertwined with healthy tissue that DIPG cannot be excised without causing life-threatening damage.

- Radiation: Radiation can prolong a DIPG patient's life an average of three to six months, depending on how early the disease is identified, but radiation has serious side effects, which can compromise much of that time and cause future cancers.
- Chemotherapy: Chemical agents have a difficult time crossing the "blood-brain barrier." The blood–brain barrier refers to the unique properties of the microvasculature serving the central nervous system. The barrier tightly regulates central nervous system homeostasis and protects it from toxins, pathogens, inflammation, injury, and disease that might otherwise enter through normal vasculature.[1] This makes it difficult to effectively treat DIPG with chemotherapy.

At the leading edge of mainstream oncology is the biopsy process Dr. Arrillaga told us about — taking a tumor sample to sequence the tissue and then looking for chemical agents to which the tumor's genes are most susceptible. Even with a promising match, however, the blood-brain barrier remains a major obstacle. In an attempt to bypass this barrier, a process called "convection-enhanced delivery" was invented to deliver chemotherapy directly into a brain tumor. Dr. Mark Souweidane has been working with this technique, and exploring this possibility would take us into the realm of clinical trials, also the purview of "immunotherapy." Immunotherapy is relatively new, and it seeks to train the patient's own immune system to recognize and attack the tumor.

The more science learns, the more it appears that DIPG is the result of dozens of gene mutations, if not hundreds. Some of these are not even "mutations" per se, but normal genes that aren't functioning properly. How genes function — their "expression" — plays a big role in cancer.

1 Paraphrased from: www.ncbi.nlm.nih.gov/pmc/articles/PMC4292164/

The study of gene expression falls into the field of "epigenetics.[2]" In DIPG, exactly which genes are mutated and/or malfunctioning can vary greatly between patients, but by virtue of tissue samples from DIPG victims, researchers have identified a handful of genes that are commonly associated with the tumor, and these have been the subject of many clinical trials.

In time, we would learn much more about all of this, but the moment's burning question was, "Why does this happen?" We found very little information about the causes of DIPG. Mainstream medicine is vague on this subject, having found no obvious hereditary links, and drawing no clear connections to specific environmental factors. This seemed oddly noncommittal — almost evasive — because these two factors, especially the latter, are the only possible candidates.

These were some of the topics we scratched during the early days of our search for information related to DIPG. We also found a host of patient stories, ranging from accounts of little children battling valiantly by one means or another against this implacable foe, to one bereaved parent's disconsolate epistle which amounted to, "abandon hope, all ye who enter here." To battle DIPG is to be stuck underwater between a rock and hard place. If there is a demon-king of cancer, DIPG lays a strong claim to the throne.

---

2 "DNA modifications that do not change the DNA sequence can affect gene activity. Chemical compounds that are added to single genes can regulate their activity; these modifications are known as epigenetic changes." https://ghr.nlm.nih.gov/primer/howgeneswork/epigenome

7

PANIC ATTACK

"Which of yourselves in which moment do you trust and listen to?" NF

The phone rang at 3:00 a.m. like a jolt of electricity. With extensions on either side of the bed, Wendy and I picked up together.

"I can't breathe," Neil gasped. "I'm...having....trouble......breathing," he stammered, panting between each word.

"You'll be okay Honey," Wendy told him reflexively. "Just try to relax. Call 911. That's what it's for. Stay still and meditate on something you love to help calm your breathing. Take the ambulance to the hospital, and we'll be there as fast as we can."

"Okay," his breath shook, then he managed a smidgen less breathlessly, "I will." Just being in touch seemed to calm him a little.

"We'll be on the road in less than five minutes," I told him, "so call Mom's cell phone if you need to talk. We'll call Evie."

"I called her," Neil exhaled.

"Okay, good," Wendy said. "You'll be okay! We love you!"

"We'll see you in less than two hours," I promised.

We pulled on the same clothes we'd been wearing, got a drink of water, and grabbed some granola bars, then we got in the car and headed back to Boston. The highway ahead stretched empty before us. For the entire length of Route 95 we passed no more than one or two tractor trailers and a handful of cars. The emptiness invited recollection:

Years ago, when Neil was five or six years old, he would occasionally cry out in the middle of the night. We'd go to his room, and he would be muttering unconsolably about a monster coming to get him. We would hold his little body, shaking like a leaf, his skin warm and clammy.

"Neil! It's just a dream," we would try to rouse him. "Wake up Little Buddy!"

But he would just moan and shiver, never showing the least sign he had heard us. This would go on for minutes, but eventually, he would calm down, and we could lay him back down and cover him up.

These episodes happened several times over the course of many months. He never seemed the worse for the wear, and he never recalled anything about what happened or about us being with him. Except for one time:

"I can't breathe!" he cried loud enough to wake us up with a start, and when we went to his room, he was wide awake.

"I can't breathe," he gasped, struggling for each breath and his eyes round with fright.

Wendy sat on his bed and held him, rocking. "Shhhh-hh," she soothed him. "Take it easy, Honey. You're all right. Take it easy. Try to relax and breath slowly."

"Should we take him to the ER?" I wondered aloud, remembering the time we took Evie to the ER to stitch up a split in her forehead, the result of horsing around with her Grandfather in a restaurant, of all things.

"Let's give him a moment," Wendy said.

With persistent gentle coaxing, Wendy calmed Neil down until he was able to breathe normally. We stayed with him a long time until he fell back to sleep, breathing peacefully. Wendy slept with him the rest of the night, and the next day, she made an appointment with the family doctor.

He prescribed an asthma inhaler in case this should ever happen again. It never did.

My mind roamed this memory. Was it some sort of premonition? Wendy, too, was lost in thoughts, so we drove in silence as the highway stretched black and empty before us. As much as we knew it would take us to Boston, what lay ahead was a frightening mystery. Alternate sighs punctuated our silence until Wendy spoke.

"What are you thinking about?"

"I was remembering the time Neil couldn't breathe," I said wistfully.

"Yeah," Wendy sighed. A few moments passed, then she raised her hands and looked up as if invoking the heavens: "How on Earth did this happen?!"

"It was those dammed vaccines," snarled up from my throat unbidden. "The moment he told us, I knew something bad had just happened. You remember that day?"

Wendy sighed again. "How could I forget?"

It was late August 2014, and Neil eagerly anticipated his first semester at Northeastern. All he needed to complete his entry requirements was to get a physical exam. He asked if he could drive himself to the appointment and get a little more practice at shifting the manual transmission in his Grandmother's old Beetle.

Why not, we thought. We had to let him start handling his own business, and he was just going into town to see our family doctor — Neil's "pediatrician" for many years.

"Sure," we told him. "Take the car."

He returned roughly an hour later.

"How did it go?" Wendy asked him.

"I'm in great shape," he exclaimed, and almost as an afterthought, he added, "They gave me a couple of vaccinations."

His innocent words struck me head to toe with a dreadful foreboding. "What?!!"

"They gave me the HPV vaccine and something for meningitis," Neil said.

"Dammit," I shouted, slamming my hand on my desk so hard the room shook. "God dammit!"

My outburst startled both Neil and Wendy.

"Were they required by Northeastern?" I demanded.

"I don't think so," Neil replied quietly.

"I wish they hadn't done that," I said. "I wish you'd called us."

"Don't worry about it," Wendy tried to smooth it over. "It's done. He'll be fine."

Neil departed the room with less bounce in his step. I was sorry to upset him, but deep down, I could not shake my worry. For two or three years, the nurses at Dr. Slattery's office had asked if we wanted to give Neil the HPV vaccine, and each time, we said, "No." Now that he was no longer a minor, it seemed Neil had been caught in the web of Rhode Island's "Vaccinate Before You Graduate" program.

"I think something really bad may have just happened," I told Wendy.

"I know," she shook her head.

Half an hour later, I called Northeastern to ask if the vaccines were required.

"No, neither of those is required."

I was so upset at the time I wrote a note to Dr. Slattery to vent my frustration:

Letter Excerpt, August 26, 2014:

Dr. John,

My son Eugene, "Neil," returned home from his physical

to inform us he received two vaccinations during his visit [one for HPV, the other for meningitis], *neither of which we approved nor does his college require. Of course he is now 18 and thus we are no longer his "guardians," but when the question of HPV vaccine has come up in the past, we flatly refused. The potential for adverse effects outweighs the "benefits" by an order of magnitude.*

I am stunned and disappointed these vaccines were administered to Neil without having him consult us, and now there is nothing I can do to intervene against this unwarranted and dangerous assault on his immune system. Words cannot express my disappointment.

Dean Fachon

Why Was I So Upset? In the last few decades, the pharmaceutical industry has created dozens upon dozens of new vaccines, many of which are effectively mandated, becoming staples in the recommended vaccine schedule for children to combat diseases they are ever less likely to contract. Evidence mounts that our immune systems are being overstimulated. For any given vaccine, some portion of those taking it will have an adverse side effect. If enough vaccines are forced on enough people, virtually everyone will suffer some sort of collateral damage, begging the question of whether the results justify the cost, both in suffering and dollars.

Occasionally, evidence of harm caused by a vaccine will reach the ears of the public, as in the ongoing debate about autism. The medical establishment has been quick to denounce any suggested linkage as "conspiracy theory," shaming vaccine-injury victims or their families into silence. If they do come forward, they are swallowed up

> by the "National Childhood Vaccine Injury Act." Signed into law by President Reagan in 1986, the act's name would make you think it's about protecting children. Not at all. In Washington, DC's typically cynical style, the act was given a warm and fuzzy name, but it is less about protecting children than it is about protecting the pharmaceutical industry: The industry, and those who administer its vaccines, are held blameless for any negative side effects. They have been given an immunity far stronger than anything a vaccine can provide.
>
> A quick review of the act's sister program, the "National Vaccine Injury Compensation Program," shows the lay of the land: Vaccine-injury victims have only one recourse for their grievances, the "Vaccine Injury Court," a Byzantine legal process designed to discourage most from ever trying to seek justice and to otherwise confound those who do. Victims can apply to the court for compensation (funded by taxpayer money) if they can prove injury. The standards of proof are almost impossible to meet, and the limit for compensation if one manages to succeed is $250,000. How much is a human life worth?
>
> On that day back in August of 2014, I was desperately concerned about how those two vaccines, HPV and meningitis, might interact with Neil's immune system. Was it just a coincidence that one of the vaccines was intended to prevent a disease of the brain, the other to prevent cancer, and a little more than a year later, Neil is incubating one of the rarest and most intractable brain tumors there is?

These thoughts were flooding my mind during the early morning darkness on Route 95.

"I can't shake the feeling those vaccines sparked this tumor," I sighed heavily.

"I know," Wendy commiserated, "but we can't do anything about that now. Let's stay focused."

We merged onto the "Southeast Expressway," normally packed bumper to bumper and now an empty ribbon connecting to Boston while leading us into uncharted territory. At some point during the ride, Evie called to say she had taken a cab to the Mass General ER and was sitting with Neil.

"He's doing better," she assured us.

"Thank you Sweetheart," Wendy sighed with relief. "We'll be there soon too."

THE ER

Evie was sitting beside Neil in a private room when we arrived at the ER. We hugged all around, and Neil seemed much like his old self, although a little abashed.

"Sorry about this," he said. "Usually, the sirens and lights are just passing by. I was embarrassed they had to come for me."

"No worries, Buddy," I told him. "That's what 911 is for. So, what's going on?"

"They've taken some blood and done a chest X-ray," he told us. "We're waiting for the results."

As we sat waiting for a doctor to return with Neil's test results, we tried to combat our shared apprehensions. The room had a TV, so we turned it on just in time to see an infomercial with the catch phrase, "Work Less, Play More!"

"Now, that's serendipity," Wendy smiled as she reached into her tote bag and pulled out *Work Less Play More,* a bound notepad with various sport ball patterns printed on the back side of each sheet. Once you were done with a sheet, the idea was to crumple up into a ball and take a shot at the recycle bin. Wendy handed Neil the book, and he tore out a page with a football on the back, crumpled it, and tossed it into the bin.

"Touchdown," I declared, and Wendy mimed like a cheerleader.

On the next sheet, Neil wrote some notes to himself — things he needed to do to tidy up his school affairs. He knew his school year was over.

Evie had some distractions in mind as well. She brought *Zen Pencils,* a book of inspirational cartoons. One particular cartoon was of a caped boy, sword and shield in hand, leaping to attack a dragon. The dragon blasts the knight to the ground and stomps off. The next frame shows the boy sitting up, and the caption reads, "Nothing in the world can take the place of persistence!" The boy goes after the dragon, grabs its tail, climbs up its back to its head, and drives his sword into the dragon's brain. In the final frame, the boy stands atop the slain dragon. The caption reads:

> "Persistence and determination alone are omnipotent!"
> —*Calvin Coolidge*

"My goodness," Wendy chuckled softly. "That's you, Neil. Do you remember that costume?"

She was referring to the Halloween when he was four years old. He wore a knight costume and carried a play sword and a shield. The shield had an emblem of a dragon.

"Yup, that was my second favorite costume," Neil grinned.

Perhaps it was just a coincidence, but medieval knights were a recurring theme in Neil's life. He liked to play "knight" as a young boy, and he dressed as one for Halloween. His middle and high schools both had knights as their mascots, and he dressed up as Link for Halloween at Northeastern. Then, of course, there are the knights on a chess board, pieces Neil loved for their ability to jump other pieces and launch unexpected attacks. Now, he stood face to face with the deadliest dragon he would ever face. To defeat it, he would need all his knightly courage, strength, faith, determination, and persistence — as would we all.

The attending ER physician eventually returned. Neil's tests were all negative as far as he was concerned. It was a panic attack. Since Neil had recovered his composure, he was discharged. The university was closed for spring break, so we stopped off at each of our kids' apartments to gather their things, then we brought them both home.

Excerpt from ER doctor's report, Mass General Hospital, March 5, 2015:

Patient is awake and alert. Patient is nontoxic appearing. Very anxious, shivering and tearful.

AND FINALLY TEARS

Being spring break, many of Neil's friends were home too. He touched base with a few and asked them to come over that afternoon. It was a pleasant day, and looking out the study window, I could see the boys playing Frisbee on the front lawn. A few minutes later, I went out to say hello and found them sitting on the ground in a scrum around Neil.

"I can't play Frisbee," he sobbed softly and looked up, tears streaming down his cheeks.

He couldn't move quickly enough, he couldn't throw with any accuracy or strength, and he couldn't grip fast enough to catch the flying disk. His body had the ability, but his brain wasn't able to relay the signals.

"Oh Pal," I tried not to choke up. "Hang in there. We'll figure this out!"

His friends, though visibly shaken, tried to add their encouragement, and it seemed best for me to just let them be. I went back into the house, the moment underscoring just how quickly DIPG moves. From one day to the next, it can squeeze here and there, causing a cacophony of symptoms that come and go with escalating repetition. We had to move as quickly as possible, but not without applying as much reason as possible. I, once again, cursed the delay in Neil's diagnosis, but as frustrating as it was, we had to push forward. Thankfully, a growing army of knowledgeable supporters jumped on board to help guide us.

8

THE REAL HUNT BEGINS

"Get clues together and solve them.
Plot them on a map, and go for it!" NF

The first order of business was figuring out how to free up Neil's digestive tract — to get it moving properly so it could be recruited to help fight his cancer. Nutrition can be powerful medicine. "You are what you eat" is not just a slogan, and to this end, Charles sent Wendy a list of books about diets to help in the fight against all types of cancer:

- *Defeat Cancer: 15 Doctors of Integrative & Naturopathic Medicine Tell You How*
- *Anticancer: A New Way of Life*
- *The Cancer-Fighting Kitchen: Nourishing, Big-Flavor Recipes for Cancer Treatment and Recovery*
- *Natural Strategies for Cancer Patients*

Between Charles's book list and some books we already owned, Wendy had some excellent resources to begin adjusting Neil's diet. She began by applying "Gerson therapy." Decades ago, Dr. Max Gerson documented scores of disease cures, including cancer, with diet and juicing alone."[3]

The Gerson Therapy is a natural biological treatment

3 Dr. Robert Jay Rowen, page 28 of the foreword to *Defeat Cancer: 15 Doctors of Integrative and Naturopathic Medicine Tell You How*, The BioMed Publishing Group.

> which uses the body's own healing mechanisms for the elimination of debilitating ailments. It was introduced to the Western industrialized nations more than sixty-years ago by Max Gerson, MD. This revolutionary dietary program was so far advanced at the time of its development that no scientific rationale was available to explain why it produced reversal of chronic and infectious diseases. But because it actually cured patients with advanced tuberculosis, diabetes, migraines, heart disease, cancer, arthritis, skin disorders and numerous other life-threatening conditions, the Gerson Therapy has long since established itself as a major contributor to the medical armamentarium.
>
> At the core of the Gerson Therapy is its diet, which includes organically grown fresh fruits and vegetables and thirteen glasses of freshly squeezed juice daily, taken at hourly intervals. The organic fresh fruits and vegetables provide the patient with elevated levels of minerals, enzymes, beta- carotene, vitamins A and C, and other antioxidants that scavenge free radicals, as well as [providing] naturally occurring phytochemicals that scientists have discovered are true preventers of chronic degenerative diseases... No meat is allowed.[4]

"Juicing" is central to Gerson therapy, and as luck would have it, an organic juice bar called Raw Bob's had recently opened in town. We became regular customers.

FROM ACROSS THE SEA

While Wendy took great strides in re-tooling the kitchen, our transatlantic correspondence increased dramatically.

4 *The Gerson Therapy*, Preface and Introduction excerpts, Charlotte Gerson and Morton Walker, D.P.M.

To: Dean Fachon
From: Raffaele
Subject: Re: Urgent request
Date: March 5, 2016

Dear Dean,

The diagnosis of DIPG is in fact a very bad one. I think you got everything very clearly. Having the head in the fog is the appropriate feeling right now. I am so extremely sorry.

As explained by Dr. Arrillaga, DIPG unfortunately is a tumor that cannot be removed and where treatment options are extremely limited. Radiation is always used to slow down the process, even in small children. As you know, I have been on Faculty as a pediatric cancer doctor at the DANA-Farber and Children's [Hospitals] for several years and cared for children with cancer, including DIPG. Therefore I know the team there very well, and I have worked closely with one of the best, if not the best neuro-oncologist in the world, who happens to be the lead investigator on DIPG trials. His name is Dr. Mark Kieran, and I could write to him if you would like to meet with him in Boston for a second opinion. Although he usually sees children and adolescents, I am sure he'd be happy to help if I ask him. He is the first person who set up a trial to do a biopsy in DIPG and do the molecular scan, to which you are referring in your message. In fact, new treatments and personalized options are needed and Mark has led the way in this. The Neurosurgery team of the DANA-Farber is the one for the Brigham and Women's Hospital and the same of Children's Boston. They are the world leaders in DIPG biopsy. In fact, I think Mark

> Kieran would be among the experts who see the most DIPG cases in the world. If there is a trial open, it will be at DFCI/Children's and if there is not, Mark would know where to go and who to ask. I think Boston and the US are the places I would go to for this disease, and I don't think there is anything abroad that I would consider to be a better alternative or solid option at this time.
>
> My personal opinion, is that a biopsy done by a good neurosurgeon who thinks it can be done and explains clearly what risks this might entail, would be important to consider. DIPG in adults is extremely rare, and it may be for Neil that something specific to his situation can be found. Everybody is different, and until you have looked at the tumor itself, it is impossible to say how best to fight it.
>
> Please let me know if you want me to talk to Mark Kieran about Neil, and I'll contact him today. If you want me to do so, please send me Neil's full name, date of birth and his MGH medical record number (if you have it on hand, its usually on a blue plastic card that is given, but no need to delay your reply if you don't). I am asking about the medical record number as the DANA-Farber and MGH work together as a group (Partners).
>
> Warmest wishes, and big hugs from Chantal and I to Neil and all of you,
>
> Raffaele

Raffaele's response was an answered prayer. Neil needed a good second opinion, and he needed it soon. Now, he could get one from a foremost authority on DIPG.

"I've got some great news," I announced. "Raffaele knows the right people — one of the best DIPG experts on the planet — Dr. Mark Kieran at Dana-Farber — and Raffaele would be happy to contact him directly on your behalf."

Neil sighed with relief. "Tell him 'Yes, Please! Absolutely!' "

To: Raffaele
From: Dean Fachon
Subject: Re: Urgent request
Date: March 5, 2016

Raffaele,

Yes, we would very much welcome such an important referral! We are supposed to meet with a neurosurgeon next week. Dr. Arrillaga will let us know when. We are exhausted today – after a 3AM panic-attack took us to the MGH emergency room, but Neil is doing better now, and we're trying to remain positive and assess all possible avenues. Your advocacy means the world!

Thank you again,
Dean

* * *

To: Dean Fachon
From: Raffaele
Subject: Re: Urgent request
Date: March 5, 2016

Dear Dean,

I am extremely sorry to hear of the stress and pain this has already caused Neil and your family. I wrote to Dr Mark Kieran now, with all the details. I think he is frequently traveling the world, but count on me to make sure Neil's situation comes to his attention, or the attention of his incredible team, as soon as possible.

Chantal and I are both thinking of Neil and you. We want to be there for Neil and your family in this incredibly difficult time. We deeply care. I am available to Neil and you all to chat on the phone anytime, if this could help in any way.

In these very challenging times, it is always important to make sure Neil and you sleep, eat and drink sufficiently. It's always stupid to say, but making sure that the bases are covered is important. Get in touch with all your support people, wherever they might be. Ask for help, and never be ashamed to do so. This is a time for your network of friends to step in and help you, but make their contributions the way Neil and you want. Keep people that are not helpful away, and don't hesitate to ask for people to respect your privacy.

Please give Neil and each other a big hug from Chantal and me. We are there, far away in miles, but very close in our hearts. I will be in touch as soon as I hear from Mark.

Warmest thoughts,
Raffaele

Raffaele's advice was a soothing balm, reinforcing many of the steps we were already taking. We were on the right track, and as promised, Raffaele reached out to Dr. Kieran immediately, with prompt results:

To: Dean Fachon
From: Raffaele
Subject: Re: Urgent request
Date: March 6, 2016

Dear Dean,

Dr Kieran replied within minutes of me getting in touch with him. It will certainly make you feel good to know that Dr Arrillaga from the MGH had been in touch with him already. In fact, she contacted him before Neil and you met with her. They discussed Neil's case, and what options are available. I think the messages that you heard from Dr Arrillaga reflect Dr Kieran's thoughts as well. Dr Kieran has not reviewed the entire set of images from Neil's MRI, but only selected representative images, and I think this is not a big issue. The features of DIPG are clear and the neuro-radiologists at MGH would have no issue whatsoever to make that call.

What the above discussions with Dr Kieran show, I think, is that your team at MGH is excellent, and deeply invested in finding the best options for Neil. The fact that they immediately, and even before your visit, were in touch with a key leader in the field and specifically DIPG proves that.

If Neil and you want to meet and discuss with Dr Kieran at the DANA-Farber in Boston, this would be no problem. He would review the entire MRI and you would be able to ask all your questions to him directly. He is available if this is what you want and need, but it is up to you. I am happy to help you connect with his personal assistant and get an appointment scheduled.

Let me know if/how I can help, and if there is anything else you would need to discuss. I am available anytime.

Warmest thoughts,
Raffaele

"Woo Hoo," I shouted, drawing Wendy, Evie, and Neil to the study.

"Thank God for Raffaele," Wendy almost cried when I shared the news. "That has to be the best referral Neil could possibly get!"

"Amen," I agreed.

"I'd sure like to know if he thinks this could be something besides DIPG," Neil grimaced in consternation. "But if Dr. Arrillaga already spoke with him, how much different will his suggestions be, do you think?"

"Well, now you'll find out," Evie smiled. "Make a list of your questions."

"Ayup," Neil nodded.

"He'll also know about clinical trials," Wendy added.

"I'm looking for those too," Evie smiled.

"I'm down with that," Neil gave his sister a hug.

After this brief celebration, we returned to our respective computers.

THREE CLINICAL TRIALS

As emails continued being exchanged like a volley in tennis, Wendy looked for more information on alternative therapies. Being a writer for *Natural Awakenings* magazine, she had contacts in the naturopathic arena. She would reach out to them. She also found a clinic in Monterey, Mexico that offered a nutritional program coupled with an array of nontoxic therapies. With a monster like DIPG, we had to look inside AND outside of the box!

Evie, as promised, took the lead in researching clinical trials. A scientist by nature, she quickly found *ClinicalTrials.gov* and searched for "DIPG." Of the trials listed, there were three in particular that seemed like realistic possibilities:

1) Memorial Sloan Kettering in New York City was testing Convection-Enhanced Delivery (CED) to deliver chemotherapy directly into the brain, bypassing the blood-brain barrier.
2) The University of Louisville was preparing to test an immuno-

therapy process intended to train patients' immune systems to recognize and attack DIPG cells.

3) The Burzynski Clinic in Houston was preparing to test antineoplaston therapy. This was the only clinical trial that did not require candidates to take conventional treatments in advance.

There was Memorial Sloan Kettering once again, along with an immunotherapy trial which sounded intriguing — at least the concept seemed very intuitive. It was also surprising to see the Burzynski Clinic mentioned on the government's clinical trials website. Perhaps the tide against Dr. Burzynski was turning. I forwarded Evie's findings to Raffaele.

ANECDOTAL EVIDENCE

I first learned about Dr. Burzynski years before when I was researching alternative cancer treatments for my mother. My findings were all over the map, but I was sufficiently curious to purchase a documentary produced by Eric Merola: *Burzynski — Cancer Is Serious Business.*[5] Dr. Burzynski did not have a cure-all, but he had treated many patients with "incurable cancers" — brain tumors in particular — with remarkable success.

My mother ended up taking standard chemo over the course of several months. In the process, she lost her hair and suffered stabbing pains and numbness in her hands and feet, which never really improved. She enjoyed another year with her family before the cancer returned with a vengeance. Could she have done better with a different therapy? We'll never know, but I never forgot about Dr. Burzynski, and I never dreamed my interest would become so much more "targeted."

"I have something you should watch," I told Neil that afternoon. Wendy and Evie were out running errands, so he and I settled onto the sofas in the living room, and I loaded the documentary into the DVD

5 *Burzynski – Cancer Is Serious Business*, a documentary written, directed and produced by Eric Merola. At the time of this writing, the video could be found on the Internet.

player. The documentary opens with the following words displayed on a black background:

> "This is the story of a medical doctor and PhD. biochemist who has discovered a genetic mechanism that can cure most human cancers. The opening 30 minutes of this film is designed to thoroughly establish this fact – so the viewer can fully appreciate the events that follow."

After giving said "viewer" a few moments to consider this bold claim, the scene shifts to a congressional subcommittee at which testimony is being given by Sargent Rick Schiff, a decorated former member of the San Francisco Police Department. The date is February 29, 1996:

> "[At the age of four, my daughter] Kristin developed a highly malignant brain tumor that spread throughout her spine and her brain. The doctors told us we had really two options. Take her home to let her die, or bring her in for massive doses of chemo and radiation simultaneously. In either event she was going to die. They were quite certain of that, and very quickly.
>
> Believing her only chance to be the standard rout, we gave her the chemo and radiation. It burned her skull so bad she had 2nd-degree burns and her hair never came back. To change her diapers we had to wear rubber gloves because her urine was so toxic, and it burned her. At the end of six months, miraculously she survived the standard treatment, she still had cancer. We were told, "Sorry, we've done everything we can. Now she's going to die, probably within a couple of months."
>
> My wife and I, choosing not to accept that, started reading. The first book I picked up, the third chapter discussed Dr. Burzynski. As you may guess, I have some expertise in

> fraud. In fact I'm quite certain there are enough attorneys in the room that I could be voir-dired (impaneled) as an expert in fraud. And I conducted my own investigation. I have no doubt the man is not a fraud. I have no doubt that he does what he does out of earnest belief that his [Antineoplaston] medicine works. Now you're in a position to judge for yourselves whether it works or not, but it's well established by the FDA that it's non-toxic.
>
> Eighteen months later, we took my daughter off the Antineoplastons. She had not died; she had no signs of tumor; she remained free for 18 months of cancer. [Then], within a month, the cancer [returned and] was wide-spread in her brain. We put her back on Burzynski's [treatment], by the way, at the objections of our doctors who for some reason felt it had failed her. We put her back on. Within nine weeks the tumor was completely gone. She died last July of neurological necrosis. Her brain fell apart from the radiation. The autopsy showed that she was completely cancer free. Out of 52 cases of that disease, ever, no one died cancer free. Just Krissy.
>
> So she didn't die of a terminal illness. She died of my inability to care for her properly, and she died from bad advise. She died because there is a government institution that disseminates false information and is not looking out for the welfare of the People..."

"What the heck," Neil shook his head.

"Sit tight," I told him. "Wait until you've seen the whole thing."

The documentary continues with Eric Merola — the film's maker — interviewing a doctor and several patients who've had firsthand experience with Dr. Burzynski. Of particular interest was Jessica Ressel, a young woman who was diagnosed with DIPG in March of 1996. She was eleven at the time. Her MRI scans looked remarkably similar to Neil's, although her tumor was smaller when they found it. Her diagnosis was confirmed by two hospitals. Neil sat up straight. What followed could not have been more germane. Jessica and her parents were unenthusiastic about radiation treatment — not when it would only buy a few months and have side effects that would undermine her quality of life:

> "The thing is with the radiation," Jessica says, "what it would do to you from what I understood, was they would shoot the beam through your ears, and the beam would burn your healthy and your cancerous cells, outside in, so all your hair around your ears would be gone...and you would become deaf..."
>
> "What she would have to go through in those extra months, that would be horrible," says Jessica's dad. "I wouldn't want to go through it. Why do it?"
>
> "You're handed a death sentence anyway," says her mom, "so what was the point of the radiation?"
>
> "Then you have to say," concludes her dad, "modern medicine doesn't have an answer. Let's find our own."

The Ressels sidestepped radiation and started searching for something else. Their search landed them at the Burzynski Clinic, where Jessica underwent treatment with antineoplastons beginning in May of 1996. One month into treatment, Jessica's tumor seemed to disappear from her scans, but given the aggressive nature of DIPG, it showed up again soon thereafter. Dr. Burzynski increased Jessica's dose, and once again, the tumor seemed to disappear.

This cycle repeated three times during which Jessica's dose of antineoplastons was gradually doubled. In May of 1997 — one year later — her tumor disappeared and did not return. In 2001, Jessica was declared cancer-free. She had a "complete response" to the antineoplastons. At the time she was interviewed by Eric Merola, Jessica was twenty-four years old. She was married with a five-year-old son, and she had another child on the way.

By this point in the documentary, Neil was on the edge of his seat. The film went on to compare two studies for brainstem gliomas: In one study, a total of one-hundred-seven patients received standard radiation and chemotherapy. In the other, forty patients received Dr. Burzynski's antineoplastons. Of the one hundred seven patients treated with standard therapy, less than 1 percent were cancer-free after treatment, and that patient survived less than five years. Of the patients treated with antineoplastons, eleven of the forty were cancer-free after treatment. All eleven survived five years or more. In Dr. Burzynski's own words:

> "So the good news is that the cancer can be cured. The worst type of cancer can be cured. For good. The people who are surviving, they live normal lives. No side-effects from treatment, no symptoms, no sign of tumors. Back to Life. We started some of them as children, and they have their own children. There is no impairment of fertility. They just live normal lives. The best thing however is that we know that we can help, not everybody, but some of these patients. Well, about 30% of patients can survive over five years, and a number of them can live over ten years without any sign of cancer."

Following this simple, rancor-free statement, the film shifts to interviews with other patients who ended up with Dr. Burzynski. These were patients who had undergone treatment at some of the world's most prestigious cancer centers and been declared beyond hope. Many of these patients were then successfully healed by Dr. Burzynski's treatment. Not all, but many.

From all Neil's years of chess training, he had developed an ability to focus with tremendous intensity. He was absorbing each moment for later analysis, but some obvious questions crossed his mind.

"So why aren't we hearing about this at Mass General?" he asked.

"Why isn't this common knowledge?" He effectively begged the next voice-over from the film's producer:

> *Eric Merola:* "Unlike other clinical trials which are supported by billion-dollar pharmaceutical companies, and which are often assisted by large tax-funded research grants from the National Cancer Institute, the United States government currently prohibits any taxpayer money to be granted to Dr. Burzynski's FDA-approved clinical trials...Given the existence of a treatment that is curing cancer at a rate that traditional medicine could only dream of, and doing so without any damaging side-effects, most would assume that every penny of our tax dollars allocated for cancer research would be thrown in Dr. Burzynski's direction."

"Why not?!" Neil interrogated the TV.

> *The film cuts to Dr. Julian Whitaker:* "The problem that we face, however, is that a huge financial house has been built on the paradigm of purging the body of cancer cells. Burzynski's discovery means that the foundation, the walls and the roof of that house need to be replaced. Think about it, you know you've got thousands of doctors in oncology and in oncology-residency programs, you've got the pharmaceutical industry pumping out chemo-therapeutic agents every month. There are all kinds of machines that deliver radiation, you've got all this stuff in the war on cancer, and it's trillions of dollars. I find it very interesting that we have all these walks for the cure for cancer, you've got all the wrist-bands, you've got all the donations, "we're going to find a cure this decade." All this money keeps pouring in, and it all goes to the same guys."

"And their pitch never ends," I paused the video. "The cure is always 'just around the corner.' I've been hearing this song for five decades!"

> *Eric Merola's narration elaborates:* "The pharmaceutical industry is arguably the most profitable industry on our planet, with its profits being triple that of all of the 'Fortune 500' companies. Rising profits means rising stock prices. The only way this industry can sustain this profitable momentum is by continuing to introduce new patented drugs. And since the pharmaceutical industry relies on the FDA as its gatekeeper to introduce these new drugs, it's in [the industry's] best interest to ensure the FDA remains as compliant as possible. And since the FDA is also an office of the United States government, it's in the government's best interest to preserve one of its most powerful industries."

So, a picture was coming into focus — a picture suggesting collusion between "big pharma" and the FDA. Merola cites the former editor-in-chief of the New England Journal of Medicine, Dr. Marcia Angell, on this very topic:

> "In 1992, Congress put the fox in the chicken coop. It passed the Prescription Drug User Fee Act, which authorizes the drug companies to pay 'user fees' to the FDA for each brand-name drug considered for approval... In effect, the User Fee Act put the FDA on the payroll of the industry it regulates...But while it's a small investment for the drug companies, it's a lot of money for the agency, and it has drastically changed the way it operates...Consequently, the part of the agency that reviews new drugs gets more than half its money from the user fees...The agency's coziness with industry is underscored by the composition of its 18 advisory committees – outside experts who help

> evaluate drugs. Incredibly, many of these advisers work as consultants for drug companies. The FDA behaves as if the pharmaceutical industry is its user, not the public." [6]
>
> *Eric Merola then continues his narration:* "By 2010, the fee revenue paid by the pharmaceutical industry to the FDA had risen to over half-a-billion dollars annually. Pharma now [at the time of the film's making] pays over $1.4 million for most cancer drugs submitted to the FDA to ensure a timely approval.
>
> Meanwhile, Dr. Burzynski, his patients and other supporting scientists have made every conceivable effort to get the FDA, and thus the government, to cooperate in the research, review and approval of Antineoplastons – since 1977."

"This stinks," Neil shook his head. "Burzynski seems to have a real breakthrough!"

I held up my hands. "It gets worse."

From that moment forward, the documentary delves into a history of complaints brought against Burzynski by the Texas Medical Board and the Food and Drug Administration. They have launched investigation after investigation, including raids on Burzynski's clinic to seize patient records. From the mid-1980s onwards, there have been grand jury proceedings, congressional hearings, and jury trials. These actions, ostensibly taken to protect the public from Dr. Burzynski's predatory practices, came to naught. One by one, Burzynski won dismissals and acquittals. The complaints brought against him were so weak it prompted the judge in his first trial, Judge Earl A. Corbitt, to later comment to Merola:

> "I'd never heard of Dr. Burzynski. I didn't know anything about him. I never was quite clear what the [Texas Med-

6 Marcia Angell, M.D.: "Taking Back the FDA," *The Boston Globe*; February 6, 2007

ical] Board's problem was. The board did not bring any expert witnesses to contest points that were raised by Dr. Burzynski. Now, without an expert witness to render an opinion in certain areas, I can't give any credence to opinion raised by a layman, and Dr. Burzynski brought in Dr. Nicholas Patronas (a Georgetown University expert, and a member of the National Cancer Institute's team that analyzed seven of Dr. Burzynski's cases):"

> "The basic conclusion was that in five of the patients with brain tumors that were fairly large, the tumor resolved. Disappeared. It's amazing. The fact that they are living, it's impressive and unbelievable." Dr. Nicholas Patronis

Judge Corbitt continues: "[Dr. Patronas] was quite a witness: He said he had never seen anything like what Dr. Burzynski was able to accomplish with his antineoplastons in brain cancer... [Dr. Burzynski] had one young boy there who had been treated, he was about 12 at the hearing – strapping lad, a good sized boy – but when he first started on treatment, when he was about four years old – I think his name was Paul – he was given up on by his original doctor. For all I know, the kid may still be alive."

(Indeed he was. At the time of Neil's diagnosis in 2016, Paul Michaels was 34 years old.)

Neil took it all in: Jessica and Paul's stories and others like them; stories of those who were less fortunate; Judge Corbitt's troubling criticisms of the TMB; excerpts from official memos between Dr. Burzynski and the TMB/FDA tag team; and records of official court proceedings and congressional hearings. Time and time again, it seemed the crimes Dr.

Burzynski was accused of committing — being a charlatan and a scam artist — were actually being committed by the TMB/FDA tag team themselves, and done with impunity. Rather than pursuing medical advancement or justice, they seemed more concerned with discrediting Dr. Burzynski and depleting his resources. Ultimately, their legal actions were failures, but they were quite effective at crippling Dr. Burzynski's reputation and his practice. Through it all, Dr. Burzynski continued to treat patients who had nowhere else to turn.

"What the heck," Neil exclaimed again as the documentary ended. "How do they get away with this!" This was a new experience for Neil — seeing agencies entrusted with protecting the public's safety apparently doing just the opposite. It was difficult for him to process, and that's saying something. He shook his fists!

"I know," I agreed, "it's maddening."

"Let's get in touch with Dr. Burzynski," Neil looked at me, anger giving way to a sense of exciting possibility.

"I will," I told him. "In the meantime, do your own research. You'll find a chorus of Burzynski naysayers. You need to dig deep and decide for yourself what's believable."

"I know one thing," Neil frowned. "At this point, I don't think I'm too interested in radiation."

He headed back to his room to start doing some research, and I went back to the study and my computer to request information from the Burzynski Clinic and do some more digging myself. I wanted to find current information about the clinic, and I discovered the saga between Dr. Burzynski and the Texas Medical Board was continuing, with trial dates looming. I also discovered the "Burzynski Patient Group" website. As the name suggests, this is a site where many of Dr. Burzynski's patients can congregate and share information — including treatment success stories. The tagline under the page title reads, "We are Living proof." It was refreshing to find this resource amongst a morass of condemnation. I sent the link to Neil, Evie, and Wendy, then I resumed my correspondence with Raffaele.

CHEMOTHERAPY TRIALS (AND TRIBULATIONS)

To: Raffaele
From: Dean
Subject: Re: Urgent request
Date: March 6, 2016

Raffaele,

While this time is very stressful, please know we are experiencing a tremendous outpouring of love and concern from our family and friends near and far. If Love could cure disease, we would all be healthy. Of course, love is an important ingredient, but so too is finding out as much as possible to make good decisions. To that end, you are a God send! While we wait for further appointments, we are also taking great pains to feed Neil a diet that cuts out sugar, wheat, and most dairy, and we are increasing his consumption of green leafy vegetables and healthy fats and foods that are generally alkaline, which is widely held to be a good anti-cancer regimen. Given the odds in this situation, we are also trying to evaluate alternative treatments. Of course, most alternative approaches are dismissed by mainstream medicine, but the circumstances make it critical to understand every option.

Thank you again for your warm wishes and advocacy! We are sharing your hugs, and we would be grateful if you would share some from us with your family. We look forward to hearing from you when you receive word from your colleague. If anything crops up here in the meantime, I will be in touch.

Thank you again!
Dean

* * *

To: Dean
From: Raffaele
Subject: Re: Urgent request
Date: Sun, 6 Mar 2016

Dear Dean,

Dr Kieran is happy to see you. Please contact his office tomorrow (Monday) AM to set up an appointment. It will be crucial to have Neil's MRI images sent to Dr Kieran at DANA-Farber in advance. Ask the person you speak to about the best way to do this image transfer. Mrs Katelyn Nkomo is usually the person most experienced in getting this done. Mention I suggested you contact her to get the MRI images uploaded.

Regarding Evie's link about the phase I/II trial for intra-arterial infusion of Erbitux/Bevacizumab,

1. Let me first say that Evie did a great job in finding the trial via the website ClinicalTrials.gov. This is very good and reliable website. As she and you certainly saw, there are several trials out there enrolling patients with DIPG. The big issue is that none have at this time shown promising results. Some are trials on medications that are using new mechanisms, and some deliver the medication by new means. Some also try known methods in other ways (hyperfractionated radiotherapy). This shows that while we are learning more and more about the biology of these diseases, treatments are lagging behind.

2. Just for background: phase I/II trials are safety/efficacy trials run with limited prior evidence. The idea is to get an understanding if it's safe and feasible to inject those medications this way. The trial is open to children and adolescents with many different types of brain tumors – all of the glioma-type, not only DIPG. Actually, DIPG might constitute the very small minority of cases this trial will enroll, and it is not targeted to those patients.

3. I think the idea to inject chemo straight into the brain is attractive, although it seems to me there could be some limitations for DIPG. First, local delivery of medications has been trialed for many years in many brain tumor types, but none has shown good results in DIPG. Second, while other types of gliomas are well localized and more typical masses, and might therefore benefit from being infused directly into close blood vessels with chemotherapy, I am not sure that this is desired in DIPG. In fact, usually DIPG is very diffuse (as in the name) and injecting chemotherapy closely could harm the normal brain tissue around the tumor significantly. I would be worried about this and how to get the infusion done properly, and its effectiveness.

4. I would think that such trial would be particularly attractive if the medications given are truly hitting Neil's specific tumor vulnerabilities. This brings us back to the biopsy. If Neil's tumor can be biopsied and the "molecular scan" shows that it could be sensitive to the medications offered in the trial, I would give it a good thought. Otherwise, I think it would worry me to be unfavorable on the risk:benefit ratio.

5. Personally, I would ask the expert on DIPG, Dr Mark Kieran, when you meet him, whether this option would be a good thing for Neil. I would ask him about any valuable trials he knows around the country as well, of course.

Regarding alternative medicine, please remember that in the pediatric cancer community we are extremely open-minded about options and things that might help, whatever those might be. At the DANA-Farber, there is in fact an Alternative Medicine Department, called the Zakim Center for Integrative Therapies. I pasted the link below for you. There may be something you'll find helpful.

Love is a key ingredient, and diet is absolutely too. What is important is that you always discuss openly with the oncologists what you are considering as alternatives. As prescribing physicians it is always important for us to know of possible interactions. It is sad that people refer to things as being from "mainstream" and "alternative" medicine. I prefer "complementary medicine," which is the term we use in Europe, to highlight approaches that can work hand-in-hand. So, my recommendation is be open and inquisitive. Ask all your questions and make sure caregivers know about anything Neil plans to take to help his condition. It's time for people and approaches to work in a team, all for the best care of Neil and patients like him.

Don't hesitate to let me know if you want to discuss or if I can do anything else.

Warmest thoughts,
Raffaele

"Hey, Neil!" I shouted from my seat at the computer.

"Yeh Dad," came a muffled voice from upstairs.

"Can you come back down?"

"Be right there," he replied, and a minute later, he joined me in the study. "Whaz'up?"

"Take a look at this," I pointed to Raffaele's email on the screen.

"What's it say?" Neil shook his head no. "My eyes are too goofy from staring at screens."

"Well," I began, "Raffaele was impressed with what Evie found so quickly."

"Kudos Evie!" Neil smiled.

"But it's a mixed bag for chemotherapy," I continued. "While there are several trials enrolling patients with DIPG, none have shown any promising results so far."

"Dr. Arrillaga sort of said that," Neil nodded. "But 'there's always a chance.'"

"Sure," I agreed. "Especially if the chemo can be delivered more effectively, like with the Convection-Enhanced Delivery method being trialed at Memorial Sloan Kettering."

"Injecting chemo directly into the tumor."

"Basically," I agreed. "But where healthy cells are so intertwined with disease, Raffaele worries that 'injecting chemotherapy closely could harm the normal brain tissue around the tumor significantly.'"

"Ugh," Neil grunted. "That's discouraging."

"It might be more attractive if your tumor matches up to a chemo they're using."

"Which brings us back to the biopsy," Neil completed the thought.

I nodded, reading more from Raffaele's note, "'If Neil's tumor can be biopsied and the molecular scan shows it could be sensitive to the medications offered in the trial, I would give it a good thought. Otherwise, I think it would worry me to be unfavorable on the risk-benefit ratio.'"

"Hmm," Neil sighed sardonically, "that's a bit of tangle, isn't it. Sort of like DIPG."

I grimaced a little at his gallows humor. "At least it's more grist for the mill."

"Indeed," Neil nodded thoughtfully, then he trundled back upstairs.

Raffaele's caution moved Memorial Sloan Kettering down but not off of Neil's short list. For the moment, however, Raffaele's connection with a foremost authority on DIPG was more crucial to pursue — especially since Dr. Kieran was right there in Boston. Between that and Raffaele's open-mindedness to "alternative" approaches, it felt like we were finding solid ground upon which to gain traction — real hope.

After praying a silent "thank you" for Raffaele and his insights, I sent a quick update to our growing group of family and friends who were pulling for Neil. Another blessing. Then, it was back to scouring the Internet for more possibilities. I found an article discussing genetic issues and DIPG, so I sent the link to my sister (who has a PhD in microbiology) and Evie:

To: Evie, Suzanne
From: Dean
Subject: Research on gene errors that seem to cause DIPG
Date: March 6, 2016

Childhood Brain Tumors Linked To Newly Discovered Mutations

"A recent study published in the online edition of the scientific journal Nature Genetics of rare, lethal childhood tumors of the brainstem has revealed that almost 80% of tumors contain gene mutations that have previously not been associated with cancer. According to early evidence, gene alterations also implicate other aggressive pediatric brain tumors. The results provide a significant insight into a poorly understood tumor that has a mortality rate of over 90% in patients within two years."

http://www.medicalnewstoday.com/articles/240977.php

(Note: The article, written in 2012, uses plain language and provides some helpful insights.)

Finally, I discovered the Hoxsey Bio-Medical Center in Tijuana, Mexico and reached out to them:

To: info@hoxseybiomedical.com
From: Dean Fachon
Subject: DIPG tumors
Date: March 6, 2016

Hello,
Have you treated any pediatric patients with DIPG tumors? If so, do you have any information on results or testimonials?
Thank you,
Dean Fachon

Surprisingly, I received an almost immediate reply from someone at Hoxsey: "Yes, we do treat DIPG. You can call the clinic and talk to a patient advisor."

I thanked them and made a note to do more research on their work.

EIGHT HUNDRED POUND GORILLA

It was after 10:00 p.m., and I was ready to wrap up when Neil padded back into the study. "Hey Dad," he said, "Can we talk?"

"Of course Buddy." I shut down my computer and smiled up at him. "Always."

"So I've been researching Dr. Burzynski," he said. "It's like nothing shown in the documentary ever happened. There's almost nothing but blogs that are anti-Burzynski!"

I shrugged my acknowledgment. "It's a curious thing, how all the negative rants end up at the top of the search engines. It takes money to claim that position."

"Seriously," Neil nodded. "But if Burzynski is really the fake these guys claim, how come the FDA and the Texas Medical Board can't prove it? They've got the resources, and they've sure tried hard enough!"

"Bingo," I smiled. "No hiding an eight hundred pound gorilla from you!"

"It's like the court stuff never happened," Neil huffed. "Not as far as these bloggers are concerned, and they dismiss Dr. Burzynski's success stories as pure fiction."

"Pretty much," I agreed. "If anything, the naysayers want people to think Burzynski's cures were no more than coincidence — the 'latent benefits' of 'standard care' kicking in."

"Or his patients were misdiagnosed in the first place," Neil added. "Like they never really had cancer." Then, he paused quizzically, as if calculating a chess move. "How can these people justify second-guessing when most of Burzynski's patients have already been treated at big-name hospitals and been told there was nothing more to be done?"

"I know, I know, " I nodded. "Any excuse, so long as Burzynski can't take the credit."

"The excuse I like best is 'spontaneous remissions' — that the cancers just disappeared," Neil observed, shaking his head. "Statistically speaking, that might happen once in a hundred thousand patients, so Dr. Burzynski must have treated hundreds of thousands of patients to have so many with spontaneous remissions."

"Which is impossible," I agreed. "I'd be surprised if he's treated ten thousand patients, total. But the way the anti-Burzynski crowd works, if one argument doesn't stick..."

"...they just pick another," Neil finished.

"Like playing Russian roulette," I said. "But the revolver is always pointed at Burzynski, and they rotate from one argument to the next until something hits."

"They even condemn him for billing his patients," Neil said.

"I seem to recall reading that insurance companies may have covered his treatment years ago," I said. "But now he's pretty much blackballed."

"What's he supposed to do?" Neil asked. "Unless he can afford to run his clinic for free, he has to bill his patients." He rubbed his chin in a gesture reminiscent of pondering a chess board. "And so the bloggers accuse him of robbing his patients' life savings."

"As if 'standard care' were free," I guffawed. "It's probably more expensive, but since insurance covers it, most patients never know the real cost."

"Which leaves that gorilla," Neil shook his head sadly.

"The truth doesn't matter," I lamented. "Not when it conflicts with the mainstream narrative. It's the projection of righteous indignation that counts. They use it to discourage people from even reaching out to Burzynski."

"These bloggers are just carrying on where the FDA and the Texas Medical Board failed," Neil said, his face screwed up in disgust. "As strategies go, it's slimy." A moment later, he smiled mischievously. "Have you contacted the Burzynski Clinic?"

"I sent them a request for information this afternoon," I told him.

"F-A-A-A-N-TASTIC!"

I chuckled. His response was right out of the "SLTP" playbook:

> SLTP, the "Student Leadership Training Program," was a leadership camp Neil attended each summer during high school. His first two years, he was a camper, then he became a counselor. "F-A-A-A-N-TASTIC!" was the theme word his first year. If someone asked any of the kids how they were doing, they were coached to respond with gusto, "F-A-A-A-N-TASTIC!" No replies like "Good," "Okay," or "I'm hanging in there." Too lukewarm. To instill enthusiasm, one should exude enthusiasm! That was an unspoken tenet of SLTP's founder, Jim Fitzgerald. Neil loved SLTP

and the friends he made there. It was about being inclusive, about embracing life and being a leader — not by shouting orders from up front, but by setting the best example you could and then getting out of the way. In that fashion, everyone gets to contribute.

Neil was keeping my spirits up by showing me that his were undaunted. The optimist in Neil was almost omnipresent, and I gave him a hug. "Now go get some sleep!"

"Goodnight," he gave me a hug and padded back upstairs.

Before going to bed, I rebooted my computer and researched spontaneous remissions of patients with DIPG. The search yielded only one reference:

Complete remission of a diffuse pontine glioma
H G Lenard 1 , V Engelbrecht, G Janssen, W Wechsler, C Tautz

"A patient is described in whom a large diffuse glioma of the pons extending into the midbrain was diagnosed at the age of 2 years. Biopsy showed a fibrillary astrocytoma. After shunting of a hydrocephalus, the clinical symptoms abated without conventional therapy. Repeated MRI studies showed a continuous decrease of the tumor which was no longer visible when the patient was 6.6 years old. In reviews on spontaneous remissions of oncologic disorders we were unable to find a case of a biologically benign brain stem tumor. There is one isolated report on a similar case, though without histologic documentation."

https://pubmed.ncbi.nlm.nih.gov/10029356/

SIT TIGHT

Despite so much happening, Neil still wanted to visit his Grandmother in Florida for spring break. He had fond recollections of playing games with his Grandparents (including chess with Grandpa Ferd); of picking oranges and squeezing fresh juice; of visiting wildlife sanctuaries to see all the birds and occasionally spy an alligator; and of swimming in the pool for hours on end. He so looked forward to getting away that he called Dr. Panis to get his clearance for flying. Subsequently, Dr. Panis sent me a note.

To: Dean Fachon
From: "Panis, Walter , M.D."
Subject: plane tickets
Date: Mon, 7 Mar 2016

I just spoke with your son. It is fine for him to fly. I want him to continue with PT and I told him I'd like to see him again.

Walter Panis, MD
Neurology and Physical Medicine and Rehabilitation
Department of Physical Medicine and Rehabilitation
Harvard Medical School

As much as a visit to Florida would give Neil — and all of us — a much needed break, further delays seemed too risky. I heard some noise in the kitchen and found Evie brewing tea.

"We can't go to Florida," I told her. "Dr. Panis said it's fine for him to fly, but it's just not the time."

"That's too bad," she frowned. "He'll be disappointed."

"Maybe you could help me tell him?"

"Sure," she agreed, so we went to his room for a quick talk. He was sitting up in bed, his laptop in front of him.

"Hey Buddy," Evie smiled.

"Whaz'up, guys," he returned her smile, if a little lopsidedly.

"Dad got a note from Dr. Panis," she told him. "He says it's okay to fly."

"I know," he nodded expectantly. "But..."

"But maybe it's not the best idea right now," Evie frowned.

"We should sit tight," I added, "until we figure out what's next."

"Yeh, I figured as much," Neil acknowledged the time lost with a frown.

"Have you heard from MGH about getting that MRI of your spine?" I changed the subject.

"Actually, I just spoke with them," he answered. "March sixteenth."

"Huh?" I grunted. "I figured they'd be a little more anxious! This MRI is supposed to help determine if you might have something other than DIPG."

"Yeh," Neil nodded. "They must be busy. You sure we can't go to Florida?"

Evie chuckled.

I shook my head, "No!"

"JK, JK Dad. Just kidding."

"I'll put in the paperwork to get a refund," I said, leaving the kids to "kibbutz."

Let's see if this travel insurance is worth anything, I thought as I wrote a quick note to Dr. Panis: *"As you were first to identify the tumor, we thought it appropriate to ask you to complete and return the attached insurance-reimbursement form. Obviously we are not flying due to the urgency of Neil's appointment schedule, but should a window open when we can travel, it's good to know there should be no complications from his current condition."* He returned the completed the forms almost immediately, adding, *"Please be in touch with any questions!"* A true gentlemen and advocate.

CONNECTING THE DOTS

Despite the delay getting a spinal MRI, we had other dots to connect. To that end, we reached out to Dana-Farber first thing Monday morning to pursue Neil's appointment for a second opinion with Dr. Kieran. As anxious as we were, this process would also take time to work through. To begin with, Neil had to register as a new patient, then Dana-Farber would need his records transferred from Mass General — all more quickly said than done:

> **To: Evie, Dean, Wendy**
> **From: Katelyn Nkomo**
> **Subject: Second Opinion**
> **Date: March 7, 2015**
>
> Hi Dean, Wendy and Evie,
>
> Here is the new patient letter that I mentioned on the phone. Below is a link that you can use to upload MRI's. As I mentioned, MGH may be willing to put together this package of records and send it over to us directly.
>
> Thanks,
> Katelyn (Saylor) Nkomo
> Administrative Specialist
> Pediatric Neuro-Oncology Program
> DANA-Farber/Boston Children's Cancer and Blood Disorders Center

Neil had some trouble working with this online form, so Evie downloaded a PDF version and sent it to Neil. Once completed, he relayed it back to her, and she forwarded it to Ms. Nkomo at Dana-Farber.

> **To: "Nkomo, Katelyn"**
> **From: Evie Fachon**
> **Subject: Re: Second Opinion**
> **Date: March 7, 2016**
>
> Hi Katelyn,
>
> Attached is a new copy of Neil's new patient form in .pdf format. Please let us know when you have a case num-

ber for him so we can pass that on to MGH. We'd like to get all of the materials over to you today if possible. If there's anything else that we need to do please give us a call! Thank you for all of your help!

Best,
Evie Fachon

* * *

To: Evie
From: Katelyn Nkomo
Subject: New Patient form
Date: March 7, 2016

Hi Evie,

Yes, this copy worked. I called MGH about an hour ago to talk through sending records. I think Eugene has been seeing an adult neuro-oncologist, which is why their office thinks that they can link the records with a medical record number from DANA-Farber, [but] I left a message [at MGH] because we are going to need actual CD copies of Eugene's MRI's. We are the pediatric side of DANA-Farber and we use a different system. I'm waiting for [a call-back] but wanted to update you with the progress we are making.

Thanks,
Katelyn (Saylor) Nkomo
Administrative Specialist
Pediatric Neuro-Oncology Program
DANA-Farber/Boston Children's Cancer and Blood Disorders Center

So, the two hospitals could not share records electronically — at least not between their adult and pediatric divisions. To expedite the transfer of Neil's records, we decided to use "sneakernet" — to bring Neil back to Mass General, find the records department so he could sign the appropriate release form to get a CD copy of his MRI, and bring it to Dana-Farber.

On the heels of this "revelation," Neil received a call to schedule a "consult" about taking a biopsy.

"I just heard from Dr. Cahill's administrative nurse at MGH," Neil announced. "He's the neurosurgeon who performs their 'stereotactic' biopsy procedures. He'll see me on the ninth."

"That's quick," I said. "But you'd think they'd want that MRI of your spine, first."

"Oh well," Neil shrugged. "It's just a consult, not the surgery. We can dovetail the appointment with a visit to the MGH records department, then a drop-off at Dana-Farber."

"Good tactics," I smiled.

We were excited to meet with Dr. Cahill, but as much as we respected MGH and Dana-Farber, we had come to think that none of the treatments suggested thus far was likely to buy Neil more than a few extra months. Such a prognosis was difficult to accept.

STRONG "ALTERNATIVE" CONTENDER

While we looked forward to meeting with Dr. Cahill, we also pursued our meeting with Dr. Kieran. We prayed he would suggest something more hopeful. This is when the Burzynski Clinic's information package arrived.

> **To: Dean Fachon**
> **From: Sonnet Smith**
> **Subject: Burzynski Clinic Information Packet**
> **Date: Mon, 7 Mar 2016**
>
> Greetings,
>
> We sincerely thank you for considering the Burzynski Clinic for your cancer treatment. We will do our very

best to assist you with your needs. I have attached the following documents:

1. Welcome Packet - This includes general information about our clinic, statistics, and information about our Personalized Gene Targeted Therapy program.
2. Admissions Forms – This includes medical forms you need to fill out and send back as soon as possible in order to establish an appointment at our clinic.
3. Foundation Medicine Patient Consent Form – The company we use for genomic testing is Foundation One. Please click on the link for additional information: http://www.foundationone.com/
4. Travel & Hotel Accommodations – This has a listing of nearby hotels, transportation, and other local Houston businesses you may wish to know about for your travels.

For those who may qualify: Antineoplastons are naturally occurring peptides demonstrating ability to re-program cancer cells without destroying normal cells. Due to their low-toxicity and anti-cancer activity, Antineoplastons represent a revolutionary avenue in cancer research. Antineoplastons are components of a complex biochemical defense system that controls cancer in the human body and are reproduced synthetically for medicinal use. Please click on the link for additional information: www.anpcoalition.org

Medical Records and other information that is required:

- All pathology reports
- Oncologist/treating doctor notes (especially chemotherapy flow sheet & last dictation)
- Operative/surgical reports

- Radiology reports (CT, PET, MRI, Echocardiogram, etc. and Mammograms if applicable)
- Laboratory reports (most recent CBC, CMP, UA, and Tumor Markers)

We look forward to providing you with best care possible and encourage you to call us with any questions that you may have.

Best regards,
Sonnet Smith
Admissions Specialist, The BURZYNSKI CLINIC
"Tomorrow's Cancer Treatment Today!"
9432 Katy Freeway, Houston, Texas 77055

The information package from the Burzynski Clinic was comprehensive and professional. Neil wanted to learn more. We all did. What could the Burzynski Clinic do specifically for him? Neil also wanted to understand the biopsy procedure. More than anything else Dr. Arrillaga had mentioned, sample tissue analysis seemed to offer a glimmer of hope beyond the short-term reprieve radiation would buy him. To help evaluate this procedure, Wendy's brother Steve — a former professional in the medical instrument industry — discovered an article he thought we should see:

Biopsy of brain stem gliomas: Changing trends?
Journal of Neurosciences in Rural Practice, 31 Mar 2014,

In recent years, there has been a trend toward reconsidering stereotactic biopsies for children with MRI characteristics of diffuse non-enhancing lesions in the brain stem suggestive of a diffuse intrinsic pontine glioma.[8,9,10] Recent studies have shown that molecular biology like 1p19q loss and, O6-methylguanin-DNA-methyltransfer-

> ase (MGMT) status is often correlated with the outcome and response to newer chemotherapeutic agents. Also, in future, tumor genetic profiles are expected to play a role in treating these tumors. These would require tissue sampling with a biopsy and molecular analysis, with the aim of finding a solution for future generations. This often puts the treating neurosurgeon in a difficult situation to decide whether to do biopsy or not. The moral and ethical reasons for biopsying these tumors, with an aim of helping understand the molecular genetics of these tumors for future generations, have to be carefully weighed against the existing suffering of the child with a malignant brain stem glioma and the family, with further aggravation of this suffering with a biopsy procedure.
>
> *http://europepmc.org/article/PMC/4064173*

While not exactly encouraging, if nothing else proved more promising, Neil was absolutely willing to be altruistic. While immunotherapy was intriguing, these two paths, biopsy or Burzynski, were at the forefront of our minds for the moment. It was time, once again, to seek Raffaele's insights.

> **To: Raffaele**
> **From: Dean**
> **Subject: Status update for Neil**
> **Date: March 8, 2016**
>
> Raffaele,
>
> The house is a flurry of activity – phones ringing, keyboards clacking, and screens flashing with articles and cancer videos. We have an appointment tomorrow with

Dr. Cahill at Mass General to discuss a biopsy procedure. The questions I've put together include:

- Where in the skull and how big an opening? "Key hole?"
- Would this be a "needle biopsy" or a more invasive procedure?
- What is the potential risk of loosing motor function?
- What is the potential benefit in terms of improved survivability from the condition?

We are also pursuing a visit with Dr. Kieran, but there is some difficulty in getting Neil's records transferred. The hospital systems are different and it can take 2 weeks or more to get a physical CD from MGH patient records. We'll try to make some progress tomorrow when we go to Boston.

Meanwhile, given the very poor prognosis for DIPG, we are looking at alternative therapies and have found other avenues that seem worth pursuing. The first is Dr. Bursynski's antineoplastons, which have a significantly better track record with DIPG than any other treatment. While controversial, widely criticized, and restricted by the FDA, it's difficult to dismiss what Dr. Bursynski has accomplished. Below is a link to a summary of his work and the controversy swirling around him:

http://www.truthwiki.org/dr-stanislaw-r-burzynski-the-burzynski-clinic/

That's news from this side of the pond. I hope all is well there, and thank you again for your support!

Hugs to all, and God Bless,
Dean

I also reached out to Dr. Jim Bass, a friend who practiced radiology in Boston.

To: Jim Bass
From: Dean
Subject: Urgent request
Date: March 8, 2016

Dear Jim,

I hate to bother you with bad news, but I'm writing to reach out for assistance. We have just learned that our son Neil has a DIPG brain tumor. We had an appointment with a neuro-oncologist at Mass General last Friday, and we have a lead into DANA Farber for a second opinion. Either way, the prognosis is terrible, so we are looking outside the box. One name that frequently pops up in regards to DIPG is Dr. Burzynski. He is considered a disreputable pariah by many in the medical world, but the results he has had with this tumor appear vastly better than what mainstream medicine is willing to acknowledge. I don't know if you would have the time to dig around to help sort the wheat from the chaff, but if you have any thoughts or suggestions they would be greatly appreciated! I hope all is well with you and your family!

Thank you,
Dean Fachon

* * *

To: Dean
From: Jim Bass
Subject: Re: Urgent request
Date: Tue, 08 Mar 2016

Hi Dean,

I am certainly no expert in oncology. However, I have spent several hours trying to review the data from his clinic as well as other clinical trials. He published a paper on DIPG in 2014, which would be very compelling if true. However, I have some concerns about the paper. My first concern is that although he has been doing this for 30 years, he has yet to produce a convincing scientific trial that antineoplastons are truly effective. The National Cancer Institute has done some studies on them, without any convincing efficacy. They have also been studied in Japan at some length, also without convincing efficacy. His paper included MRI images of the brain which purported to show significant tumor resolution following treatment. I have some concern about how those images are presented. First, the before and after images are not obtained at the same levels through the tumor. They are close, but clearly not identical levels. This would allow the images post-treatment to appear to show shrinkage just because sections had been taken through a smaller section of tumor. Like CT, MRI images are displayed with a certain "window and level" which determines the contrast within the apparent image. The images that he presents in that paper are windowed quite differently before treatment than they are after treatment. The windowing is consistently set to give much more tumor contrast in the pre-treatment images and altered to make the tumor less conspicuous in the post-treatment Films. That observation is consistent for all of the images in that paper. When publications use that sort of image "trickery" I have concerns about the integrity of the data.

> The treatment is certainly extremely expensive. I found multiple websites of people fund-raising to get money to be treated at his clinic. Many of those seem to reach an initial goal of $200-$300,000. Within a few months, they have gone through that money, and seek additional funding.
>
> There are certainly a large number of bloggers and reporters who essentially consider him a scam artist. Unfortunately, my brief review of the data would suggest that they may be correct. I wish that I had better news for you, and I wish that his treatments did represent a remarkable step forward in treatment. We are so sorry that Neil and your family are facing such a difficult situation. I would be more than happy to discuss this more if you have any further thoughts or observations. I hope that your visits to DANA-Farber and Children's Hospital go well. Please let us know if there is anything else we can do for you guys.
>
> Jim

Jim's detailed response was incisive and sobering. I wondered, however, if he was fully aware of the tremendous harassment Dr. Burzynski has endured throughout his career. At one point, this harassment included prolonged confiscation of his patient records. This alone could help explain the quality issues that have cropped up with the information Dr. Burzynski was able to publish. Dr. Burzynski has also gone on record stating that the independent trials Jim cited did not follow his recommended dosage guidelines. Thus, the results were undermined. Many doctors have voiced amazement at Dr. Burzynski's results, but their voices have been drowned out. It seemed unlikely Jim would realize the sheer volume of effort expended to derail Dr. Burzynski and discount his patient success stories. We would be mindful of Jim's caution flag, but there were two sides to this story. With this in mind, I discovered two websites I thought our "home team" should read:

Excerpt from:
Antineoplastons – an alternative treatment for cancer?

31 December 2012, Chris Woolams

In 1991 a group of investigators from the National Cancer Institute went to the Burzynski Research Institute in Houston and reviewed his best 7 cases, where patients – mainly with astrocytomas and glioblastomas – had experienced complete responses to the drugs. The NCI recommended a Phase II clinical trial, which began in 1993 and was overseen by such eminent institutions as the Mayo Clinic and Sloan-Kettering Cancer Center. However, only nine patients were assessed, and the final report concluded that the results were insufficient to recommend antineoplastons for wider use.

Burzynski was extremely unhappy, especially when he discovered that the doses used had been far lower than those he was giving his own patients. Indeed, he published a letter stating that the levels used during the clinical trial were previously established by him to be ineffective!

Meanwhile Burzynski undertook his own studies in his clinic. In a study of 36 patients (all with brain tumors, some of highly malignant glioblastoma multiforme) he produced the following results:

- 9 (25%) had a complete response, i.e., disappearance of the tumor on an MRI scan.
- 7 (19.5%) had a partial response i.e. more than 50% reduction on MRI scan.

- 12 (33.3%) were stabilized.

In his report Burzynski noted the general consensus in the medical community is that these brain tumors cannot be cured by chemotherapy, and the response rate is only modest. However he, himself, achieved a claimed complete tumor resolution, or over 50 percent tumor reduction, in 16 of his 36 patients. These research findings have never been confirmed by independent sources.

https://www.canceractive.com/article/antineoplastons-an-alternative-treatment-for-cancer

Excerpt from:
Cancer Diaries, Part Three: Burzynski, the Modern Prometheus

Rick Archer, July 2013

The reason that Burzynski terrifies the Medical Establishment is that even his so-so batting record FAR SURPASSES conventional cancer treatments. Until Burzynski came along, NO ONE survived these types of cancer. Burzynski doesn't cure everyone, but he does cure a few. That suggests that he really is on to something.

*And from a segment of this document called "**Final Word:**"*

The U.S. Patent Office issued 11 copycat patents on medical therapies that Burzynski had already patented himself. These patents were issued to Dvorit Samid, Burzynski's former lab assistant who had nothing to do with their original discovery.

Question: Why would the U.S. Patent Office assign fraudulent patents to some of the most powerful institutions in American government?

Possible Answer: Because Burzynski already held the original patent. All Burzynski would need now would be to plow his way through the excruciatingly expensive Phase III "efficacy" trials.

If Dr. Burzynski's antineoplastons are approved, it would mark the first time in history that a single scientist, not a pharmaceutical company, would hold the exclusive patent and distribution rights on an industry-shifting medical breakthrough.

When that happens, the game is over. Checkmate to Burzynski, Nobel Prize for Medicine certain to follow.

Note that all of this NCI [National Cancer Institute] patent chicanery was taking place while these same government agencies were spending $60 million dollars of taxpayer money trying to put Dr. Burzynski in jail.

Now ask yourself this: Why would anyone spend $60 million dollars trying to put Burzynski in jail?

If this man really is a quack doctor with an ineffective treatment, then he is a nobody. Word of mouth drives his business. If no one survives for long, then his business dries up automatically.

Did they spend $60 million to protect the patients?

Hell, no. Even if every single one of Burzynski's patients were doomed (which they aren't), everyone agrees Burzynski's treatment is a dramatic improvement over chemo because it doesn't hurt anybody. So that can't be the answer either.

The most obvious conclusion is that if Burzynski was in jail, he could not fight the criminal theft of his discovery.

People ask me, "Rick, does Burzynski's treatment work?"

And I am going to say this again, "Why would anyone spend 14 years and $60 million dollars trying to put Burzynski in jail?"

There is your answer right there. If Burzynski did not represent the greatest possible threat to the entrenched interests, then they would not go to these extremes.

According to Dr. Chen, the absurd $60 million dollar, 14-year spectacle of one useless trial after another was nothing more than a smoke and mirrors attempt to muscle the doctor out of the picture so the NCI could steal his treatment.

"Under the capitalist sun, there is nothing sacred. Money talks."

Do these people have no shame? Were they born without a conscience? I cannot begin to understand how they turn a blind eye to the suffering of the people crying for a cure to cancer.

I have spent the past three Chapters attempting to illustrate that the United States cancer treatment and pharmaceutical drug industries are rife with corruption and conspiracy.

The situation is so bad it seems like the industry itself has cancer.

I rest my case.

Rick Archer
August 2013"

https://ssqq.com/stories/cancerfight03.htm

Together, these articles were further encouragement. While we had yet to hear back from Raffaele, our overall impressions of Dr. Burzynski and his clinic were still positive. These are sincere people using ingenious and nontoxic medicine, working against odds stacked heavily against them, to successfully treat some of the most intractable cancers. Dr. Burzynski could offer no guarantees, but his antineoplastons had saved many cancer patients who had otherwise been deemed "incurable."

JUGGLING

While interest in the Burzynski Clinic was rising, we had other balls in the air. Getting that second opinion from Dana-Farber was next in hand, and Evie reached out to Katelyn Nkomo regarding the status of transferring Neil's records. *"I just wanted to let you know that I'm still trying to get through to Neil's doctor at MGH. I've left a couple of messages with them today and haven't been called back yet, but hopefully they'll get back to me soon! Apologies for so much delay."*

As Evie's "hurry up and wait" update went out, I received a response to the email I'd sent Dr. Slattery on March 6: *"I am so sorry to hear this news. In this situation there is really no wrong way to do anything. I would certainly try all the options you are considering. There's a lot to be said for alternative treatment options, and it is good to pursue ones that look promising. Keep in touch and I will try to do what I can to help you and your family."*

So, we had some degree of local backup. Thank you, John.

As part of the day's normal search pattern, I discovered another resource which detailed alternative cancer therapies: Cancer Compass, an Alternate Route (*www.cancercompassalternateroute.com*). We found a wealth of information at this website — information which helped us to cross-reference other resources. As the day drew to a close, I reached out to family and friends with an update:

> *Dearest Family and Friends,*
>
> *Home at the 'Fortress' we have been going non-stop – organizing an additional consult at DANA Farber; scheduling an*

MRI for Neil's lower back; scheduling an appointment with a neurosurgeon to discuss the risks/benefits of doing a biopsy; and we have also been scouring the Internet for alternative therapies. We found one in particular that has shown real potential with the exact type of cancer Neil has. This treatment uses "Antineoplastons." The Internet is full of information about them and the man who invented them, Dr. Stanislaw Burzynski. He is widely ridiculed by much of the medical establishment, and the FDA and Texas Medical Board have tried for years to shut his clinic down, but they have been curiously unsuccessful. Dr. Burzynski soldiers on, and his 'anecdotal' results are eye-opening. Sadly, if you 'search' his name, the first few pages of results point to quackery, but dig a little deeper, and the picture changes – not rainbows and unicorns, but a tough battle being fought on many fronts with some surprising success.

Anyway, you can see we are trying very hard to sift as much information as possible. If you have the time, please do some research and let us know what you think. At this point, we are thinking very seriously about taking a trip to the Burzynski clinic to see it first hand and get a preliminary evaluation. There is nothing to lose. Otherwise, we are having a busy-good day. Neil woke up sort of logy, but he seems pretty good now. He has lost some strength and coordination, but as long as he isn't playing tennis you wouldn't notice too much. We are keeping our chins up. Hugs and kisses to you all!

Love you very much, and God Bless,
Dean

TAKING STOCK

The following morning — in advance of our return trek to Boston — I received a reply from Raffaele:

To: Dean Fachon
From: Raffaele
Subject: Re: Status update for Neil
Date: Wed, 09 Mar 2016

Dear Dean,

Thank you for the news.

For the appointment with Dr Cahill, I think you have all the questions to ask absolutely spot-on. As I said before, getting a biopsy to "profile" the tumor, trying to find its vulnerabilities, is really key in my opinion. It opens the avenue to specific drugs that can be used.

I am sorry to hear about the administrative delays of getting an appointment with Dr Kieran. It used to be much simpler, but that's the problem with huge institutions. While they have great advantages, admin tends to grow disproportionately, and things then slow down their effectiveness. Good luck with all those steps. Again, I think Dr Kieran knows Neil's case and has been involved.

Regarding Dr Burzynski, he has been around for decades. Recently, I started a fresh review of the claims, successes and side-effects, because I had another patient pursuing this avenue. I focused on patient reports and published studies (any of them in any shape or form). I found reports of individuals who said it worked for them (plenty of video advertisements online), but no scientific evidence to support Dr Burzynski's ideas and his treatment. And there have been reports of some medical consequences. At the end of the day, I can only encourage Neil and you to form your own opinions and decide what is best for him.

> Hope all goes well for the appointment with Dr Cahill.
> Big hugs to Neil and all of you.
>
> Raffaele

"So I heard back from Raffaele this morning," I told Neil as we sat down at the breakfast table. "He confirmed our list of questions for Dr. Cahill, and he commiserated about the delays getting the appointment with Dr. Kieran."

"What's he say about Burzynski," Neil cut right to the chase.

"Well, he's not too big on Burzynski," I shrugged. "'No scientific evidence to support his ideas.' But he acknowledged a volume of anecdotal evidence."

Neil nodded in between doing reps of an eye exercise. "I'm certainly interested."

"Raffaele also said, "At the end of the day, I can only encourage Neil and you to form your own opinions and decide what is best for him.'"

"Well I'd be interested to see you eat a good breakfast," Wendy smiled as she set a bowl of fresh berries and yogurt in front of Neil. He set his eye apparatus aside and dug in.

Taking stock of the situation, maybe the light at the end of the tunnel wasn't just a freight train. It even felt like we might just be starting to get ahead of this thing.

JUMP SHOT

The late morning ride to Boston was uneventful, and Neil slept a good part of the way. We dropped off Evie at school to attend to some school business, then Wendy, Neil, and I headed for MGH. We were getting to know our way around the complex, so parking was quick, but we still had to track down the records department. To get there required traversing many long hallways and riding too many elevators. If a hospital could have a "cubbyhole," the records department at Mass General's was it, a hidden nook tucked in like an afterthought to squirrel away secrets. The office itself was pedestrian in comparison to the plush waiting rooms for the doctors. Neil signed in and sat in one of the chairs opposite the service desk until he was called. When he got his turn, he explained what he needed, and they had him sign the requisite form to get a copy of his records. The clerk explained it would take an hour or so to fulfill Neil's request, so this gave us plenty of time for his appointment with Dr. Cahill.

We quickly found Dr. Cahill's domain, and we did not have to wait long before the receptionist ushered us into his office. "Dr. Cahill will be right with you."

Indeed, he arrived almost immediately. He seemed a bit disheveled, as if he were squeaking us in between procedures, but he was very open and enthusiastic about what could be learned by taking a biopsy.

"We use a stereotactic procedure," Dr. Cahill began to explain.

"We've heard something about it," Neil nodded, "but please give us the details."

"The patient's head is held immobile in metal brace that serves as a stable platform for controlling the surgical instruments," Dr. Cahill began. "We cut back a small flap of skin and drill a small hole in the base of the patient's skull — low and behind the ear — and we use imaging technology to precisely guide a needle-like probe into the tumor to select a small sample."

"How big is the hole?" Neil quizzed further.

"Like a keyhole," Dr. Cahill explained. "Not big. And it gets concealed when the flap of skin is sewn back."

Neil nodded.

Wendy and I grimaced a little. "What about the hole in his skull?"

"It fills in over time," Dr. Cahill assured us. Then, he continued, "We take several small samples through the same opening."

"Several," we all cringed as one. "That sounds risky!"

"Well, the pathologists want as many samples as they can get for research," Dr, Cahill quickly countered. "But I don't let them get carried away. Generally, the risks are minimal."

"What is 'minimal' exactly?" Neil asked. "Could I die?"

"Not likely," Dr. Cahill shook his head. "There is some risk of internal bleeding, maybe two to five percent. And there is some potential for mild nerve damage."

"Could you put that in context" Neil persisted.

"Think of it like this," Dr. Cahill replied, "if you play basketball, it might throw off your jump shot."

"Uh huh," Neil cringed a little. "I guess that equates to my tennis forehand. And the upside?"

"With samples, we can see if your tumor matches favorably to available chemotherapies," Dr. Cahill said. "If there's a good match, we can fight the tumor."

Dr. Arrillaga had already explained about finding a chemo-match and what that might mean. We also knew something about the issues of delivering chemo across the blood-brain barrier, but there was one other thing Neil really wanted to ask Dr. Cahill:

"Dr. Arrillaga believes there's a small chance this could be something other that DIPG. She puts the odds at about one percent. What do you think?"

"Yes, there is a small chance," Dr. Cahill agreed. "I'd put it closer to ten percent."

"Ten percent," Neil raised his eyebrows. "That's significant!"

"The biopsy would tell for sure," Dr. Cahill concluded.

"Well, that gives us plenty to think about," Neil said. Then, after a pause, he added, "I'm not quite ready to sign up today, if that's okay."

"I understand," Dr. Cahill agreed as his phone started ringing. "It's a difficult situation," he nodded, muting his phone. "The sooner you decide, the better. I wish you the best of luck with whatever you do. Let Dr. Arrillaga know or call my office if you want to go ahead with the biopsy. We can work you in quickly."

We thanked Dr. Cahill, shook hands all around, and left his office. He certainly did give us plenty to think about, and Neil was very quiet as we wended our way back to the records department.

"So what do you think," I finally asked.

"I think ten percent is ten times more than one percent," Neil said matter-of-factly. "I'd like that disparity nailed down."

"Yup," I agreed. "You should get that MRI before they start drilling holes."

"Agreed," Neil nodded emphatically.

"Hopefully, Dr. Kieran can shed more light on the odds," Wendy added.

"But we still need that MRI," I frowned. "The clock is ticking."

"I'm doing okay," Neil said reassuringly, smiling at Wendy to acknowledge her nutritional ministrations. "We still have some time." After a pause, he continued, "And I don't mean to seem selfish. I'm all for research. They can take biopsy samples if nothing else is more promising, but I want the best hope for survival. I'll take a ten percent chance of surviving another year or two over a one hundred percent chance of an extra three months."

"Amen to that," Wendy and I both agreed.

When we arrived back at the records department, Neil's CD was ready and waiting.

"Thank you very much," he said to clerk, and we retraced our steps to the car.

We drove from Mass General to Neil's apartment so he could check his mailbox, then we picked Evie back up.

"How was the appointment?" she asked as she slipped into the backseat next to him.

Neil filled her in as we navigated to Dana-Farber. We were lucky and found a short-term parking spot near the entrance. Evie hand-delivered the CD to the Pediatric Neuro-Oncology Department, then we drove home early enough to avoid rush hour traffic, which makes almost any trip to Boston a good one.

CLOGGED PLUMBING

Despite the radical changes Wendy had made to Neil's diet — including a few intense days of juicing, which we hoped would help loosen things up — Neil's GI tract was still balking. He needed more help. Fortunately, in her experience writing for "Natural Awakenings" magazine, Wendy had been introduced to different types of holistic health therapy, many of which hearkened back to tried-and-true remedies of simpler times. For constipation, that includes enemas. As serendipity would have it, next to her most recent magazine article, Wendy noticed an advertisement for "colonic hydrotherapy" (i.e. industrial strength enema). After discussing it with Neil, she lined up an appointment for the following day.

Neil's colonic hydrotherapy would prove somewhat explosive, so much that he blushed sheepishly when asked about it, but that's what it took to start moving the food that was stalled in his gut — pounds of waste getting increasingly toxic and polluting his body. He was so blocked that a second session was needed the following day, with comparable results. Finally unblocked, the hydrotherapist suggested Neil add coffee enemas to his in-home health regimen. These were also recommended in Gerson therapy, so it seemed like an excellent idea which Neil fully embraced.

> Capable of removing circulating toxins and partial metabolites, the coffee enema stimulates the bile ducts. This happens because the coffee administered by means of a cleansing enema stimulates an enzyme system in the liver known as glutathione S-transferase (GST) that removes a vast variety of free radicals (electrophiles) from the bloodstream.
>
> Electrophiles are atomic particles with one or more electrons in unpaired spins which have an affinity for other electrons. They want to get involved where they should not. As charged particles, these free radicals damage membranes of cells and inflict disturbances in cellular metabolism.
>
> Under the influence of a coffee enema, the GST enzyme system increases activity to 650 percent above normal and removes electophiles from the bloodstream....
>
> During the time coffee is being held in the gut, all the blood in the body passes through the liver at least five times...

> The palmitate compounds and the caffeine, theobrmine, and theophylline in coffee cause dilation of the liver's blood vessels and bile ducts, relaxation of smooth muscles, stimulation of intestinal peristalsis, and elevation of bile flow.
>
> Basically, the coffee enema "frees the body from becoming poisoned by its own wastes." [7]

Figuring out how to administer the coffee enemas was a bit of trick. As with any young man, Neil needed his privacy, so we had to come up with a method of getting everything prepared — a process of brewing a special coffee, chilling it back down to body temperature, putting it in a gravity feed container — then delivering it to Neil so he could take care of business. This process took some getting used to, but coffee enemas would become an important part of Neil's daily health regimen.

The hydrotherapist also recommended adding probiotics to Neil's diet. Probiotics are the good bacteria that should be plentiful in a healthy gut biome. They assist in the breakdown and absorption of food, vitamins, and nutrients, and they strengthen the immune system. Probiotics would become an important supplement in Neil's arsenal.

ADVANCING DIALOGUE

While Wendy and Neil continued to fine-tune his home care, I reached out directly to Dr. Burzynski. I wrote an old-fashioned letter, which I would "overnight" to his clinic:

> *March 9, 2016*
>
> *Dear Dr. Burzynski,*
>
> *I first learned about you and antineoplastons about five or six years ago. At the time, your story was of great inter-*

7 "The Gerson Therapy," Charlotte Gerson and Morton Walker, D.P.M. Introduction and page 44.

est because it fit into the pattern of how our corporate-government deals with outliers who threaten the status quo. You are suffering under a withering blitzkrieg of perception modification. Unable to squelch your work, our "corpogov" is instead trying to contain it by vilifying you and conducting clinical trials with watered-down antineoplastons to make them look at best on a par with other experimental cancer treatments, thus blending antineoplastons into a smothering background of promising treatments that don't quite seem to make a game-changing breakthrough.

The frustration you feel must be almost intolerable. I am frustrated on your behalf, but little did I ever think how much more frustrating this situation could be until I learned I have need of your help, or more correctly, my 19-year-old son has need of your help. Last Friday, March 4, 2016, we learned that Neil has a DIPG tumor. This diagnosis was made at Mass General Hospital in collaboration with doctors at DANA Farber. We have seen Neil's MRI, and we were stunned – an otherwise perfectly healthy young man full of promise, a sophomore at Northeastern University holding down a 3.9 GPA, with an illness like this? It was inconceivable just one week ago. Sadly, the treatment being proposed by MGH/DF is hardly better than doing nothing at all. They want to take a biopsy in hopes they might find a match with some drug that could knock the tumor back for awhile. Then too radiation. Mights, maybes and radiation – a poor prescription – pitched with all possible sincerity, but nonetheless likely to be almost ineffective.

Since learning of Neil's condition, my wife, daughter and I have undertaken to provide him the best possible care. To that end, we immediately started him on a modified Gerson diet of high-alkaline foods. Of course, I also thought of you, and fortunately I saw the documentary by Eric Merola years ago, and Ty Bolinger recently announced a new docu-series, "The Quest For the Cure," so I have compelling materials to show my family about the possibilities outside mainstream medicine. We are all of a mind to bring Neil to Houston for a consultation.

Thank you very much for all you have done and continue to do! Your perseverance in the face of mountainous adversity is an inspiration. I hope to hear from you at your convenience.

Sincerely yours,
Dean Fachon

I showed Neil the letter, and he gave a me thumbs up. "I'm going to show Evie the documentary."

"You absolutely should," I agreed. "Mom too. Although she may recall having seen it when we were researching treatments for Maga."

Neil nodded soberly.

I sent the letter to Dr. Burzynski the following morning, and the day after that, I received an email from his Executive Secretary, Ms. Carolyn Powers: *"We received your Fed Ex letter. I have opened and read it. I have also scanned it and emailed it to Dr. Burzynski. He is off today, but you should hear something regarding this by Monday morning."* It did not take nearly that long. Only a few hours later, I received another email from the clinic:

To: Dean Fachon
From: Sheryll S. Acelar
Subject: Treatment at the Burzynski Clinic
Date: March 11, 2016

Hello Mr. Fachon,

My name is Sheryll Acelar from the Burzynski clinic. I am Dr. Burzynski's study coordinator for clinical trials. Dr.

> Burzynski relayed the message to me that your son is diagnosed with DIPG. We are sorry for the sad news. We would like to help your son. To speed up the process, we would need medical records as soon as possible. I understand that Sonnet Smith will help you, but Dr. Burzynski requested I reach out and see if we could get this done faster. We work Monday thru Thursday, so the best way for me to evaluate Neil's records quickly is to send them via email. Once I receive all this information, I will let you know Dr. Burzynski's recommendations. I hope to hear from you soon.
>
> Sincerely yours,
> Sheryll Acelar

I replied immediately: *We will work this as quickly as possible. We can send his written records fairly promptly, but the MRI we do not have and will need to get a CD to send to you via overnight FedEx. I will keep you posted, and thank you and Dr. Burzynski for your prompt response.*

Sheryl responded: *You're very welcome. We look forward to your email and records. I will confirm when they arrive.*

An additional note from Dr. Burzynski: Per the protocol we have, in order to be qualified for the clinical trial the MRI should not be more than 14 days prior to start of treatment. So we might have to repeat the MRI at one of the imaging centers here.

I will provide more details about arrangements if you decide to come here once I get the full records.

It was a positive reflection on Dr. Burzynski and his staff that they would engage in such a rapid volley of correspondence during "off-duty hours" with a prospective patient.

"Neil," I hollered up to his room, "I just heard from the Burzynski Clinic. They want your records ASAP, and they would welcome a visit."

"Fan-tastic!" he hollered back. "When do we go?"

"Well, they need your records first," I replied. "Everyone wants your records all at once."

At the same time this exchange was occurring, Evie received an email from Katelyn Nkomo at Dana-Farber: *"Hi Evie. I picked up the information you delivered. The MRI's are uploaded and ready for review. Dr. Kieran is out of town but will be back on Monday and should be able to review the information."*

Evie forwarded this to me and asked if I could pick up the ball because she needed to head back to school to get organized for the coming semester.

"Of course," I agreed, and sent a quick note to Katelyn: *"This is Evie's Dad. Evie is getting busy with school and asked me to take over. If the MRI files have been uploaded, do you still need the CD? We would like to have it, as Eugene's MGH patient portal includes only his written files... If that is possible, we will arrange to pick up the CD at your earliest convenience. Thank you for all you have done to help this process along."*

Then, I hollered to Neil yet again, "Hey Neil! Dana-Farber has your images uploaded. Dr. Kieran should be able to look at them on Monday. Hopefully we can get that CD back from them and send it on to Burzynski."

"Yee Ha," Neil hollered. "Things are starting to happen!"

BEACH WALK

While we waited for tests, relayed medical records, worked our lines of communication, and kept searching for miracles, Neil took time to tidy up loose ends at Northeastern. He needed to download and complete a medical leave form, and he needed to ask his advisor to let his professors know the situation. Although he was halfway through the semester and on track to maintain his GPA, he would have to take "incompletes" and repeat the semester upon his return. To take his mind off this added injury, we went to Cape Cod for a walk on Black Beach.

Spring was in the air, and the morning clouds had parted into a sunny,

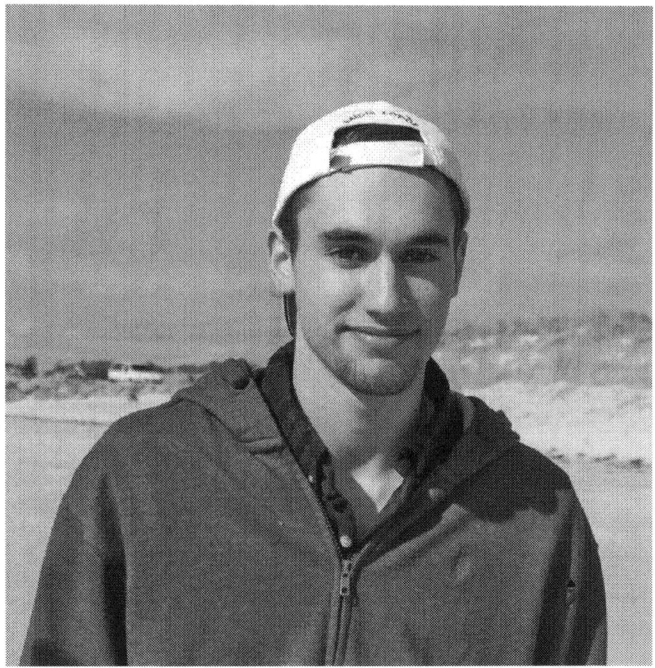

warm afternoon at low, low tide. Half a dozen sandbars stretched in a line from the bathhouse to the first breakwater. The beach was speckled with small rocks and pebbles, rounded from eons of tumbling. The gentle waves hushed up to the shore, and we ambled along, finding flat stones to skip and wading out to a sandbar, the water crisp and invigorating at our ankles. As we approached the stone breakwater, a few jovial women were gathered with a small pack of dogs who came running to greet us. One little long-haired mix had the biggest grin I had ever seen on a dog — so happy to see new people. We were drawn in, Neil especially, to a rescued greyhound, and we petted the dogs and exchanged pleasantries.

"Why does the ocean move?" asked one lady, then she paused. No replies. "You would too if you had crabs all over your bottom."

It was the Black Beach Dog Park and Comedy Club.

Half an hour later, we climbed over the breakwater to peek toward the inlet, then we meandered back towards the bathhouse, stopping to take a few photos.

We were barefoot, so when we got back to the car, we sat on the rocks and rubbed our feet dry and sand-free, then we for headed home, picking up some "fish chowdas" at Crabapple's on the way. Neil would have loved a "chowda," but he was completely committed to his new diet.

THE SEMESTER BEGINS

The following day, I drove Evie to the train station in Providence. She wanted to head back to school a day early to make sure she had everything organized for the coming semester. I parked in front of the station and leaned over to give her a hug.

"Remember," I told her. "We may be right back in Boston first thing next week to pick that CD back up."

She nodded and got out of the car. Hoisting her backpack from the rear seat. "Just let me know what you need me to do," she nodded.

"We will, Honey" I smiled and blew her a kiss. "Thank you."

She did likewise, then she crossed the street to the station, striding with all the confidence in the world. I marveled at the brightness of her life. Despite everything Neil was going through, it was soothing to know she was right where she needed to be, doing her best and loving it. We were lucky and proud!

When I got home, however, Neil was not having such a good day. Perhaps he was feeling the previous day's exertions and was sad to see Evie leave. He would miss her, and he may have envied her return to Northeastern. He wasn't really complaining, however. His spirits were good. He was just tired and having trouble with eyes. "Some days are a little better," he observed philosophically, "and some days a little worse."

JOURNAL RUMINATIONS

> The landscape before us is one of dispassionate probabilities, overarched by an abundance of Love and Spirit. There are no easy answers — or rather, there may be an easy an-

swer, but it is not easily arrived at — but we take solace in knowing we are just passing through this world, and it's not how long we live but how we live that matters most. Neil is living with extraordinary courage. We could not be more proud of him, and we are trying our best to support him.

Neil really needs that MRI of his spine; he needs the second opinion at Dana-Farber! Will Dr. Kieran concur with Dr. Cahill or Dr. Arrillaga? One thing is sadly probable: the biopsy path seems like wishful thinking. They want to match Neil's tumor to a drug in their arsenal, but statistically speaking, this strategy adds no time to the prognosis he would have if he took radiation alone. Of course, there's a chance Neil could be a breakthrough case, but what are those odds, and how do they weigh against the extra pain and suffering he would have to endure? And let's be clear, if he goes "all in," his survival chances are hardly better than if he does nothing. Those chances are about nil. Is the pain and suffering worth it? Or do we just take a trip to Hawaii or the rain forests of Costa Rica? (You see where I'm going with this...)

Then, there is holistic medicine, which we are trying to follow with Neil's Gerson therapy diet. Many people have beaten "incurable" disease by following the holistic path. That's not wishful thinking. It's fact, but there are no rigorous studies to point to because that's not the nature of holistic medicine. These doctors treat people and keep records, but they cannot afford to run double-blind studies or clinical trials, nor would they want to. Their mission is to treat people with the best natural medicine they know of, not experiment for the sake of proving one thing is better than another. If we follow the holistic path, there are many clinics in idyllic locations. We could take Neil for an adventure and get treatment too.

Finally, there are treatments that raise the hackles of mainstream medicine — things like laetrile, high-dose intravenous vitamin C, and Dr. Burzynski's antineoplastons. Mainstream medicine dismisses them all. At the moment, the slings and arrows are directed mostly at Dr. Burzynski, yet some of his DIPG patients have gone on to lead completely normal lives. Mainstream medicine can point to no such success.

9

BOSTON SHUTTLE

"Don't stop chasing your dreams,
or your dreams will chase you." NF

MARCH 14, 2016

First thing Monday morning, I received a call from Katelyn at Dana-Farber. Yes, we could pick up the disk of Neil's MRI. We were scheduled for a run to Boston in two days, but this couldn't wait. I told her we would do so that day.

"Looks like we're headed back to Boston today," I hollered to Wendy and Neil. "Double dipping this week!"

Then, I called Evie. "We can get the CD back from Dana-Farber today. Can you be the runner again?"

"Sure," she agreed. "I'll be done with classes by 10:00 a.m. Maybe we can stop by Whole Foods afterwards? I need to stock up on groceries and a ride would be very helpful."

"Sounds like a plan," I said. "We'll leave after rush hour — nine o'clock-ish. Mom will call you when we get into town."

"Okay! I'll be ready and waiting."

"Thank you Sweetheart. See you soon."

Then, I sent a quick email:

To: Sheryll Acelar
From: Dean Fachon

Subject: Re. Treatment at the Burzynski Clinic
Date: March 14, 2016

Hello Sheryll,

We're heading back to Boston today to get records and overnight them so you have them as quickly as possible. Neil is scheduled on Wednesday for an MRI of his lower spine. He has had some issues with initiating urination and bowel movements, so his MGH doctor (Isabel Arrillaga) wants to check for any tumor involvement in his spine. We will not wait for those results to send you everything else we collect today. Once you have his records let's touch base to set up a visit. Thank you and Dr. Burzynski.

Yours,
Dean Fachon

"Let's get an overnight envelope addressed and ready to go," I suggested to Wendy. "As soon as we get the CD, let's drop it at the nearest location."

"Already done," Wendy replied.

"Neil," I hollered up to his room. "Have you completed all the forms for the Burzynski Clinic? We need to send them with the CD and your records. I want to leave here around nine."

"The forms are all set," he hollered back. "I'll be down in a few. I hope breakfast is ready!"

Wendy made sure it was, and with breakfast tucked in and an overnight envelope addressed to the Burzynski Clinic, we piled into the car for another trip to Boston.

"And some people do this every day," Wendy mused as we merged into late morning rush hour traffic.

"A lot of people," I shook my head. "I used to drive an hour-plus each way when I worked for DEC in Spitbrook, New Hampshire. Some people drive a lot further. It makes for cranky drivers."

Wendy shook her head too, but Neil pulled down the bill of his cap, slumped in his seat, and dozed off. Wendy called Evie as soon as we got off Route 128.

"We'll pick you up at your building in five minutes."

"I'll be waiting," Evie answered.

Good to her word, she was at the curb and hopped in. Then, we wended our way back to Dana-Farber, pulling into a quasi-legal parking spot, and Evie hopped out.

"I know right where to go," she assured us. "I'll be back less than five minutes."

"I'll call if we have to move," Wendy told her.

Evie disappeared into the lobby and reemerged a few minutes later with a small flat package in hand.

"They had it ready and waiting," she smiled, handing the package to Wendy.

"Good stuff," Neil smiled, as Wendy tucked the package into the overnight envelope and sealed it securely. We drove to the nearest FedEx drop box, deposited the envelope along with a silent wish for "God speed," then we took Evie to get groceries.

There was a queue at Whole Foods, and parking was a matter of waiting for an attendant to motion us into a spot being vacated. In the store, Evie filled a carriage and then some, while Neil picked out a "green drink." Wendy paid for the groceries as a thank you to Evie.

"I guess you really did need a ride," I said to Evie as we loaded bags in the back of the car. "No way you could've walked with all this!"

"I needed to stock up," Evie hugged us. "Thank you!"

"Thank you, Sweetheart!"

When we got back to Evie's apartment, Neil gave her a big hug, and Wendy helped bring up the groceries, then we said our goodbyes and departed. As soon as we got home, I notified Sonnet at the Burzynski Clinic to expect a package: "*The forms, records and copy of my son's MRI have been sent via FedEx. There is only one question left incomplete on the forms – the physician who would assist with any ongoing treatment when we return home. We have two possibilities in mind – Neil's neuro-oncologist at MGH or his childhood pediatric physician – but neither has been consulted about this possibility. We'll "cross that bridge when we get to it." If there are any questions, please contact me. Otherwise, we look forward to learning Dr. Burzynski's preliminary assessment."*

TRIPLE DIP TRIP

On Wednesday, March 16, we resumed our Boston commute, first to see Neil's physical therapist, then to Mass General for the long-awaited MRI of his spine. If any tumor growth showed up, Neil's diagnosis might be something less dire than DIPG. It might also help to explain his sluggish GI and urinary tracts. Finally, we would wrap up Neil's appointment-schedule with a visit to Dr. Panis.

"Where should we park?" I asked Neil as we neared Mass General.

"Just go to the hospital," Neil replied. "Dr. Hergot is a block away. We can walk. That will be easier than lucking into a parking spot on the street."

"Are you sure?" Wendy asked. "That's a lot of walking."

"It's a nice day," Neil smiled. "I'm up for it."

We parked on the roof level of the hospital garage and took the elevator down to the street, then we walked. Along the way, Neil regaled us with "Husky Hunt" stories and other adventures around Boston. Neil's capable stride and happy conversation made us feel almost normal. Five minutes later, we arrived at the therapist's office. Wendy and I sat in the waiting area while Neil and his therapist had a brief meeting. She advised him to continue his exercises, wished him the best of luck, and they exchanged farewell hugs.

Back at Mass General, the oncology wing of the imaging center was a few floors above Dr. Arrillaga's office. We had a few minutes to spare before Neil's appointment, so we sat in the hallway overlooking the city, and Neil tried to give her a call. They had been playing "phone tag," and this time was no different. He left a message, and we passed the time by looking out the windows. City buildings loomed above and hulked below.

We could see our car on the roof of the parking garage, like a "Matchbox toy, and pedestrians resumed the appearance of ants, just as we would have looked to anyone peering down a few minutes earlier. Perspectives. It made me think of the dimensional shift we were caught in. Like Alice falling down the rabbit hole.

The appointed hour arrived, and Neil walked into the waiting area to check in. As luck would have it, Dr. Arrillaga returned his call at just the same moment, so he stepped back into the corridor to speak privately. He wanted to ask, once again, about his prognosis, in clinical terms, without any hedging. She reaffirmed her assessment: The disease would likely run its course in three months if he did nothing. With recommended treatment, she thought he had six months. She encouraged Neil to do the biopsy. Even so, she acknowledged it could cause some minor damage, but she felt the risk was worth it. After recovering from that procedure, she advised immediate radiation over the course of several weeks, then he would hopefully get a few Cinderella months of reprieve — time in which to have an adventure. And say his goodbyes. She urged Neil to move quickly. Every day of delay was a day lost.

If he followed this course, Neil realized the months he might gain would be taken up in part by the treatments themselves, not to mention recovery. And then what if his "brain trust" decided to throw chemo into the mix? For someone accustomed to analytical thinking, this path left Neil bemused: "Just to gain a few months?!" Fear alone seemed to auger for the path being proffered, and then surrender to death, but Neil's intuition demanded something more; he believed there had to be something better. He wasn't sure what it was, but he knew he was all but dead set against radiation, and that alone cast a shadow over the MGH program.

Within minutes of finishing his conversation with Dr. Arrillaga, a nurse called Neil in for his MRI. He spent well over an hour in the torpedo tube — bombarded by a constant din of bangs, clacks, and whirs — and he emerged a bit frazzled. Nonetheless, he was eager to see Dr. Panis and introduce us to him. His office was also within walking distance, but time and energy constraints suggested we take the car. The drive was short, but finding the correct turn-in for the parking garage was confusing, and we had to make a U-turn. Not fun, but once in the garage, we snagged a convenient spot near the entrance — not too much walking. That was fortunate, because getting to Dr. Panis's office was somewhat like finding the records-department at MGH. We all had a laugh about that, but soon enough, we were at the door to his office.

The waiting area had just enough seats for the three of us, and the receptionist recognized Neil immediately.

"Dr. Panis will be right with you," she smiled warmly, which indeed he was.

"Hello Eugene," he greeted Neil as he opened the door to his inner sanctum and gestured us in.

"Dr. Panis," Neil smiled, shaking his hand. "Meet my parents."

Dr. Panis was roughly the same age as us, with Robert Redford's hair, a warm handshake, and smiling eyes suggesting a playful, caring soul.

"It's a pleasure to meet you," Wendy said, avoiding the obvious subtext (but not under these circumstances).

"Thank goodness someone finally had the presence of mind to order an MRI," I wasn't shy about saying.

"Easy dad," Neil chided.

Dr. Panis nodded sympathetically, then he motioned Neil to sit down. "Let's have a look at you."

Dr. Panis checked Neil's mobility, strength, and reflexes in all of his limbs; he checked Neil's eye movement in all directions (separately and together); and he checked Neil's balance and gait. When he finished his physical exam, Dr. Panis proclaimed, "You seem to be doing well — no significant change since when I first saw you two weeks ago!"

"That's good," Neil smiled. "We've been working on it. Mom's flipped my diet completely," and he smiled gratefully at Wendy. "The biggest frustration is seeing double sometimes, when I'm tired."

"You might try an eye patch," Dr. Panis suggested. "Use it when you're fatigued and your left eye really wants to wander."

"That sounds like a good idea," Neil nodded in agreement.

We nodded, too, and at Neil's urging, Wendy gave Dr. Panis a brief overview of Neil's diet. While trained in traditional medicine, Dr. Panis was open-minded and listened intently, applauding her efforts. He also encouraged our search "outside the box" for other treatment options — like the Bursynski Clinic. Dr. Panis took the time to just listen and talk, to acknowledge the tragic hand Neil had been dealt, and to assure us of his full support. He told Neil to be as active as possible, and toward the end of our meeting, he gave Neil his personal mobile phone number so he could call anytime. Open door. What a good way to end the day! We thanked Dr. Panis, feeling grateful to have a such a wonderful advocate amongst the cadre of doctors on Neil's "treatment team."

That helped make the mood light as we drove home. On the way, we stopped at the drugstore to pick up an eye patch, which Neil tried on immediately.

"Arrgh Cap'n," he grinned.

"Hide the women," I chuckled, and Wendy rolled her eyes.

Once home, it was back to the computer to resume our research and exchange emails in the anxious quest to advance Neil's treatment. Wendy also had Neil's special-needs dinner to prepare.

Excerpts from report by Dr. Panis, March 16, 2016:

> He is doing remarkably well mentally considering his diagnosis. They were given a prognosis of a very short time without treatment. It was recommended they do a biopsy. Radiation could be tried. Experimental agents could be used. However they were also told that although this would increase his survival it would not be very long....He is changing his diet a bit.
>
> We all spoke. It was very frank. They were looking into alternatives including a clinic in Houston, functional doctors and nutrition, etc.

On examination he looked very well. He continued to have the persistent double vision… I told him I would be available for them for any questions or issues…

ONE STEP FORWARD, TWO STEPS BACK

To: Dean Fachon
From Sheryll Acelar
Subject: Records
Date: March 16, 2016

Hi Dean,

I hope you are well. We received your son's scans and the medical records and Dr. Burzynski has them. The Protocol for Eugene's type of tumor requires an enhancement that is measurable, but since the scans and reports state that the mass is non-enhancing, it decreases the chances of him being enrolled in the clinical trial. Dr. Burzynski stated that there is another way and this is to do a PET/CT scan of Eugene's brain to see if the mass is metabolically active which will allow him entrance to the clinical trial. This PET/CT brain has to be done at least 14 days prior to starting the treatment. Dr. Burzynski will let you know when will be the right time for this test.

Also, Dr. Burzynski informed me that the FDA requires separate batches of the medications be prepared for patients in clinical trials. Our pharmaceutical plant is working on this now and it should finish the products in 3 to 4 weeks and at such time we will begin admission of patients

If you have any questions, please feel free to ask me.

Best,
Sheryll

"Non-enhancing?" "Metabolically active?" If these terms had been mentioned before, they'd escaped me. How could the tumor be anything other than metabolically active, especially one that would take our son's life in three months?! Clearly, we had more to learn, but this email hit me like a roadblock, just when I thought we were catching some real traction with the Burzynski Clinic! I told Neil about it, my chagrin too apparent.

"I'd say that's more of a caution light than a roadblock," he bucked me up. "I'll take whatever tests I need to."

Speaking of more tests, Mass General called Neil later that morning to inform him the spinal MRI they had just taken was no good. "They have to redo the MRI."

"Redo it," I exclaimed. "Why?!"

"Something to do with contrast," Neil shrugged.

The seconds were too precious to lose on something like this. "When?" I asked anxiously. "Do we head back tomorrow?"

"No," Neil looked down with a shake of his head. "They have me scheduled for Thursday, March 31."

"That's two f#&!ing weeks," I howled, clenching my fists. "Dam! I guess that tells us how important it is to figure out whether you could have something besides DIPG! They just want to start drilling!"

"Take it easy," Wendy waded calmly into my tantrum. "It is what it is."

"I hate that expression," I said ruefully.

"Be that as it may," she continued. "We take it in stride and keep plugging along, putting irons in the fire. The right opportunity will become self-evident in due course."

"C'mon dad," Neil put a hand on my shoulder. "It's not like I'm chafing at the bit to start radiation. Or do the biopsy. Mom's right," he smiled. "We need to learn more. I'm good with that. We are doing FAN-TASTIC!"

He got me again. My anger melted away, and I hugged him. "Okay. Put it on the calendar and let's forget about it for now."

HEALTHCARE PROXY

For all our efforts to take things in stride, it was depressingly clear we needed a plan if worse came to worst — if Neil's cancer progressed and he was unable to voice his medical questions and choices. Having some sort of control would be vastly preferable to being shut out, unable to access his records or make any decisions on his behalf. The Health Insurance Portability and Accountability Act of 1996 (HIPAA) saw to that. If Neil were incapacitated, the state would take over. The very notion was horrifying. To put this worry behind us, on March 17, 2016, Neil executed a "Massachusetts Health Care Proxy." Although never known for his penmanship, Neil really struggled to sign his name. The clock was running. The proxy named Wendy and I as Neil's "Health Care Agents."

I also touched base with Raffaele:

To: Raffaele
From: Dean
Subject: Re: Status update for Neil
Date: March 17, 2016

Raffaele,

We've had a few days of good family time, but today we were back at it. The meeting last week with Dr. Cahill was somewhat confusing. Where Dr. Arrillaga said she was 99% sure the tumor is a DIPG. Dr. Cahill put the odds at 90%. We are hoping Dr. Kieran will help make things more definitive, but whichever end of the scale it ends up, the prognosis with current interventions runs from very poor to very very poor, offering hardly any more chance that Neil would live much longer than if he does nothing at all. Or if he does live a little longer, it would be at the expense of enduring the treatment and its side effects, likely offsetting the extended time.

There are risks with any course of action, so the question really becomes, where is the greatest potential benefit? The answer is found in alternative medicine, where several approaches have been very successful in dealing with cancer, but as regards DIPG, Dr. Burzynski has the best track record by far. Yes, much of that evidence is anecdotal – partly because the FDA at one time seized all his patient records – but Dr. Burzynski also has a large and well-respected following amongst many alternative medicine practitioners. That's not a fluke. Yes, I have heard of potential side-effects from antineoplastons, but I have also witnessed first-hand the guaranteed side-effects of radiation and chemo therapy.

We have made no decisions, but we have sent Neil's records to the Burzynski Clinic and will probably go for a consultation. Otherwise, we continue to work with Neil's diet and surround him with love and compassion – to celebrate Life in the Spirit of Christ! As ever, we welcome your continued support.

Dean

10

THE "IN-BETWEENS"

"What kind of stuff can be learned on a busy sidewalk? Watch the people around you. Feel their stories." NF

Although our lives were taken over by urgent communications and appointments — and excruciating delays — as our daily routines became more established, we found time in between to "take the world in" with greater intention and intensity.

THE FAMILY WE CHOOSE

Grappling with Neil's situation would not have been possible without our family and friends, and we could not have been more fortunate in our neighbors — Tim and Sherri, Carl and Donna, and especially the Grady family:

At the age of four or five, Neil met Andrew Grady when they enrolled in a Taekwondo class for beginners. As serendipity would have it, shortly thereafter, we moved to the home I grew up in, just up the street from the Grady's. From fourth grade through junior high school, Neil and Andrew walked together to school, sharing good and not-so-good experiences that forged a tight bond. When it came time for high school, they went separate ways, but they would still "hang out" after school — shooting hoops, lifting weights, and taking Hera (Andrew's possessive German Shepherd) for long walks and talks to match. Those walks often occurred in the wee hours of the morning when everyone else was asleep — everyone save for the occasional coyote on the prowl around our neighborhood, which would drive Hera nuts. If Neil wasn't at home, nine times out of ten he was "down at the Grady's." Even if Andrew wasn't there, his mom Cindy treated Neil like another son. She loved "kidding" with him. Cindy is also an exceptional cook in the grand Italian style, which means she feeds her family well, including "adopted" children. Neil loved Cindy's cooking!

As often happens, a strong connection between childhood friends leads to a friendship between the parents as well. Wendy and I would often end our evening walks by stopping in to see Cindy and Ted. Their door was always open, and we would just knock and walk in. We were always greeted with warmth and generosity, no matter what might be happening in their lives. Old-fashioned neighbors. The Grady's were crushed when they first heard of Neil's illness. They offered to do anything they possibly could, and they meant it.

One evening, on a solo stroll after dinner, I decided to stop by their home. As soon as I opened the door, I was greeted by a marvelous aroma from the kitchen, followed instantly by Hera barking madly in her guardian-voice until she recognized me. Then, she whimpered plaintively, as if saying, "Where the heck have you been," beating me with her wagging as she fishtailed around my legs.

"Hey," Cindy greeted me with a hug. "How you doin'?"

"Hangin' in there," I answered with a shrug, just as Ted came up from the basement with a bundle Cindy asked him to grab from their big freezer — doubtless the foundation for some upcoming family feast.

"Hey Dean," he handed Cindy the package and gave me a gentle thumping hug. "Have a seat," he motioned to their kitchen table, a place where we've had many good times together. "Want a seltzer?"

Before I could answer, Cindy chimed in, "Want some chicken and homemade gnocchi? The gnocchi I made yesterday. The chicken just finished baking."

"Oh," Ted purred, "you gotta try this chicken!"

"I knew there was something good cooking the moment I opened the door," I smiled and shook my head no, "I just had dinner."

"Well have a little more," Ted grinned and pulled out a chair.

"I have some pepper biscuits to send home with you too," Cindy added.

There was no refusing this tag team, so I sat down with a chuckle. "Just a taste."

"And a seltzer," Ted adopted a head waiter pose. "We have lemon or grapefruit."

"Lemon," I smiled, and there quickly appeared a seltzer with a glass of crushed ice.

A moment later, Cindy brought a plate of chicken in sauce, buttered gnocchi, and a saucer of freshly ground Parmesan. "Welcome to Italy," she smiled. "The chicken was baked in olive oil with marinated artichoke hearts, sliced Kalamata olives, diced tomatoes, and a dash of salt and pepper."

"What, no gah-lic?" I arched an eyebrow like Neil would have done.

"Of course garlic!" Cindy scoffed. "You have to ask?"

I wasn't hungry, but my appetite had no trouble reviving as I "tucked in" for a dose of homestyle comfort with Ted and Cindy seated on either side.

I sprinkled some Parmesan and dug in. "Wow, this is good," I managed between bites.

"What did I tell you?" Ted kissed his fingers. "Magnifico!"

I chuckled appreciatively, then they gave me time to just enjoy eating while they caught up with each other on events of the day.

"You want more?" Cindy asked when my plate was clean.

"Wow," I nodded. "I would, but now I'm really stuffed."

"It's good for you," Ted chuckled.

After a pause to savor the moment, Cindy asked, "So, how's it going; anything new?"

"Well," I sat back, "you know we're looking at everything we possibly can, but the Boston hospitals are pretty much telegraphing not to expect much more than stalling this thing a few months."

"Did you contact that clinic you mentioned?" Ted asked.

"The Burzynski Clinic," I nodded, pushing back from the table as

Neil's situation came rushing back to the front of my mind. "Burzynski is a pariah to mainstream medicine, but he's a hero in alternative medicine. He's had some success with DIPG. Anecdotal, but it's tough to dismiss."

"Well, you're doing your homework," Cindy commiserated. "You'll do the right thing."

"I just can't imagine losing Neil," I said, each word like the stroke of an old-fashioned hand pump, drawing tears up from a well I tried to deny.

In an instant, Ted and Cindy were hugging me from both sides, a scrum of sniffles and wet cheeks. They just held me. That was the first time I'd really managed to cry since our shared nightmare began, in the familial embrace of Neil's favorite adopted parents.

HITTING THE GYM

Despite delays and uncertainties, we were making important progress in many areas. For one thing, Neil's bowels were finally moving normally, which made him feel better than he had in weeks, much as the rhythm of our lives had become more routine. With this came the opportunity to include more exercise in Neil's regimen, as Dr. Panis had suggested.

"You wanna go to the gym?" I asked him late one morning.

His eyes lit right up. "Absolutely!"

Neil needed no urging. He loved "working out" and had been to my gym, "American Health Fitness," a few times in the past. He still had a card, so we "hit the gym."

A typical gym visit would begin with Neil stretching and doing some simple hand-eye coordination exercises. Next, he'd spend fifteen minutes on an elliptical trainer just loping along. After that, it was time for some weight lifting. He would sometimes use free weights and sometimes the circuit machines. He wouldn't push much weight so much as challenge his coordination, range of motion, and symmetrical muscle function.

Neil's favorite part of our workouts was the pool, especially on days when we had it completely to ourselves. At its deepest, the pool was four feet, so we could stand opposite each other at the far ends and throw a tennis ball back and forth. He loved diving out for the ball, as if stretching for a tennis volley, and he had me throw to alternate sides so he could work both hands. Some days, he struggled, and some days, he caught the ball firmly. Those were good days when he could catch with either hand.

JUICING UP

Work out or not, we would often cap our mornings with a trip to Raw Bob's to get a fresh juice drink. After several visits, this habit was becoming expensive, so we decided to start juicing at home. We could save some money, and Neil would have plenty of fresh juice available throughout the day, which is what Gerson recommends.

Step one in juicing is getting the correct equipment — not inexpensive, but we would have it "forever." First up on the list was a heavy-duty mixer. A regular blender could never stand up to the rigors of grinding enough veggies to make a few pints of juice every day, so we needed something with commercial-grade strength. Fortunately, there was an unused "Vitamix" in the family, so we commandeered it. Then, we needed a press to remove the pulp from the juice. After some research, we found a mechanical press made of surgical stainless steel that had a large capacity. We were in business.

A typical day of juicing would actually begin the day before. Wendy would stock up on fresh organic produce — things like cucumbers, celery, carrots, chard, romaine lettuce, kale, cilantro, beets, and occasionally an apple — whatever was fresh and looked good. With the ingredients on hand, I would fire up the Vitamix and start adding the veggies, using the machine's plunger to push them down into the blades and grind everything into a slurry. We followed no exact recipes but took cues from some of the drinks we liked at Raw Bob's.

With the ingredients turned into a thick slurry, next came the pressing (which required setting up the press in advance). Our press has a tall, perforated cylinder that affixes to a catch pan with a drain nozzle. A short food-grade plastic hose connects to the nozzle, and the other end leads to a stainless steel bowl in the sink, so liquid is gravity fed. Next, the cylinder gets lined with an ultrafine mesh cloth, then we pour in the slurry, using a rubber spatula to get everything out of the mixer. As soon as the slurry is poured, liquid starts to ooze through the mesh and the cylinder's perforations, collecting in the catch pan and finally draining into the bowl. Now comes the fun part — the pressing itself. A tight-fitting plate affixed to a threaded rod gets pushed down the cylinder — like a piston — by spinning a T-handle on the rod's opposite end. The rod is held tight in a threaded mount that spans the top of the cylinder. As the pulp gets pressed down, a torrent of juice begins streaming out all sides of the cylinder into the catch pan and then into the bowl. A good pressing would fill a two quart bowl to the brim, leaving a solid puck of veggie fiber about an inch thick at the bottom of the cylinder. Juice for the day! Last came the disassembly and cleanup, which was tedious but had to be properly done to get ready for the next day.

AN "HERBAL" BOOST

Among her many friends, Wendy wanted Neil to meet Mary Blue, a "community herbalist" and owner of Farmacy Herbs, a cozy shop in Providence. Mary is an expert on traditional herbal healing, and Wendy scheduled a consult to see if she could recommend some immune-boosting herbs that might be helpful for Neil. Surrounded by shelves of dried herbs, bottles of tinctures, and natural medicine books, Mary served Wendy and Neil a mild tea while she asked Neil about his illness and its effects on his body. After listening intently, she discussed which herbs could boost his immune, nervous, and endocrine systems, and which herbs could support health in the liver, blood, and brain.

Neil thought a tea blend of these herbs would be great to try, so he and Wendy watched as Mary scooped measured amounts from various jars — dried dandelion leaf, red clover, nettle, tulsi, lemon balm, and other herbs — into a food-grade plastic bag. She closed the bag and turned it in her hands while shaking it gently to mix the ingredients, then she explained how the tea should be steeped and how frequently Neil should take it.

In addition to Neil's blend of tea, Mary mixed a tincture derived from extracts of ashwagandha, St. John's wort, poke root, and other herbs. This tincture would support Neil's adrenals, lymphatic system, and other functions. Adrenal glands, located on top of the kidneys, produce hormones that help regulate the body's response to stress. A lymphatic system functioning properly is critical for fighting infections and helping the body to destroy old or abnormal cells. When Mary finished the tincture, Neil gave it a taste.

"That's Warrior Juice," he dubbed the bitter concoction, but he would faithfully take one tablespoon three times a day from then on.

Mary's also suggested Neil take curcumin capsules. Curcumin — a spice derived from turmeric — is a strong anti-inflammatory, which can be effective in treating many diseases. In the case of brain cancer, curcumin would traverse the blood-brain barrier and might help to turn on "sleeping genes" that promote apoptosis. Curcumin could also help to promote neurogenesis — the formation of new nerve cells. Mary wrapped up the meeting by referring Neil to a renowned naturopathic oncologist in Connecticut, Dr. Jody Noé. Naturopathic oncologists work with conventional oncologists in an integrative model of cancer co-treatment, which Dr. Noé helped pioneer. Naturopathic oncologists are versed in botanical medicine, homeopathy, diet, nutrition, nutraceutical supplements, and traditional oncology.

When Wendy and Neil returned home, they looked online for more information about Dr. Noé:

> "Dr. Jody E. Noé obtained her Doctorate of Naturopathic Medicine from Bastyr University in Seattle, Washington. Previous to this, she was awarded her Bachelor's and Master's of Science degrees from Old Dominion University in Norfolk, Virginia. Dr. Noé has held several faculty positions and is a founding member of the Botanical Medicine

> Academy. She is president emeritus for both the Oklahoma and Vermont Associations of Naturopathic Physicians."

"She's impressive," Neil nodded when Wendy showed him her findings. "Let's talk to her too." Wendy called Dr. Noé's office to schedule an appointment on March 23.

FRESH AIR

Between food prep, trips to Boston, the barrage of emails, constant research, various appointments, and visits to the gym, we kept ourselves busy. Even so, sometimes minutes seemed like hours — waiting to get a second opinion, wondering if Neil would qualify for a promising clinic trial, and the endless hunt for any shred of new information that might help. It was like being smothered in a haystack while searching for the proverbial needle, so when Dr. Kieran called from Dana-Farber, the breath of fresh air was glorious. He wanted to touch base in advance of Neil's appointment, and we spoke candidly for several minutes. I immediately shared this news with Neil and Raffaele:

> **To: Raffaele**
> **From: Dean**
> **Subject: quick update**
> **Date: March 18, 2016**
>
> Raffaele,
>
> I just spoke with Dr. Kieran! He corrected me on the recovery time for the biopsy. Assuming no complications, it would be a few days, not two weeks. Otherwise, he confirmed the diagnosis and suggested the real benefit from doing the biopsy is that in 1/3rd of the cases there may be a drug that can have some impact. However, the blood brain barrier still negates much of the

potential effectiveness, even when a drug is identified. He spoke of a trial in England where they are delivering chemo directly into the pons, but that was not by way of suggesting we should look into it so much as informational. Basically he admitted unabashedly that where DIPG is concerned, they are flying in the dark. Neil's case is of note because he is so much older than the typical patient, thus his tumor may behave differently.... I wonder if anyone has tried hormone therapy to shrink these tumors... Thinking out loud.

Thank you again for lending an ear...
Dean

THE SOUL OF COMPASSION

Raffaele replied at length to my latest emails.

To: Dean
From: Raffaele
Subject: Re: quick update
Date: March 18, 2016

Dear Dean,

I am happy you spoke to Dr Mark Kieran. Thank you for the update. I am answering both emails you just sent, and I want to share some personal thoughts. These are my opinions and not medical recommendations. I want to share how I feel because I deeply care about Neil and you. I will always distinguish my opinions from the facts that are purely professional data. My opinions are just that, and you can take them or leave them. You need to do what Neil feels is best for him, but I want to help your thought process.

I think the question of the biopsy – that Neil's neuro-oncologist seems eager about – is crucial. Unfortunately, there is little data to make a wise and solid decision. I deeply appreciate Mark for his honesty, and I always have. He tells the truth as it is. As I told you previously too, there is a possibility that Neil's tumor is different because he is suffering from it at an older age. Whether this is good or bad is not possible to say. It cannot be excluded that Neil's tumor could be vulnerable to a specific drug, but there is no way of knowing before the biopsy. So the decision is very personal and comes down to what Neil feels is the best for him. Here comes my own opinion, and what I would do if I had DIPG: I personally feel very strongly about research, as you can imagine. If I had this disease I would always try to give something to the labs working on finding a cure that helps them. It might not help me, but others. So, personally, and this is just my personal opinion, I would do the biopsy. Even if there is only a small chance to find a drug that might slow the growth of the disease, I would want that opportunity.

Back to medical facts and thoughts: Radiation therapy has been shown to slow down the tumor growth. Radiation does not cure the disease, but it gives patients time, and it is the only proven therapy known to work albeit imperfectly. Sometimes it is 3 months, sometimes 6 months, but I have seen cases up to 1 year. In the majority of cases, the symptoms get better after radiation. Here again is my personal opinion: If something buys me time, I would do it. If I can enjoy even weeks with my family, do something I always wanted to do or take a trip, I would want that time.

Regarding prognosis, I think the numbers given by Neil's neuro-oncologist are factually correct, although again they are based on the study of DIPG affecting children much younger than Niel. It is exceptional for DIPG to affect a young adult. Nobody knows (without biopsies) how the tumors evolve. Little is known, but what is known suggests it is an exceedingly bad disease. I understand that both love and logic suggest looking for alternatives, and that is exactly what anyone does.

Regarding the trial in the UK with the injection of chemotherapy directly in the affected region, this study is not very different from the study Evie found on the Internet. It is an option, and worth considering. I would look at everything. Personally, I have the same thought Mark did: I would check it out, and see if there is anything new or DIPG-specific that is convincing. Again, I would always try to join a study, but that is my bias.

To your specific question, hormonal therapies have been tried, but historically lead to no improvements. Many people think it made things worse. In fact, to grow tumors in the laboratory, researchers use hormones. Depending on what hormones are used, the tumor growth is boosted.

Regarding, the Bruzynski clinic, here are the facts: the theory of antineoplastons has been around for decades. http://www.cancer.gov/about-cancer/treatment/cam/patient/antineoplastons-pdq

Many patients (including some I have cared for) have gone there and, disappointingly, I have not seen many successes. Furthermore, no clinical trial/study has shown credible (to me) results of any kind (good or bad). The National Cancer Institute and many others (including the local Medical Board) have issued warnings, but I have also seen many reports on the Internet of cures, and this has always intrigued me. It seems that it is impossible to know if this works, and for whom it will work. Certain antineoplaston trials were done elsewhere (Mayo Clinic for example) and failed to show similar results to those obtained by the Burzynski clinic. It seems that certain patients have gotten standard chemotherapy as well as antineoplastons. Taking it all together, I can only say I would give this as much consideration as all the other approaches. My personal opinion is the following:

I would give everything deep thought and ask as many questions as I can. When something is unproven, I usually take the common sense approach and ask

- Is it dangerous? If it isn't, I would look at it very carefully.
- How many DIPG patients treated? How many cures/ responses?
- How did patients feel during treatment?
- What is the treatment exactly, and what does it involve?
- What are the side effects? Any long term side effects?

If a trial asks for other tests to be done, I would ask why? CT/PET scans are done to measure the metabolic activity of tumors. It is a nuclear imaging test that measures the uptake and metabolism of radioactive glucose (or some other tracer). As I do not know what antineoplastons do, I cannot say whether this is a helpful to guide therapy or not. The only thing I can say is that DIPG are usually active tumors, but there have been studies that show that PET activity does not correlate with survival in DIPG. This is why neuro-oncologists do not generally use CT/PET scans to help with therapy decisions, but I can not comment on what should be done to evaluate somebody for trials at the Bruzynski clinic. My personal opinion is that whatever Neil feels comfortable with and would like to do, that is the right thing to do. I alway support my patients in their choice, unless I feel there is something dangerous or unethical. That is why I always tell my patients to ask as many questions of anyone else offering them therapy as they ask me. And safety comes first.

I spoke to several colleagues (France, Canada, UK) to hear if there is anything else new or helpful. They have not heard of anything, but I keep my ears and eyes open all the time for Neil. I also spoke to a colleague who is specialized in alternative medicine. He suggested things from hypnosis for stress relief, to herbal therapy and aromatherapy – many things you already know. Unfortunately, he is not aware of other therapies to treat DIPG, but he will keep eye and ears open too. If anything comes up, we will be in touch asap.

As you very importantly point out, it is central to never forget the importance of love and family. This disease is terrible, but fighting it should never abolish whatever plans Neil and you might have to make his life as beautiful, as loving and as fulfilling as possible. I have lost patients, friends, neighbors and family members to

> cancer, but I always remember and focus on the power of love that gave them strength. They continue to live in my heart thanks to the love that made life beautiful, even when all else was dark.
>
> I always encourage my patients to make plans that make them happy, that give them comfort, that allow them to receive and give love. Medicine (alternative or not) should not take away all that matters, and treatments that have less than certain chances to beat the disease should not stop anyone from realizing dreams or unfulfilled wishes. All of us do not know when our time will come, so we should all fight back at whatever wants to harm us, but also never forget to make every day count for the things that make us who we are. These might be different things for all of us. For some it is love, family and the beauty of nature. For some it is swimming in the ocean or climbing mountains. For some it is listening to music. For some it is reading poetry. For some it is riding horses or petting a rabbit (that is usually what my patients prefer to do). For some it is praying. Nothing should take this away from anyone. I am sure Neil and you are aware of this, but I needed to say it.
>
> Hope all of this helps. Warmest wishes to Neil and all of you.
> Biggest hug, and much love,
>
> Raffaele

Wow.

I printed this out and shared it with Neil. He took fifteen minutes to read it, then he read it again. When he finished, he smiled through his tears. "Raffaele is all heart. He sent us his heart."

"He really did," I agreed. "He opens every door and leaves them all open. 'Follow your heart' was never said with more compassion." I hugged Neil. "Anything is possible."

To: Raffaele
From: Dean
Subject: Never dismissed...
Date: March 18, 2016

Raffaele,

None of the thoughts you so graciously share are EVER dismissed. Your lengthy email was formatted and printed for all of us to share. Obviously we are holding nothing back from Neil, and he was very moved by your words. There is no easy quick answer – no definitive "right" answer. We are on a journey. One day we hope to thank you in person, but for now you are in our prayers of thanks. No doubt we will be in touch soon.

Love and God Bless,
Dean

To this day, Raffaele's compassion stirs deep feelings of gratitude. He was a central pillar for us all, sustaining our efforts to juggle Neil's immediate care and supporting our search for a miracle among the stars.

With that thought in mind, the light from the Burzynski Clinic, if remote, was very bright, so I replied to Sheryll's cautionary email.

To: Sheryll Acelar
From: Dean Fachon
Subject: Re: Records
Date: March 18, 2016

Sheryll,

I know the clinic is under tremendous constraints, but in cases like my son's, where the treatment offered by the "best hospitals in the world" is nothing more than palliative – more like a Hospice prescription – is there a mechanism to petition the FDA to make an exception? I will most certainly pursue this route if it means the difference between a genuine glimmer of hope and capitulation. Any advise or information you can share would be greatly appreciated.

Thank you again,
Dean Fachon

CLOSING IN

We were finally closing in on the desperately needed "second opinion" from Dr. Kieran. To urge things along, I sent a quick email to Katelyn at Dana-Farber: *"I had a good phone conversation with Dr. Kieran, and he is happy to meet with us. That would be a big help for Eugene. Is there be a time next week when we could possibly sneak in?"*

She promptly replied: *"Would you be available to come in on Tuesday 3/22 from 12:30-1:30? Dr. Kieran is traveling the second half of the week so I'm hoping we can find a time in common to set this up."*

That would be perfect." I told her. *"Unless we hear otherwise, we will be there at noon."*

"That's good news," Katelyn answered. *"We are all set for a 12:30-1:30 appointment on 3/22. Please come to the Jimmy Fund Clinic located of the third floor of the DANA building (44 Binney St). Dr. Kieran will see you and Eugene then!"*

As eagerly as we anticipated this meeting, we never knew when a new lead would turn up. Such was the case when Charles discovered a clinic in Germany — *IOZK: Immun-Onkologischues Zentrum KÖLN* — which was using immunotherapy to assist patients' own immune systems in combating cancer. We forwarded Katelyn's and Charles's emails to the kids and suggested they make a list of questions for our upcoming meeting with Dr. Kieran. We shared a draft of our thoughts as well:

> What is your degree of confidence in the diagnosis?
>
> What are the other disease-options for the remaining possibility?
>
> Let's run through all the treatment options from a statistical point of view:
>
> 1) Radiation – (dosage, duration, frequency and recovery)
> 2) Biopsy and molecular profiling
>
> Are you familiar with Dr. Souweidane's work with "interstitial infusion?" Does it hold promise? Are you using this method? If not, would you recommend contacting his clinic?
>
> Are you familiar with "IOZK – Immunologisch Onkologisches Zentrum Köln" (immunotherapy to assist patient's own immune system in recognizing cancer)? Are there any other clinics doing this? What if any promise does this approach hold in the short term for DIPG patients?
>
> Given Neil's record and MRI-results, can you speculate on a time-frame for when this tumor might have begun?
>
> In your experience, what role can nutrition play in combating this condition? Do you have any specific recommendations?
>
> Are there any clinical trials we should look at?
>
> Are you familiar with any alternative treatments that, no matter how controversial or "wacky," we should investigate?

> When was the first known case of DIPG diagnosed? Since then, how many cases have there been? In that time, have there been any known cases of remission that lasted 5-years of more? Spontaneous, or while being treated. Any names?

This list of questions would grow and change, and we would keep juggling all our options, but everyday living would happily intervene in the meantime: Andrew Grady called Neil to check in, and a few minutes later, he announced plans to have Andrew and two other friends come over to play board games the following day.

"SETTLERS OF CATAN"

On the afternoon of Sunday, March 20, Andrew, Josh, and Matt knocked on the back door. These three had been friends with Neil for many years — Andrew the longest, as previously mentioned. Neil and Josh went to public school and had played soccer together for several years. As for Matt, Andrew had introduced him to Neil in their early high school days. Matt had not seen Neil since he'd gotten home, but the two had a special bond. Matt too had once wrestled with a brain tumor, now successfully treated and in remission. That was big.

"Come on in," Wendy hollered, and the three trooped into the kitchen, big feet and big smiles, each hugging Neil in turn.

"So how goes the battle?" Andrew asked.

"It goes well," Neil nodded. "We're making steady progress."

Andrew smiled broadly, and Matt chimed in, "Glad to hear it!"

"Excellent," Josh agreed.

"So what are you thinking you want to play?" Andrew asked.

"What do you want?" Neil replied, eyebrow arched in challenging jest.

"Not chess," Andrew shook his head, and both Josh and Matt shook their heads no in agreement.

"We've got *Carcasonne*, *Ticket to Ride*, or *Settlers of Catan*," Neil replied. "And of course we have the ever popular *Monopoly* or *Risk*."

"Not *Monopoly,*" Matt shook his head.

"Poker," Josh interjected, and for a moment, they gauged each other's interest. If they'd been someplace else besides our kitchen, poker would have taken the day.

"I've never played *Settlers of Catan,*" Matt broke the stalemate. "What's it like?"

After a brief explanation, they winnowed the choice down to *Settlers of Catan* or *Ticket to Ride.*"

"Dealer's choice," Andrew grinned at Neil.

"*Settlers,*" he tipped his head toward Matt, then Neil fetched the game while the boys took seats around the dining room table. They all "shot the breeze" as Neil and Andrew set up the game, then it was time to explain the rules amidst the jokes flying back and forth. Wendy and I let them be for the most part, but it's amusing to watch games being played — especially with the snipes these guys would come up with — so we poked our noses in from time to time to catch the action. In his typical style, Neil seemed to be playing a circumspect game until he was ready to pounce. Matt, on the other hand, was establishing an early lead in road-building and settlements. As the game progressed, it was clear he would be "the man to beat."

One aspect of *Settlers* is that temporary alliances can occur: At the beginning of each player's turn, he rolls the dice, then resource cards are distributed to all players according to the territories they control. Once the player draws and cards are distributed, he is allowed to trade cards with any other player: "I'll give anyone two 'lumber' cards for an 'ore' card." That sort of thing. Once trading is done, the player can pay cards to the bank in exchange for a piece with which to build on the board — roads, settlements, and cities. Josh, Andrew, and Neil worked together to hold off Matt's steady advance, but he was completely unphased.

"I only need one card," he goaded. And he drew it.

"Dang," Andrew quipped. "It's not polite to win the first time you play!"

"You guys suck," Josh frowned briefly, then he held out his hand to Matt. "Good game."

"GG," Neil chuckled.

Matt grinned like the Cheshire Cat — radiating his trademark good humor — and they all had a good laugh.

They lingered around the table another ten or fifteen minutes, joking mostly, but also quizzing Neil on the latest developments, then it was time for goodbyes.

"You look good," Matt told Neil with a hand on his shoulder. "Keep it up."

"I intend to," Neil hugged him. "Getting a second opinion at Dana-Farber tomorrow."

"Good luck," Matt nodded, giving him an extra squeeze.

"I'll see you again soon," Andrew promised with a hug and a pat on the back. "Good luck tomorrow!"

"Good luck," Josh hugged Neil too. "See you soon."

"Thanks for coming over," Neil beamed. "It was great seeing you guys! Let's do it again."

"I'm not sure Josh could take the strain," Matt quipped to another round of chuckles, then they were on their way out the door.

It had been a good day, and Neil turned in on that note.

KEEP RATTLING THE CAGE

Late that same Sunday evening, I received a reply from Sheryll to my query about petitioning the FDA.

To: Dean Fachon
From: Sheryll Acelar
Subject: Re: Records
Date: March 20, 2016

Hello Dean,

I received Dr. Burzynski's response after he read your emails. The antineoplastons will work on a non-enhancing tumor, but we are tied by FDA regulations in how we treat patients and must follow a strict protocol. Unfortunately, we can no longer make special/compassionate exceptions with clinical trials. The best way to proceed is for Eugene to get a PET/CT scan. This will have to occur within 14 days of starting treatment. A consultation can still be done if you wish, but you would have to return home and wait until we are fully ready.

Looking forward to meeting you and your son if you choose to come.

Take care
Sheryll

Unwilling to take no for an answer — not where Neil was concerned — I rattled the cage a bit more.

To: Sheryll Acelar
From: Dean Fachon
Subject: Re: Records
Date: March 21, 2016

Sheryll,

I feared as much. There are no mainstream treatments – including biopsy and molecular profiling – that offer any hope of a cure, let alone a significant chance of extending Neil's life more than another few months. Can you tell me who I might contact at the FDA to request an exemption? I cannot sit idly by while the best chance Neil may have is apparently being withheld due to misguided regulations...

Thank you!

And that wrapped things up for the day.

11

THE "SECOND OPINION"

"You need to pick what really interests you and learn about it, get behind it and make it your responsibility." NF

While pushback from the Burzynski Clinic was discouraging, the long-needed "second opinion" was at hand, and that became our primary focus. I sent a quick note to Katelyn: *"We look forward to meeting Dr. Kieran today at 12:30. Just to confirm, we will park at the garage off Jimmy Fund Way, come to the Jimmy Fund building and then to the Pediatric Neuro-Oncology center and ask reception to notify you we are there."*

She replied: *"You will come to the DANA building. We have a building called the Jimmy Fund Building (confusing) but the clinic is not there. Come to the DANA building, third floor. When you park in the garage, if you take the elevators up to the first floor lobby, you can stop at the security desk and they will direct you. When you arrive at the Jimmy Fund Clinic, you will check in with the front desk and they will notify Dr. Kieran you are there."*

"That's an affirmative." Then, I sent a quick note to Evie: *"We will pick you up on the way to DANA Farber. Besides adding your academic acumen to the discussion, if you could take notes of the meeting, that would be a huge help! Bring your favorite notebook and pen. See you shortly."*

As excited as we were, Neil once again managed to snooze for much of the ride to Boston. We arrived in plenty of time to get Evie and navigate traffic and construction to the clinic. Once parked, we did as Katelyn instructed, stopping at the security desk to get our bearings, then we took the elevator up to the clinic.

The elevator doors opened on a scene that was completely unexpected. Save for its panoramic windows, the Jimmy Fund Clinic could not have been more different from Mass General. Instead of looking down on a world in miniature, we looked directly across at the "Jimmy Fund" building, the construction of which — including images of smiling patients signing their names on the girders — is featured in so many movie theaters. The clinic itself was filled with the piping voices and laughter of children, not the hushed voices one might expect. Everything is set up for children, from educational displays à la the Boston Children's Museum to overstuffed chairs for lounging, and all in a myriad of bright colors. There were books and toys in one area, and opposite the check-in area was a "breakout" room for private meetings or more important things like puppet and magic shows. The passion for caring about little patients was powerfully present. Regardless of having outgrown it long ago, Neil fell in love with the magic and wore a huge grin as he walked up to a receptionist and said a cheerful, "Hello!" He signed in, then we sat down to listen and watch. All the activity made our wait seem like just a few minutes, then Neil was called.

We took a deep collective breath, and with notes and notebooks in hand, we were led from the children's oasis through a door and down a hall to a spacious and comfortable office. Dr. Mark Kieran greeted us warmly, especially Neil. Having Raffaele in common made the atmosphere relaxed right away, and Dr. Kieran's caring demeanor — not unlike Dr. Panis — gave us confidence we were in a good place.

After the pleasant greetings, Dr. Kieran gave Neil a thorough examination, similar to what Dr. Panis had done. He and Neil discussed the onset of his symptoms, dating back to the first "concussion," then Dr. Kieran brought Neil's MRI up on his computer and discussed the images in detail. Before we asked any questions, Dr. Kieran launched into a detailed assessment of Neil's condition and the possible avenues of treatment:

- It is very unlikely that Neil's condition is due to multiple sclerosis. The manner in which connecting cells in Neil's pons are being pushed apart is characteristic of DIPG.

- Incidences of DIPG are globally distributed, so it's very difficult to link them to a common cause.
- In general, it is believed that DIPG symptoms would not be present for more than three to six months. It's hard to tell whether Neil's case falls within this window because of the confusion caused by concerns of concussion.
- Constipation doesn't fit in with the rest of DIPG symptoms — those movements aren't controlled by the pons.
- One percent of patients have a tumor of the neurons, as opposed to the glial cells.
    - » This would be a PNET tumor
- There are three types of DIPG tumors thus far identified:
    - » The PDGFRA mutation (platelet derived growth factor). This type of tumor has experimental drug options; it also shares an "H3 mutation" with the second type of tumor.
    - » The ACVR1 mutation. This type usually occurs in six-to-seven-year-old girls.
    - » The third kind of tumor does not have any specifically identified mutations, and its occurrence accounts for roughly 20 percent of cases.

While understanding the nuances of each mutation was too esoteric for us, just hearing about them put a stronger spotlight on the rationale for a biopsy. From there, Dr. Kieran took up the subject of immunotherapy. "The theory behind it is to wake up the patient's immune system to fight the cancer itself."

Current approaches to immunotherapy include:

- Developing generic vaccines to inoculate the general public (as in the case of the HPV vaccination, which Neil and so many others have received to stop the spread of human papillomavirus, and thus, ostensibly, prevent cervical cancer).

***Note:** Many children around the globe have been injured by the HPV vaccine, including some reported deaths. A great deal of effort has gone into rationalizing these reports, but the linkages cannot easily be dismissed.*[8]

- Developing personalized vaccines by taking biopsies from individual patients to identify their tumors, then extracting some of the patient's own immune cells and using special techniques to help train those cells to recognize and combat the cancer. The trained cells are then reintroduced into the patient in hopes his or her immune system will pick up the training and replicate cells that can fight off the cancer.
- Finally, developing "immunomodulating" treatments, which help to trigger the patient's immune system into combating his or her cancer.

Dr. Kieran said this last technique has had exciting success treating melanomas — one of the most virulent types of cancer — but he also cautioned that side effects can include some very difficult-to-manage autoimmune disorders.

While each of these treatments sounded promising in its own way, they were not all equally available at the time. It takes being in the right place at the right time, a luxury of which Neil had little to spare.

Dr. Kieran also discussed the treatment options Dr. Arrillaga had suggested, and he reviewed some clinical trials Neil might want to investigate:

- In Kentucky, the University of Louisville was beginning an immunotherapy trial to develop a personalized vaccination program using the patient's blood cells.
    - » To enter this trial, a diagnostic biopsy might be re-

8 "Serious Injuries From Merck's Gardasil HPV Vaccine Significantly Underreported, Study Shows," the Defender, Children's Health Defense, May 2021.

quired, and radiation therapy would likely be required to participate.

- » Healthy cells would be harvested before radiation. The radiation therapy usually lasts six weeks with daily doses.
- » Dr. Kieran acknowledged that 5 to 10 percent of patients who take a full course of radiation will eventually develop a secondary tumor.

- IOZK (Immun-Onkologisches Zentrum Köln) — the same clinic in Germany that Charles discovered— which was exploring a "multilayered" approach to immunotherapy.
- Convection-enhanced delivery (CED) — inserting a catheter directly into the affected area of the brain to inject chemotherapy. There was a study being done in Leeds, England, with the following provisions:
    - » Cannot be done if there has been a biopsy because drugs will leak out.
    - » You have to bank on the chance the tumor has the mutations which are affected by the primary DIPG-targeted drug being used.
- Dr. Kieran also mentioned a CED trial being conducted in New York at Memorial Sloan Kettering (the same trial Evie discovered on *ClinicalTrials.gov*), but it appeared they were using traditional chemotherapy, as opposed to the DIPG-targeted drugs being used by the research group in Leeds.
- M.D. Anderson also had some sort of immunotherapy vaccination program to investigate.

In the course of our meeting, Dr. Kieran provided us with as much information as he possibly could. In so doing, he addressed the bulk of our questions before we could ask them. He also offered to help oversee Neil's progress if he elected to enroll in a clinical trial.

As our meeting drew to a close, I asked if I could pose one more question, which might be a bit touchy.

"Of course," he smiled warmly.

"One word," I replied. "Burzynski."

"Don't do it," was his emphatic response. "Hobo piss."

That seemed pretty definitive, but then Dr. Kieran continued to recount a curious "anecdote:"

> Some years previous, there had been sufficient interest in the stories coming out of Houston that a small group from Dana-Farber, including Dr Kieran, approached Dr. Burzynski to discuss the possibility of running a clinical trial. However, this early negotiation was terminated when an independent consulting group (required to ensure objectivity of the trial) expressed reservations about Dr. Burzynski's methods of data-collection and reporting.

That pretty much wrapped up Neil's consult. As dire as his prognosis was, meeting Dr. Kieran and hearing his insights had an uplifting effect. We spent the better part of two hours in his office, and he was as gracious and candid as the reception area was a comfort. We profusely thanked Dr. Kieran and departed Dana-Farber with a great feeling of hope: We had the best input we could possibly get in the time Neil had available.

"Just wow," Neil exclaimed as we made our way back to the elevator. "I hope you took good notes," he said to Evie.

"I did my best," she nodded.

"I really like the idea of immunotherapy," Neil continued. "It makes intuitive sense."

"That's one of the trials I found listed on the government website," Evie pointed out.

"Good work," I nodded appreciatively.

"Immunotherapy is very interesting," Wendy said. "Let's take a close look"

"I'll start as soon as I get back to my apartment," Evie promised.

After dropping her off and getting back on the highway, I had to comment: "'Hobo piss' or not, it's curious that Dana-Farber approached Dr. Burzynski about running a clinical trial."

"Indeed," Neil agreed, the same neon light flashing in his mind. "That is curious."

That evening, before going to bed, Neil mentioned it again. "If he just wanted to warn us off Dr. Burzynski, why do you suppose Dr. Kieran told us that story?"

"I don't know," I shook my head. "Being honest to a fault. But if they were intrigued enough to reach out to Burzynski — even tentatively — that's significant."

Neil furrowed his brow in an expression he'd often worn at the chess board, then he smiled, "Goodnight Dad."

I gave him a hug. "Goodnight."

Neil padded off to bed while I sat back at my computer, suddenly full of more questions. Why did Dr. Kieran tell us that story? Was he just being honest to a fault? And what about Neil's so-called "concussions?" He was never knocked out. Did this series of head traumas cause the DIPG, or did the DIPG cause the injuries by dulling Neil's reflexes? Or were there other contributing factors? The HPV/meningitis vaccinations still loomed in my mind. While mainstream medicine would scoff at any correlation, I was haunted by the possibility. Regardless, according to Dr. Kieran, the symptoms of DIPG would typically be present (in small children, at least) within three to six months of the tumor's onset. Thus, he felt Neil's condition could have been recognized in November of 2015, if not sooner. The loss of those months is something we will always lament.

> ***March 22, 2016 DANA Farber visit, excerpts from Dr. Kieran's report:***
>
> I brought up the MRI scans on the computer screen to demonstrate to Eugene and his family...the fact that he has

a signal that is diffusely expansive the pons, that is bright on T2 and FLAIR, dark on T1. There is no obvious enhancement. It appears to obey the pontomeduliary boundary and encircles the basilar artery. <u>These are all completely consistent with a diffuse intrinsic pontine glioma...</u>

The 3 concussions that he suffered in August through October complicate the neurologic assessment, as some of the symptoms he was having are likely related to those 3 traumas. <u>Certainly, by November, there is clear evidence of cranial nerve dysfunction suggesting the tumor has likely been in place since that time...</u>

In addition, we discussed the fact that at the age of nineteen, it is unusual to have a newly diagnosed DIPG, although certainly it can be seen at this age in a small number of patients. Overall, I, therefore, would consider this diagnosis to be consistent with DIPG. Whether the natural history of the disease would behave exactly the same as it does in children, where the median age is more around six, is hard to say as the number of patients with DIPG at age nineteen is too small to make a firm conclusion..."

12

MORE JUGGLING

"My mind is here, then it's there, then it's over there and back again, all within a split second." NF

First things first, I had to let Raffaele know about our meeting with Dr. Kieran:

> **To: Raffaele**
> **From: Dean**
> **Subject: Great meeting with Dr. Kieran**
> **Date: March 22, 2016**
>
> Raffaele,
>
> Just a quick note. A long day, but fruitful. We finally met with Dr. Kieran, and it was a very good meeting. He spent two hours with us, answering questions and opening new possibilities for consideration. He also discussed his experience with Dr. Burzynski. Very interesting, and for now he puts a cautious perspective on Antineoplastons. We are also looking hard at immunotherapy: Dr. Kieran is familiar with a clinic in Germany; he is familiar with some trials in the US; and he would be happy to assist in selecting a trial and overseeing progress if Neil decides to go that route. Given the dim outlook with radiation and even molecular profiling for drug therapy,

immunotherapy seems a more hopeful and progressive possibility. We're just sinking our teeth into it and will keep you posted, but suffice it to say we were all very impressed and pleased with Dr. Kieran. Thank you for making that referral! Meanwhile, Neil is doing reasonably well – fairly stable since we took him out of school almost three weeks ago. Wendy, Evie and I are also doing better – finally getting restful sleep once again.. Thank you!

God Bless,
Dean

Then, Evie was quick to start gathering details on the clinical trial in Kentucky:

To: Dean Fachon
From: Evie Fachon
Subject: Immunotherapy in Kentucky
Date: March 22, 2016

Just found this;

Phase I/II: Decitabine/Vaccine Therapy in Relapsed/Refractory Pediatric High Grade Gliomas/Medulloblastomas/CNS PNETs

The main purpose of this study is to determine the safety of using the combination of decitabine and a cancer vaccine plus Hiltonol. The vaccine will be made from the subject's blood cells and is designed to interact in the subject's body with cells that are programmed to fight specific tumor proteins NY-ESO-1, Melanoma Antigen Gene-A1 (MAGE-A1) and Melanoma Antigen Gene-A3 (MAGE-A3). The decitabine will be given to increase the

> amount and activity of these cancer proteins on the surface of tumor cells to increase the possibility that the vaccine will stimulate cells to act against the tumor cells. Subjects will be assessed to determine how these tumors respond to the treatment.

Another ball in the air. We would explore this clinical trial in depth, but as a layperson, I immediately wondered how melanoma could possibly correlate to DIPG?

Next in hand was a note from Sheryll:

> **To: Dean Fachon**
> **From: Sheryll Acelar**
> **Subject: Re: Records**
> **Date: March 22, 2016**
>
> Hi
>
> Dr. Burzynski does not recommend contacting the FDA. It could cause more problems. He also stated that it will take 4 weeks to get everything in order to run the clinical trial. The best way for Neil to potentially qualify is to repeat the MRI and do a PET/CT 14 days before we start the trial. I will let you know when that will be.
>
> If you wish to come here for a consult in the meantime, you are welcome to do so. Please let me know if you have further questions.
>
> Best.
> Sheryll

Okay, I'd leave the FDA be. That was best anyway. Then, Evie threw another ball up:

DEXAMETHASONE

To: Wendy and Dean Fachon
From: Evie Fachon
Subject: Steroid Question
Date: March 22, 2016

Hey,

What type of steroid was prescribed for Neil? I've been reading about the side-effects of steroids, and I just want to check up on what Neil might be taking. Some cancer-treating steroids can cause high blood sugar and difficulty sleeping. Long-term use can cause muscle wasting and eye problems, as well as 'Cushings Syndrome.' There's also evidence that people who have a family history of 'bipolar disorder' have a greater chance of experiencing mood disruption when on steroids.

I'm not saying Neil shouldn't take the steroids. If they make him feel better then that's the most important thing. Everything will have side effects, but they can be managed, we should try to figure that out beforehand. Let me know the name of the prescription, and I'll do some research.

Love you,
Evie

* * *

To: Evie Fachon
From: Dean
Subject: Re: Steroid Question
Date: March 22, 2016

The prescription is for "Dexamethasone" - 3 milligram dosage. He has not taken any thus far.

Thank you for sending the links and notes from the meeting with Dr. Kieran! (Way better than mine.) The Kentucky trial sounds interesting. Hopefully there will be no need for the biopsy, as per Dr. Kieran's explanation that diagnosis is a virtual certainty. The trial also says the patient must have undergone standard treatment, but in a case where standard treatment offers no significant benefit, maybe this could be waived... Lots to think about and research....

Love you, and talk soon,
Dad

* * *

To: Dean, Neil, Wendy
From: Evie Fachon
Subject: Re: Steroid Question
Date: March 22, 2016

Everything I'm reading says that Dexamethasone should be used sparingly... its a powerful steroid, but has a lot of adverse side effects, most notably mood swings, high blood sugar, weak muscles/bones and bloating/weight gain. Risk of side effects increase the higher the dose and the longer it's taken.

The reason dexamethasone is an anti-inflammatory is because it inhibits the immune system, which is why patients taking it are more likely to develop infections. This might be something to ask Dr. Kieran about if we decide to go ahead with any immunotherapy treatment; not much use boosting the immune system if the steroids are going to knock it right back down!

Just some stuff to think about.

Hope you get some good sleep tonight :^) miss you guys already!

And we missed her too. Thankfully, in light of Evie's misgivings, Neil's intuition to lay off the "dex" was a good one. And so, juggling for March 22 drew to a close. On top of Neil's normal routine, it had been a long day. A good night's sleep was all we could ask for.

13

NO STONE UNTURNED

"What does it mean to think holistically? Think big picture." NF

March 23 was the day Neil had his first appointment with Dr. Jody Noé, the naturopathic oncologist recommended by Mary Blue. It was sunny and warm outside, and we eagerly piled into the car for the drive to Pawcatuck, Connecticut, just over the state line from Westerly, Rhode Island.

Dr. Noé had a country doctor's office in the basement of an old New England home. We descended the steps to a reception window, and Neil checked in. Then, we were escorted to a cozily decorated waiting area. As we sat, Wendy picked up a large book off a shelf full of reading material. The book was a tome written by Dr. Noé herself, called the *Textbook of Naturopathic Integrative Oncology (Fundamentals of Naturopathic Medicine.)*

"This is impressive," Neil nodded as he and Wendy leafed through some pages.

A few minutes later, Dr. Noé came to greet us and walk us back to her office. She was as impressive as her book, radiating "earth mother" vibes, which she focused intently on Neil. She took him to her private examination room for several minutes before inviting Wendy and I to join the consult. Acknowledging the severity of Neil's situation, she shook her head no at any thought it was hopeless.

"The body is capable of amazing things if given the proper conditions to mend," Dr. Noé said.

"He's on a 'Gerson therapy' diet," Wendy told her.

"Gerson therapy is an excellent platform to support the immune system," Dr. Noé nodded, "but a growing young man also needs animal protein. You also need to feed him grass-fed beef, organic free-range chicken, and fresh wild-caught fish and shrimp."

Neil grinned in delight.

"We can do that," Wendy said.

"Good nutrition isn't difficult science," Dr. Noé continued, "yet you'd be amazed at how little training conventional oncologists ever get."

"Oh," Wendy shook her head with chagrin, "we've seen posters hawking candy in some of their waiting rooms — for patients to 'keep up their strength.'"

"It's hard to fathom," Neil scowled. "Everything I read says cancer loves sugar!"

"It certainly does," I agreed. "That's what gets injected for a PET scan — radioactive sugar dye. Tumors gobble it up, and the radioactivity lights up the scan."

Dr. Noé nodded, pleased we had been doing our homework. "Mainstream oncologists are schooled in surgery, radiation, and chemotherapy," she continued. "Cut, burn, and poison — all things which take a toll on the immune system," she concluded. "They might get a day's worth of training on nutrition."

"My Grandma always said, 'You are what you eat.' So what could nutrition possibly have to do with health?" Neil chuckled.

"Coming from the guy who was completely backed up," Wendy cringed, "that's a revelation."

"Hey," Neil pouted, "I'm a good cook."

"Maybe so," Wendy smiled, "but what goes in must come out." She proceeded to tell Dr. Noé about Neil's bout of severe constipation.

He just grimaced.

Dr. Noé shook her head no. "That can't happen again."

"We're doing our best," Wendy agreed. "His diet is completely organic," and she ticked off his regimen on her fingers. "Lots of cooked greens — often pureed into soups. Bone broth. Freshly juiced vegetable drinks.

Fresh fruit. Raw veggies of every color. And complex carbohydrates like brown rice, potatoes, oatmeal, and quinoa. Now we'll add meats and fish," Wendy rounded off her review.

"And you've eliminated all processed foods, especially those containing simple carbohydrates that quickly turn into sugar, along with all forms of processed sugar, like corn syrup," Dr. Noé asked rhetorically.

"Absolutely," Wendy nodded vigorously.

Dr. Noé approved. "I'd also prescribe some supplements to support your immune system and brain function," she told Neil, listing off Meriva, omega oils, vitamin D3, alpha-lipoic acid, resveratrol, CoQ10, Methyl Protect, and many others.

Wendy also described the tea and tincture from Mary Blue.

"Excellent," Dr. Noé smiled. "That's very helpful too."

Then, we launched into a discussion of the treatment options being proposed and other options being considered, including the Burzynski Clinic.

"Dana-Farber led the charge for integrative approaches," Dr. Noé told us. "And Mass General has gotten a lot better." Then, she paused thoughtfully. "I've actually met Dr. Burzynski. At a conference. He was having a very tough a time with the FDA as I recall, but he seemed to be on the right track."

"That's how it seems to us," I said, Wendy and Neil nodding too.

We discussed treatment options further, and Dr. Noé was confident she could support whatever path Neil decided to take. She was also outspoken about medical marijuana.

"Some people, younger adults, and even children," she informed us, "have had some amazing results."

"What do you mean?" Neil raised an eyebrow.

"I mean they've outlived their prognoses — sometimes by years," Dr. Noé said. "But of course that's all anecdotal. There have been no clinical trials."

"There's that 'anecdotal' again," Neil waved his hand as if shoeing off a gnat.

"Wait," I wondered skeptically. "Are these kids wandering around high all the time?"

"Effectively yes," Dr. Noé shrugged with her hands. "It beats being dead."

"Well," I muttered, "when you put it that way."

"I don't mean to be glib," she smiled apologetically. "I mention it as something to research. I can't prescribe it, but Rhode Island has a 'compassion center,' which dispenses medical marijuana. The criteria for receiving it is a demonstrable need, which Neil certainly has, and getting a referral letter from a doctor licensed in Rhode Island."

"Let's look into that," Neil appealed to Wendy. The thought of marijuana-induced euphoria doubtless had its appeal, and who could blame him. I cringed, but there was nothing for it but acquiescence.

"I don't think we'll have any problem with getting a letter," Wendy agreed. "I'll call Dr. Slattery this afternoon."

"Before you go," Dr. Noé added, "would you like a session of 'craniosacral therapy?' On the house, just to see how you like it."

"Sure," Neil smiled.

Dr. Noé introduced him to their therapist while Wendy scheduled a follow-up appointment with Dr. Noé, then we sat in the waiting room while Neil enjoyed half an hour of his skull being pampered. He enjoyed it so much Wendy scheduled a follow-up appointment with the therapist too.

It was lunchtime when we finished up at Dr. Noé's office. In keeping with her recommendation, we drove into Westerly to an old pub situated alongside the Pawcatuck River, which winds into the sea. After being seated, a waiter took our orders — gourmet hamburgers made from local grass-fed beef accompanied by fries and large salads. We discussed the meeting with Dr. Noé until our meals arrived, then all talk ceased. Given Neil's dietary constraints, fries were off-limits, but he had to indulge in honor of celebrating his first hamburger in weeks. He savored every bite of his burger and most of his fries and salad, but he drew the line at ketchup with its added corn syrup. All told, we were all very pleased with our outing.

MEDICAL MARIJUANA

As soon as we got home, Neil retired to his computer to research medical marijuana. Wendy did much the same thing, and they quickly learned how the two key compounds derived from cannabis — THC and CBD — can affect the human body, and thus, cancer cells. From Wendy's notes:

> Our bodies have many "systems" that work together synergistically, including the cardio-vascular, nervous, digestive, endocrine, integumentary, lymphatic, muscular, urinary, reproductive, respiratory, skeletal and endocannabinoid systems. The endocannabinoid system (ECS) was discovered in 1992 at the Hebrew University in Jerusalem by Dr. Lumar Hanus and Dr. William Devane, scientists who were studying how cannabis interacts with the brain. They discovered how this previously unknown molecular signaling system helps regulate a broad range of biological functions which maintain homeostasis (healthy equilibrium) in the body. The ECS is a two-way system, sending signals back and forth to support the body's ability to heal itself.
>
> CBD and THC are compatible with the receptors in the ECS. While CBD and THC have not been proven to cure cancer, they have demonstrated potential to:
>
> - prevent cancer cells from reproducing,
> - prevent the formation of new blood vessels needed by a tumor to grow,
> - prevent cancer from spreading to other organs,
> - and help promote apoptosis (cause cancerous cells to kill themselves).
>
> There are anecdotal stories which suggest cannabis oil helped patients put their cancers into remission, but

> there also are cases where it had no identifiable impact on patient-outcomes beyond offering relief from discomfort. Of course, relief itself is a blessing. Medical marijuana was legalized In Rhode Island in 2006. At the time, state-regulated "compassion centers" were established for producing and dispensing cannabis products.

With this foothold of knowledge about medical marijuana, Wendy called Dr. Slattery to request a referral letter, then she began investigating the process of actually getting a card. Wendy also gave Cindy Grady a call to get her advice.

"Once you have the card," Cindy offered, "I have a friend who works at the Slater Compassion Center." Then, she chuckled, "He'll hook Neil up!"

That's Rhode Island: "I know'a guy." When the time came, Cindy's connection would be very helpful.

JUGGLING RESUMED

As for me, the idea of treating Neil's cancer with medical marijuana was a stretch (although not impossible), so I left that up to them while I continued juggling MGH/Dana-Farber, the clinical trials Dr. Kieran had mentioned (especially the one investigating immunotherapy), and the Burzynski Clinic:

> **To: Sheryll Acelar**
> **From: Dean**
> **Subject: RE: Records**
> **Date: March 23, 2016**
>
> Sheryll,
>
> Since sending the records, we have had another consultation, this time with Dr. Kieran at DANA Farber. He has pretty much ruled out anything besides DIPG, and

he agrees with the prognosis from Dr. Arrillaga at MGH. Neil is thus far leaning away from radiation or biopsy procedures. If a CT/PET scan might improve his chance of the Burzynski Clinic accepting him into the clinical trial with Antineoplastons, we will get that test scheduled. Otherwise, a consultation-visit might still be worthwhile, if only to discuss other therapies Dr. Burzynski might suggest.

Yours,
Dean Fachon

And I heard back from Raffaele.

To: Dean
From: Raffaele
Subject: Re: Great meeting with Dr. Kieran...
Date: March 23, 2016

Thank you for the good news. I had little doubt Mark would be a valuable addition to Neil's team. I am very happy the meeting went well. Immunotherapy is currently of great interest, and it deserves great attention and consideration. I am incredibly happy Mark is willing to support Neil in giving this a good look. I would trust him, as nobody has more experience with this disease than Mark, and he is open-minded. I will continue to hunt for something I feel could help in any way.

I am also very happy to hear you are all sleeping better and things are stable for Neil. Please hug him from me. He is always in my thoughts. It must also be very tough for Evie. Siblings tend to be the forgotten victims. Please make sure that you give her as much love, attention and time to her emotions and feelings as possible. I am sure you know this but I still like to say it. Say hello to her from me please. I think of her very much in these tough times.

Warm wishes,
Raffaele

And I still needed to send a "thank you" to Dr. Kieran.

To: Dr. Mark Kieran
From: Dean Fachon
Subject: Eugene Fachon, DIPG
Date: Wed, 23 Mar 2016

Dear Dr. Kieran,

We hope your travels have been safe and rewarding. We all want to thank you for the generous time you spent with us going over every detail of Eugene's (Neil's) situation. One of your colleagues called shortly after our meeting to let us know that Neil's age would not be a problem for the immunotherapy trial you mentioned. However, that trial does appear to require 'conventional' treatment. Can you clarify whether or not this is certain? Given that conventional DIPG treatment is more palliative than a cure, Neil is leaning away from doing either the biopsy or radiation. He would prefer to pursue a very small chance of a cure to extending his life a few months. We tend to agree. The thought of losing him is unimaginable, but worse is the thought of just accepting this premature fate. If there are any trials that would accept Neil without his having to undergo conventional treatment, we would be VERY interested to learn as much as we can. We have a pretty good research team if

> you point us. If we can find a trial that looks promising to us and to you, we would hope to work with you to pursue it. Thank you again for your time and for all you do to combat the scourge of cancer.
>
> Yours,
> Dean, Wendy, Evie and Neil Fachon

I heard back from him promptly: *"In the Kentucky trial, the individualized vaccine is given after the patient receives standard therapy, in this case radiation therapy. As you indicated, this means Eugene would need to have radiation to be eligible. Another trial that may not require prior therapy is the one at Memorial Sloan Kettering in New York (a convection enhanced chemotherapy trial) and a similar trial in England."*

After reading Mark's email, I spoke to Neil.

"Hey Buddy," I ruffled his hair. "It sounds like Louisville will require radiation to enter the immunotherapy trial. The 'convection-enhanced chemotherapy trial' at Sloan Kettering may not."

"What is it with radiation?" Neil shook his head. "What good is immunotherapy if your immune system has been irradiated?"

"Wouldn't ya think," I nodded. "But I'll get in touch with Kentucky anyway. Maybe we can find a workaround."

"Sounds good," Neil remained upbeat, hoping this line of treatment could be his "brass ring."

I left Neil to his computer and returned to my own, wanting to send an update to family and friends. I described the appointments with Dr. Kieran and Dr. Noé, then I said: *"The most important thing for you to know is we are not giving up. Not even close. Neil's attitude could easily be called heroic. No crying, no sour grapes. He has moments when he's unsteady and sluggish, but since we've had him home his condition has been more or less stable. We are all in this together, and that is a great source of strength. The best thing to do is let him know he is in your thoughts, not in a tearful way, but in a hopeful way, sending positive energy."*

MORE VOICES WEIGH IN

While we tried to keep our family and friends in the loop, we couldn't touch base with everyone we knew. Even so, news of Neil's illness rippled further afield, and one day, out of the blue, Wendy heard from an old and dear friend from high school. Mary, a mother herself, and a doctor of pathology as luck would have it, called to commiserate with Wendy. After their conversation, Mary had some suggestions:

Date: Thu, 24 Mar 2016
From: Mary
To: Wendy

Hi Wendy,

I found an encouraging article about Sloan Kettering (2012 article, "Milestone Clinical Trial for DIPG Approved"). I also wanted to mention that I took steroids for my ear problem for a couple weeks and the side effects were nil. I think you should consider using them to keep the intracranial pressure down. I think the benefits may be far greater than any side effects. I will continue to research and let you know what I can find out from colleagues.

All of our love to you. Tell your precious son we think he is very brave.

Mary

Mary did not mention which steroid she took, and taking it for just a couple of weeks was probably less than a strong anecdote in favor of steroids. On the other hand, she was now the third person to mention Sloan Kettering. That was noteworthy.

Meanwhile, various members of the family weighed in on my last update. In particular, Neil's cousin Elise — a budding animation artist who moved to California to pursue her career — had something fun up her sleeve.

To: Dean, Neil
From: Elise
Subject: Re: Status update for Neil
Date: March 24, 2016

Thanks for the update, Uncle Dean. Thinking of you all constantly, sending lots of love, positive vibes and warm sunshine. I'm working on a fun surprise, so keep an eye on the mail : ^) It's taking me a little bit to organize, but I promise it'll bring smiles all around.

Wish my arms were long enough to reach all the way across the country and wrap you all up in a big bear hug. Until next I'm home, I'll just hang onto that hug and consider it as accruing hug dividends at a high interest rate.

All my love,
Elise

How sweet the sound! We had no idea what to expect. The cousins' rumor mill suggested something extra special, but we would have to wait until Neil's birthday to find out. Meanwhile, we would be busy — keeping balls in the air and cultivating a new possibility.

IMMUNOTHERAPY TRIAL

I replied to Dr. Kieran's last email: *"Thank you Dr. Kieran, Mark. It's too bad about the radiation requirement. I would think the study could benefit from having one or more candidates with intact immune systems. Can you recommend anyone in the Kentucky trial we could contact to suggest this possibility? If this path proves fruitless, I would not completely rule out Neil's going ahead with radiation under your supervision, but no radiation is infinitely preferable. One other question: Dr. Arrillaga prescribed "Dexamethasone" – 3 milligram/day dosage – in case Neil felt he needed some assistance. To date he has not taken any because of the side-effects. Is there anything he could take as an intermediate intervention to provide relief without serious side-effects?"*

Mark responded: *"Unfortunately there are no good alternatives to steroids to control swelling, although some places try Avastin (which has different side effects). Radiation is usually very well tolerated and usually makes the patients better. That is why it is considered the standard. I'm including Dr Plant on this email, and she can guide you to Dr Lucas in Kentucky. I do not have access to his contact information while traveling."*

I had hoped he would mention an alternative of the herbal variety, like curcumin. It's widely known for its anti-inflammatory properties, and Neil was already taking it at Dr. Noé's suggestion. Maybe that helped to explain the relative stability of his condition. Regardless, shortly thereafter, I received an email from one of Dr. Kieran's associates:

To: Dean Fachon
From: "Plant, Ashley"
Subject: Re: Eugene Fachon, DIPG
Date: March 24, 2016

Hi Dean,

I am one of the pediatric oncology fellows at DANA Farber. I work closely with Dr Kieran and am the liaison to the Kentucky vaccine trial. The study coordinator is Jennifer Comings. She is the best person for getting connected with the trial. She can also put you in contact with Dr Lucas, the head of the study, should you have further questions about exceptions to eligibility. I agree with Dr Kieran that it's unlikely they will allow a patient

> to enter a study without receiving standard radiation therapy first. The vaccine is still experimental, while we know radiation provides some benefit. Also the vaccine takes 4-6 weeks to make so it helps to do some other therapy while wait. Thank you, and let me know if I can help in any other way.
>
> Dr. Plant
> Ashley S. Plant, MD
> Fellow, Hematology/Oncology
> Boston Children's Hospital/Harvard Medical School
> DANA Farber Cancer Institute

Another ball in the air!

UKULELE LESSON

While communications bounced back and forth without seeming end, Neil had an unexpected visitor. Alexia, a fellow student from East Greenwich High School and a good friend from Neil's SLTP days, heard of his illness while at school. She was studying music therapy and applied music at State University of New York in Fredonia, and during her spring break, Alexia came over for a visit. She spent an afternoon teaching Neil how to play the ukulele. By the time she departed, Neil was happily strumming on this simple four-stringed instrument. He liked to play "Radioactive," a popular song by one of Neil's favorite bands, Imagine Dragons. For the next several days, it was not uncommon to hear Neil strumming softly in his room.

THE "BRASS RING"

I replied to Dr. Plant: "*Thank you! I will keep you in the loop regarding my communications in this matter. If you celebrate Easter, I hope yours is blessed.*"

She answered: *"I definitely do, although this year I am working on Easter. I hope you and your family have a good Easter as well, and may it give you comfort. Let me know if there is anything else I can help with."*

Neil was drawn to the idea of immunotherapy. We all were. It had the feel of an imminent breakthrough, so I wasted no time reaching out to the contact Ashley provided.

To: Jennifer Comings
From: Dean
Subject: Immunotherapy trial - University of Louisville
Date: March 25, 2016
CC: "Plant, Ashley"

Dear RN Comings,

I'm writing with regards to the immunotherapy trial for brain cancers being run by Dr. Lucas. Dr. Ashley Plant at DANA Farber kindly provided me with your contact information.

Three weeks ago my 19-year-old son Eugene (Neil) learned he has DIPG. This was first diagnosed by Dr. Isabel Arrillaga at Mass General and confirmed by Dr. Mark Kieran at DANA Farber. Neil and his family and friends are all stunned, but since learning of his condition we have been doing all we can to research potential treatments – conventional, experimental, and alternative. Obviously, the prognosis for DIPG is very bleak, but being older than the typical DIPG patient and otherwise very fit, we're hoping Neil will be resilient. He has remained fairly stable since his diagnosis. We have him on a strict diet, and his Naturopathic Oncologist has prescribed several supplements to support his immune system and health.

After discussing conventional therapies at length, Neil is leaning away from using steroids or taking radiation treatment because they offer little more than short-term symptom relief and perhaps a few-month reprieve before succumbing to the disease, but these "benefits" come at a significant cost to the patient's long-term health should he/she beat the steep odds and survive. That's what Neil wants to do – beat the odds and survive. He would rather aim for the "brass ring" than accept defeat. Consequently, we would like to learn more about this immunotherapy trial and discuss its enrollment requirements to assess the possibility of Neil's participation.

Thank you for your time, and if you celebrate the holiday, Happy Easter.

Yours,
Dean Fachon

THE BEST OF INTENTIONS PART 1

While I contacted Nurse Comings in Kentucky, the conversation between Wendy and Mary grew more intense. After another phone conversation, Mary sent this:

Date: 25 Mar 2016
From: Mary
To: Wendy

I think Sloan Kettering has a specialized drug and a new way to get it into the tumor. I know you are trying to do your due diligence, but having read how quickly this tumor grows and the limited but crucial area it impacts, I urge you to begin therapy very soon if you are going to choose to fight it medically. If not, I respect that. I'm just going to just say this...if it was me, I'd go to NYC and get started.

I am not trying to be pushy or a know-it-all, but I do read this type of literature daily for my work, and it is clear to me that Memorial Sloan Kettering is the most advanced at this point with this particular tumor.

I love you and I'm in complete despair for you guys. Please ask anything of me, including shut up.

I'm here. Willing to travel anywhere with you, be present to talk and share ideas, hugs or whatever is needed. Hotel on me.

Love,
Mary

Mary was certainly sold on Sloan Kettering, but based on the consultation with Dr. Kieran, we understood them to be testing a new method — convection-enhanced delivery to bypass the blood-brain barrier — to deliver standard chemotherapy directly into the brain. Previous to that, Raffaele had expressed some uncertainty about potential risks of this method for patients with DIPG in particular. Nonetheless, Mary's enthusiasm for Sloan Kettering prompted Wendy to do some immediate research on their website, then she tried to bring Mary up to speed on where we were in Neil's journey: *"Recommended radiation protocol is for six weeks, everyday M-F, to qualify for a trial at Sloan Kettering. Neil would then have to wait before he could start the experimental treatment. Should he qualify, Sloan Kettering' is "testing dosages for safety," primarily with young children. That's what I'm reading on their web site.*

We've read a lot about how this cancer can come roaring back even hard-

er after radiation. Yes, this is a nasty SOB, diffused throughout the glioma tissue. Here are some details of Neil's particular tumor from the imaging report:

> Centered within the pons, there is a T2 /FLAIR hyperintense lesion which demonstrates relatively decreased and heterogeneous T1 signal and no significant enhancement. This measures 3.6 x 5.7 x 5.1 cm (AP by transverse by craniocaudal). The lesion encases both vertebral arteries as well as nearly completely circumferentially surrounds the basilar artery with an exophytic component. These vessels remain patent. On the CISS sequence, there is a mass effect on the surrounding cranial nerves. It partially extends into the left superior cerebellar peduncle and right middle peduncle. There may be some evidence of bony remodeling along the clivus without evidence of invasion.
>
> There is also a small amount of increased linear FLAIR signal along the lateral aspect of the posterior horn of the left lateral ventricle which does not enhance and is nonspecific.
>
> There is no evidence of hemorrhage or acute infarction.
>
> The flow voids of the major intracranial vessels appear intact.
>
> The bones and extracranial soft tissues are unremarkable. (3/4/16)

You can imagine how viewing the scans just blew us away. Neil was functioning as a perfectly healthy 19-year-old in August! I ask myself everyday, "What is the cause of this? What triggered it?"

Do you know anything about treatments at the Medicor Cancer Centers in Toronto? Let's talk by phone again this weekend. When is a good time to reach you?"

The following day Wendy heard back from Mary: *"Wow, going from a normal healthy college kid to that scan! Do you think it can be a genetic thing? Your aunt had a granddaughter who had a brain tumor at this age, no? Wondering about that.*

I looked at Medicor in Toronto. There's no data on studies with large cohorts, no basic research. I'd take a pass and focus on getting Neil into Memorial Sloan-Kettering. Are you going forward with radiation? I think the radio-labeled molecule with Convection Enhanced Delivery is really cutting edge. It's a monoclonal antibody that will seek and attach to tumor cells and radio sensitize them with radioactive iodine. Radioactive iodine has been used for decades to treat people with thyroid cancer and they do great! I would be meeting with this Dr Souweidane ASAP. Neil can start his RT and he's within the age range (under 21).

I'd love to talk on the phone, but my ability to hear on the phone is very poor. I love you and want so much to be able to help you with getting through this literature. Please focus in on MSK. I really think you should get a copy of Neil's scan and send it ahead. He has not been biopsied? Ask MSK if there needs to be a tissue diagnosis (biopsy) or whether diagnosis is confirmed by scan and history of onset?

Have you talked to your local hospital(s) about the RT? I think it's time to begin if you're going to do it. I'm sorry to be so forthright but I feel a duty as a physician to say it like this. I am also your friend and a mother, and believe me when I tell you I cannot imagine what you are all going through.

I got a copy of "Walk In Their Shoes" to read and get into Neil's mindset. I adored him when I spent that short time at the Lake with him. He's the real deal."

These were powerful words, spoken with true affection, but at the same time, they were somewhat overwhelming. Wendy kept the ball rolling: *"Have you seen anything about the immunotherapy trial in Louisville, Kentucky?"*

Mary replied: *"I did not. It sounds very interesting. What is Neil's wish regarding the 6 wk RT regimen?"*

Before Wendy could answer, Neil's loving sister discovered a miracle.

WE HAVE A SURVIVOR!

Evie was back at Northeastern. Though busy with classes, she devoted every spare moment to research on her brother's behalf. She called that evening with some exciting news. When I heard Wendy pick up the line and say, "Hi Evie," I picked up too.

"I found someone who was treated for DIPG at the Burzynski Clinic," Evie told us. "Her name is Celeste. She lives in Argentina."

"How did you do that?" we both asked.

"Social media," Evie said.

"How's she doing?"

"She's doing fine," Evie said. "She finished her treatment three years ago!"

"Holy Mackerel!" we exclaimed.

Neil heard the commotion and came downstairs. "What's going on?"

Wendy handed him the phone. "Talk to your sister."

He put the phone to his ear. "What's up?" then he listened intently. We watched his jaw drop. "Wow! That's FANTASTIC! I'd sure love to talk to her!"

"I figured," Evie said, ever one step ahead, "so I asked. She'd love to talk to you too!"

"When?!"

"I'll message her and call back as soon as I know," Evie told him.

Neil was shaking a little as he hung up the phone.

"WOW!" He just stood there, his face glowing with hope.

We wrapped our arms around him. "Yeh," we nodded, wiping the corners of our eyes. This was a "lifeline."

Evie called a bit later. "Celeste can 'Skype' with us tomorrow evening at seven o'clock."

"FAN-TASTIC!"

"I'm coming home to be in on the call," she added.

"Wouldn't have it any other way," Neil grinned ear to ear.

Just the prospect of Neil speaking with a DIPG survivor — a survivor! It was momentous!

This new sense of hope was like nothing so far, and Wendy was eager to tell Mary the great news: *"Not keen on the RT. Monday night, Neil and Evie will be skyping with a woman in Argentina who was diagnosed with DIPG at the age of 24 and took antineoplaston treatment at the Burzynski clinic in Houston. She is 30 now. Evie just connected with her on facebook. At one point Evie says the woman was so bad, she was unable to walk. Dean has been in a conversation with this clinic, which has a trial coming up in 3-4 weeks. Apparently, the catch with this trial is enhancing versus non-enhancing. They would require a PET scan two weeks before the trial begins.*

Mary was quick to reply: *"Wendy, the Burzynski clinic is a scam."*

BAM! A textbook reaction. It threw Wendy for a loop. When a renegade doctor has good anecdotal results treating an intractable disease, but he garners nothing but contempt from mainstream medicine, that suggests the doctor is "over the target." If anything, Mary's total condemnation helped cement our determination to consult with Dr. Burzynski:

To: "Sheryll S. Acelar"
From: Dean
Subject: RE: Treatment at the Burzynski Clinic
Date: March 26, 2016

Hello Sheryll,

Just checking in to get the latest information on when your trial might begin. FYI, Neil has remained fairly stable in the three weeks since diagnosis. His naturopathic oncologist has him on a strict diet and regimen of immune-boosting/cancer fighting supplements. We continue to search for additional alternatives and have found one immunotherapy-based clinical trial that seems interesting, as well as the Medicor Cancer Center in Canada. We have some options, but we are not counting on the continued grace period we are experiencing. The time for decision draws near... We hope all is well with you, and we wish you and Dr. Burzynski a Happy Easter.

Yours,
Dean F.

A VISITOR ARRIVES

Amidst the erupting jousting match with Mary, a special gift arrived for Neil — a copy of *The Jester Lost His Jingle*, along with a jester doll. The book was inscribed by the deceased author's mother, Barbara Saltzman:

To Neil,

May The Jester & Pharley always bring a smile to your face & laughter to your heart. Never lose your jingle!

Love
The Jester's Mom
Barbara Saltzman
3/21/16

Barbara's son, David, was an English and art major at Yale University when he was diagnosed with Hodgkin's disease. He died on March 2, 1990, but not before leaving the world with the gift of his book. *The Jester Lost His Jingle* is a fairytale story about a kingdom that loses its sense of humor and the jester who goes in search of restoring it. In so doing, the jester discovers that "not only can laughter redeem a weary world, it can also provide the best tonic for anyone facing seemingly insurmountable odds."

The Jester Lost His Jingle was a favorite of Neil's since his SLTP days. As part of SLTP training, the kids were asked to do community service, and SLPT's founder, Jim Fitzgerald, partnered with The Jester & Pharley Phund's "Reading To Give" program to guide the kids in fulfilling this service. Neil volunteered to lead the effort in East Greenwich. Teaming up with other SLTP students in the area, their goal was to playact a reading of the *Jester Lost His Jingle* to elementary students in their classrooms. After this skit, the SLTP students encouraged their young counterparts to conduct "read-a-thons" of their own, raising money to donate *Jester* books and dolls to pediatric cancer patients at nearby hospitals. Neil organized and coordinated the planning meetings, but most of all, he loved playing Pharley, the jester's animated companion, speaking in a squeaky Pharley voice.

When Neil unwrapped this package and saw the book, he grinned, danced a little gig, and broke out in a squeaky voice, "I'm not losing my jingle!"

THE BEST OF INTENTIONS PART 2

After this happy distraction, Wendy resumed her "dialogue" with Mary: *"Our research on Burzynski indicates a mixed bag of information. We met with Dr. Mark Kieran, DANA Farber DIPG expert last Tuesday. At one time, DANA Farber actually approached Burzynski about conducting a clinical trial, but they pulled back because of incomplete reporting of data. We're still sorting through the Burzynski info and have been in touch with the clinic.*

I'm skeptical about so much. In the meeting where we learned of Neil's diagnosis, I also learned that Neil had been constipated for two months. His intestines were clearly compacted and no doctors addressed this. I don't know, but the constipation could be partly due to what's happening to the nerves in the brain stem. Just from common sense I know that when the digestive track is blocked, nutrients can't enter the body and toxins aren't being removed. The combination is deadly.

*I took Neil to a colonic hydrotherapist. It took two sessions to clear the sh*t out. The first session was very unpleasant for him, and the second a great relief. It was an exhausting process, yet necessary before we could move forward.*

Neil is now administering his own coffee enemas. The caffeine in the colon is absorbed into the blood system and goes to the liver, signaling the release of toxic bile, the creation of fresh bile, and the stimulation of peristalsis activity. We follow that up with juicing to replenish his prebiotics, electrolytes, and nutrients. He is also taking Colon X and a probiotic capsule, along with probiotic foods. He has a 19-year-old appetite, and we need to keep the proteins, good fats, carefully monitored carbs moving into and out of his system. Food is medicine.

Neil's naturopathic oncologist, Dr. Jody Noé, prescribed Meriva (curcumin) and Alpha Lipoic Acid to help relieve Neil's inflammation, and it has been working. She also prescribed Methyl Protect to support optimal methylation – addressing MTHFR. She has suggested a number of other supplements to help stabilize Neil's condition while we take a little more time to sort through all his options.

We are also looking more into convection-enhanced-delivery of chemotherapy, but I have a hard time understanding how it would be to inject something beyond the blood brain barrier – something the blood brain barrier would otherwise keep out, as in it's not supposed to go there. Our body was designed for optimal function and self- regulation. What happened inside Neil's body in the first place?

I'm also researching the endocannabinoid system. Believe me, Mary, we are not sitting and doing nothing. We are using our brains and doing what seems to make the most sense."

Mary replied: *"Nutrition is great and so is getting unblocked (un-constipated) but forget worrying about toxins. Nutrition is supplying the tumor cells, preferentially as tumors do. The tumor will kill Neil in the way brain tumors do, quicker in his case because of the terrible location. Cancer kills by taking over vital functions. In Neil's case, the vital functions are already surrounded. He will die sooner if you do nothing. He is an altruistic guy. Would he consider making himself part of MSK's data? To make a way for younger 5-7 year olds who will get this disease in the future?? They will be from ghettos and from lake forest. Peoples beloved children. I assure you in this case the disease will be quicker and more evil than the therapy. Please consider doing the radiation to KILL the existing tumor cells and make Neil eligible for the radioactive iodine plus specialized tumor toxic drug (monoclonal antibody). Their therapy is new and untested but biologically makes sense. Neil has had optimal nutrition his whole life. It was never the problem. Good nutrition doesn't kill bad cells. Please do the RT in the near future. Please. I'm on your side.*

By this time, Wendy needed to unload. We were all running on depleted reserves, and Mary was just adding more stress. We had a lot more going on than should be dismissed out of hand. Wendy was very upset, so I tried to take things down a few notches by sending Mary a lengthy email reviewing our efforts, including excerpts from communications with all the doctors we have been consulting with.

Mary replied: *"Read all your emails. Neil has a devastating tumor. It will quickly kill him if you do nothing. And nothing is totally understandable. It is a choice. What you are currently doing is nothing. Sorry and forgive me. Nutrition, acupuncture, vitamins, prayers, etc will not kill tumor cells. Radiation will. It won't cure him but it will make time and will be no worse than the tumors effect. And he can try the radioactive monoclonal antibody which is new. What if it works??? What if??? What if??? It's new, but guys, forgive me but Memorial Sloan Kettering is a major major place in cancer care. Please please please go there. Clearly they have something new and promising to offer. Again, I'm saying if it was my kid he'd be there, yesterday. Forgive my frankness, but you are dragging your feet. These other things are BS. Even Annie chose RT and chemo which she combined with acupuncture and other alternative therapies. There's no time to look around for better ideas. Vitamins don't cure cancer. This is an aggressive serious disease. Soon he will be paralyzed or you will find him gone in his bed. Please begin. RT is the way forward. Talk to your son. His life depends on your actions."*

As good as Mary's intentions may have been, they were sorely misguided. She just wasn't absorbing what we were trying to tell her: Neil did not want radiation or a biopsy, not unless they proved to be the most promising path he could be found. With his life on the line, he preferred to take a small chance at long-term survival — the "brass ring" — over a large chance of just adding a few months to his death sentence.

To: Mary
From: Dean
Subject: Time out...
Date: March 28, 2016

Mary,

What we are doing is not nothing. While you are well-intentioned, that is a painfully callous assertion. Wendy has turned our kitchen upside down and Neil is getting dietary and supplemental support like he has never had in his life. Yes, the cancer Neil has is a killer. One way or the other. But there are alternative therapies that have had MUCH better success than anything mainstream offers. People who had DIPG ten or more years ago, married today with their own kids. Evie and Neil will be "skyping" with a survivor tonight. Mainstream medicine can not point to any such success, at least none that have been brought to our attention. The treatment of cancer is an industry. There are mixed motives when is comes to finding real cures, not on the part of most researchers, but on the part of major pharmaceutical corporations that will not invest in anything if they can't make a huge profit. That is as much a fact as is Neil's deadly tumor... At this point, you have Wendy in a tailspin. With no easy answer, we are following our instincts. Your assertiveness eclipses anything even our neuro-oncologists have expressed, and Dr. Kieran is at the tip-top of the pyramid. Yes, doing nothing is a perfectly viable option, especially when death is forecast to be coming within a few months, and prolonging life another few months carries with it a potentially hefty price-tag of suffering. I'm sorry, I don't mean to be angry. This is a very very difficult time.

God Bless,
Dean

Mary replied promptly: *"I meant to shake things up a little so forgive me. I understand that you must be furious with me. Don't. I just want you to go talk to Sloan Kettering. Yes they use RT first, but the CED delivery of a radio labeled monoclonal antibody is new stuff. This line of therapy is being used so much in hematologist malignancies as well as more recently with melanomas, with huge success.*

Regarding the biopsy...I think perhaps they are more interested in a tissue diagnosis in Neil's case because he is an outlier age wise for this particular tumor. I feel they might think the possibility of a low grade glioma remains. It's a different trajectory.

The people you are finding who did well with alternative therapy probably had a low grade glioma in the first place, which have not progressed. This can happen over many years.

I again encourage you to consider the biopsy. Brain biopsy material is very scant. I see them daily at work. They will take a small sample and decide if it's high or low grade.

Radiation will help Neil feel better and put the tumor at bay for some period of time. I truly truly believe that the benefits outweigh the side effects. Or the side effects will be no worse than letting the tumor continue to cause Neil's condition to deteriorate. There just isn't time to keep weighing the options.

Have you spoken to any patients or parents of dipg patients??? Ask how RT helped or didn't. I understand that this is terrifying. I understand the love of a child. I am so sorry.

I think Anne is a good example of someone who's not super confident with traditional cancer therapy but she chose to do both. RT, chemo, acupuncture, nutrition etc. Maybe she can tell you how she chose????

I love you and my heart hurts for all of you. Please keep talking to me."

There it was, a professional pathologist playing armchair quarterback and suggesting Neil might be misdiagnosed. She also pushed the familiar skepticism of mainstream medicine: if an alternative therapy has had miraculous cures, it's probably because those patients were misdiagnosed in the first place. This could have come directly from a documentary by Eric Merola.

I replied to Mary: *"Not furious. Frustrated. Wendy has called Sloan Kettering and we hope to get more information to weigh in the balance along with so much else. Yes, the time for some decision draws near. Neil has done very well these last few weeks, but he is slowly getting worse. We have ruled nothing out. We will keep you in the loop, absolutely."*

With this, Mary finally eased up and switched gears to share some thoughts regarding the immunotherapy trial in Louisville: *"The Louisville trial sounds interesting. I follow the biology of the Sloan Kettering trial better. I think the biopsy is a good idea. His age and the non enhancing indicate this could be low grade glioma rather than high grade/dipg. Please discuss this more with Dr. Kieran. He looks very experienced and I would trust anyone at DANA Farber. The nuances will be in his play book, not mine."*

Sloan Kettering, Sloan Kettering. Charles had also mentioned Sloan Kettering back when he first learned of Neil's prognosis, and Evie found Sloan Kettering's clinical trial early on. When Mary mentioned "monoclonal antibodies" and "melanoma," we looked back at our notes and inferred she meant the "immunomodulating" study Dr. Kieran had mentioned, the one where "side effects can include some very difficult-to-manage autoimmune disorders." We did not think he was referring to Sloan Kettering, but with so much information being processed, we were getting overloaded. Dr. Kieran did mention Sloan Kettering specifically with regards to studying convection-enhanced delivery (CED) of traditional chemotherapy, and he mentioned a second CED study using "targeted" drugs in Leeds, England. And both studies appeared to require radiation.

Radiation kept coming up like a bad penny. "It will help shrink the tumor. It will buy more time." But then the tumor comes roaring back, and it's over. It seemed pointless to endure this cycle just to gain a few months.

This was a real stumbling block, but even though radiation might also be required for the immunotherapy trial in Louisville, the idea of training one's own immune system to recognize and destroy cancer cells was exciting. It made intuitive sense — to us and to Neil — so in addition to the clinical trial at the Burzynski Clinic, we would turn our attention to the immunotherapy trial in Kentucky.

14

HEAVY LIFTING

"Sometimes I have so much going on in my head all at once that I can't even begin to grapple with it all." NF

As luck would have it, in the midst of this difficult exchange with Mary, we received an email from Charles with several informative links regarding "epigenetics." Although stated previously, this bears repeating:

"The more science learns, the more it seems DIPG is the result of dozens of gene mutations, if not hundreds. Some of these are not even 'mutations' per se, but normal genes that aren't functioning properly. How genes function — their 'expression' — plays a big role in cancer. The study of gene expression falls into the field of 'epigenetics.' In DIPG, exactly which genes are mutated and/or malfunctioning can vary greatly between patients, but by virtue of tissue samples from DIPG victims, researchers have identified a handful of genes that are commonly associated with the tumor, and these have become the target of many clinical trials."

HISTONES AND CHROMOSOMES

The links from Charles required some heavy lifting just to grasp the gist of their content, but given the direction Neil was taking — away from standard therapy — the links provided some valuable insights. Some brief excerpts:

To: Wendy and Dean
From: Charles
Subject: Panobinostat-histone deacetylase (HDAC) inhibitors slowed DIPG cell growth; see last article
Date: Mon, 28 Mar 2016

First link:

NATURE MEDICINE – NEWS AND VIEWS:

An epigenetic therapy for diffuse intrinsic pontine gliomas.
By Vijay Ramaswamy,Marc Remke & Michael D Taylor
Published online, 04 December 2014

Diffuse intrinsic pontine glioma is a uniformly lethal malignant tumor of infancy with no effective therapies. A new study reveals that inhibition of **JMJD3** has robust anti-tumor activity in diffuse intrinsic pontine glioma....

(Note – The following "Abstract," published in November 2019, helps explain the significance of "JMJD3:"

"JMJD3 in the regulation of human diseases"
By Xiangxian Zhang, Li Liu, Xia Yuan, Yuquan Wei & Xiawei Wei
ABSTRACT:
In recent years, many studies have shown that histone methylation plays an important role in maintaining the active and silent state of gene expression in human diseases. The Jumonji domain-containing protein D3 (JMJD3), specifically demethylate di- and trimethyl-lysine 27 on histone H3 (H3K27me2/3), has been widely studied in immune diseases, infectious diseases, cancer, developmental diseases, and aging related diseases.)

Second link:

Frontiers in Oncology. 2015; 5: 148.
Published online 2015 Jul 1. doi: 10.3389/fonc.2015.00148
PMCID: PMC4486770

Future Clinical Trials in DIPG: Bringing Epigenetics to the Clinic

Andres Morales La Madrid, Rintaro Hashizume, and Mark Kieran

Abstract: In spite of major recent advances in diffuse intrinsic pontine glioma (DIPG) molecular characterization, this body of knowledge has not yet translated into better treatments. To date, more than 250 clinical trials evaluating radiotherapy along with conventional cytotoxic chemotherapy as well as newer biologic agents have failed to improve the dismal outcome when compared to palliative radiation alone.

The biology of DIPG remained unknown until the recent dove-tailing of neurosurgical expertise and the recognition by the scientific/clinical community of the importance of tissue sampling at diagnosis. Ideally, this sampling would be done in the context of a clinical trial and by trained neurosurgical teams to maximize patient safety. These pre-treatment tumor samples, and others coming from tissue obtained post-mortem, have yielded new insights into DIPG molecular pathogenesis.

We now know that DIPG comprises a heterogeneous disease with variable molecular phenotypes, different from adult high-grade glioma, other non-pontine pediatric high-grade gliomas, and even between pontine gliomas. The discovery of histone H3.3 or H3.1 mutations has been an important step forward in understanding tumor formation, maintenance, and progression.

Pharmacologic reversal of DIPG histone demethylation therefore offers an important potential intervention strategy for the treatment of DIPG. To date, clinical trials of newly diagnosed or progressive DIPG with epigenetic (histone) modifiers have been unsuccessful.

Third link:

"Existing drug may treat the deadliest childhood brain tumor, Stanford-led study finds" May 4, 2015, by Erin Digitale, Stanford Medicine

For the first time, scientists have identified an existing drug that slows the growth of the deadliest childhood brain tumor. The drug restricted the tumor's growth in a lab dish and improved the survival time of mice that had the tumor implanted into their brains, according to researchers at the Stanford University School of Medicine, in collaboration with colleagues at other institutions. The work is noteworthy because the disease, a brain stem cancer called diffuse intrinsic pontine glioma, is nearly always fatal and lacks an effective treatment. A paper describing the findings were published online May 4, 2015 in ***Nature Medicine***.

"There have been over 200 clinical trials of chemotherapy drugs for DIPG, and none have shown any survival benefit," said Michelle Monje, MD, PhD, assistant professor of neurology at Stanford and a senior author of the paper. "But those trials were conducted before we knew anything about the unique biology of this tumor."

While the preclinical data in the new study are encouraging, Monje cautioned that the drug, panobinostat, needs further testing in a closely monitored human clinical trial. The research team is now planning such a trial in children with DIPG. Panobinostat was recently approved by the Food and Drug Administration for treatment of a form of blood cancer.

The drug repairs a portion of the cellular machinery now known to be defective in DIPG tumor cells, the new research showed. "A key thing that is wrong with DIPG cancer cells gets corrected by panobinostat," said Monje, who also treats DIPG patients in her role as a pediatric neuro-oncologist at Lucile Packard Children's Hospital Stanford. However, the new data also showed that some DIPG cells develop resistance to the drug, which means it will likely need to be combined with other drugs to achieve the best results in humans. "I don't think this is a cure, but I do think it will help," she said.

Fourth link:

Epigenetic Drugs Could be Used to Treat Deadly Pediatric Cancer
NEUROSCIENCE NEWS
MAY 4, 2015
BRAIN CANCER FEATURED NEUROLOGY

Six years ago, Dr. Monje started to create and share cell cultures of patients' DIPG cells that could be studied in labs. In this study, she and her colleagues used cell cultures collected from 16 patients in the US and Europe to search for drugs that could kill or stop the growth of DIPG cells. By performing experiments in petri dishes and with mice, they found that panobinostat, a drug designed to change the way cells regulate genes, may be effective at inhibiting DIPG growth.

"It's astounding. In only six years, scientists have gone from knowing virtually nothing about this tumor to understanding its underlying genetics and finding a potential therapy," said Jane Fountain, Ph.D., Program Director, at the National Institute of Neurological Disorders and Stroke (NINDS), part of NIH. "This study epitomizes collaborative medicine at work. It took a dedicated team of international scientists working with patients, families and foundations to get to this point."

The scientists began their work by performing high-throughput screening experiments, an advanced method for rapidly searching for effective compounds. The screening simultaneously tested 83 known or potential cancer drugs on each of the DIPG cell lines. They found that drugs called histone deacetylase (HDAC) inhibitors consistently slowed DIPG growth. Several of these drugs block histone deacetylases, a group of enzymes that regulate genes by removing chemical tags, called acetyl groups, from histone proteins. The scientists saw similar results when they genetically blocked individual histone deacetylases in the DIPG cells.

The scientists also analyzed the genes of each cell line. After reviewing the genetic and screening data they decided to focus on panobinostat, a drug designed to block multiple types of histone deacetylases. In petri dishes, they showed that panobinostat inhibited the growth of 12 out of 16 DIPG cell lines. When the scientists placed DIPG cells in the pons area of mice they found that sys-

> temic injections of panobinostat inhibited DIPG growth and extended survival.
>
> "All roads lead to histones," said Dr. Monje. "Our results support the idea that histone modifications are the keys to understanding and treating DIPG."
>
> Located in a cell's nucleus, histones are protein complexes that act like genetic spools wound with genes on chromosomes. Enzymes, including histone deacetylases, influence how chromosomes wind around histones by adding or removing chemical tags. In turn, the tagging indirectly, or **epigenetically**, controls whether a gene on a chromosome will be used, or expressed, in that cell.

And these are just excerpts! From them, we gleaned that gene expression plays a major role in disease, and inhibiting the "Jumonji domain-containing protein D3 (JMJD3)" in particular could be significant for patients with DIPG. Additional DIPG-related mutations have been discovered, but attempts to exploit them have thus far proven disappointing. (Of special note was Dr. Mark Kieran's co-authorship of the study referred to in the second link.) Another recent discovery shows an existing drug, panobinostat, can influence gene expression to inhibit the growth of DIPG in lab animals. This finding has inspired concerted research to find additional compounds with similar properties and refine understanding of their influence.

Taken together, the links "expressed" growing excitement about epigenetics, but while newly discovered experimental treatments showed promise, they had yet to demonstrate any significant survival benefit as far as we knew. In light of this, immunotherapy still seemed more likely to offer the chance of a breakthrough for Neil, and, of course, there was Dr. Burzynski. These links from Charles helped to underscore some key points that bolstered Dr. Burzynski's approach to DIPG:

- Epigenetics is quickly emerging as a promising field of cancer research and treatment;
- Antineoplastons function "epigenetically" (*"antineoplastons are naturally occurring peptides demonstrating the ability to re-program cancer cells without destroying normal cells"*);
- Dr. Kieran's co-authorship of one study, "*Future Clinical Trials in DIPG: Bringing Epigenetics to the Clinic*," showed his interest in epigenetics, which might help explain why he'd taken an interest in Dr. Burzynski's work at one time.

EPIGENETICS, PEPTIDES, AND ANTINEOPLASTONS

The human genome contains twenty-three pairs of chromosomes with about three billion DNA base pairs. As of this writing, the precise number of genes in the genome has yet to be determined, but estimates are roughly twenty-three thousand. Within the genome are many possible permutations. Some genes are switched on, "expressing" their influence on cellular biology, and some genes are switched off, or inactive.

Epigenetics is the study of the biochemical handshakes that influence the symphony of gene expression at the molecular level: What switches genes on or off; what causes them to amplify their behavior; and what causes them to mutate? With cancer in particular, epigenetics looks at which genes promote cancer (oncogenes), and which genes suppress cancer (tumor suppressor genes). Ironically, mutations can cause genes to flip roles: tumor suppressor genes can transform into oncogenes, and vice versa. As these genes are identified and understanding of the biochemical factors that influence their molecular behaviors are refined, the objective of epigenetic cancer therapy is to promote tumor suppressor genes and thwart oncogenes to help the body heal itself.

Now, wind the clock back to 1967. As the result of many years of experiments using chromatography to separate and analyze the molecular makeup of amino acids, a young Dr. Burzynski made a breathtaking discovery: There are certain naturally occurring peptides that healthy people have in abundance, but cancer patients seem to lack.

> ***What are peptides?***
>
> Peptides are naturally occurring biological molecules. Peptides are found in all living organisms and play a key role in all manner of biological activity. Like proteins, peptides are formed (synthesized) naturally from transcription of a sequence of the genetic code, DNA. Transcription is the biological process of copying a specific DNA gene sequence into a messenger molecule, mRNA, which then carries the code for a given peptide or protein. Reading from the mRNA, a chain of amino acids is joined together by peptide bonds to form a single molecule.
>
> There are 20 naturally-occurring amino acids and, like letters into words, they can be combined into an immense variety of different molecules. When a molecule consists of 2 to 50 amino acids, it is called a peptide, whereas a larger chain of > 50 amino acids is generally referred to as a protein.
>
> In the human body, peptides are found in every cell and tissue and perform a wide range of essential functions. Maintenance of appropriate concentration and activity levels of peptides is necessary to achieve homeostasis and maintain health.[9]

In other words, peptides are key players in epigenetics. The peptides Dr. Burzynski discovered are normally present in a healthy person's blood and urine, but he noted a persistent lack of these peptides in cancer patients. This seemed to be more than coincidence. Believing these peptides could play a role in preventing the growth of cancer, Dr. Burzynski invent-

9 Zealand Pharma, *https://www.zealandpharma.com/what-are-peptides*

ed a way to extract them from the urine of healthy people and use them in an experimental cancer treatment (hence, the sobriquet, "piss doctor.").

Fast forward a few years, and Dr. Burzynski's experimental therapy was having dramatic success — no magic bullet, but significantly prolonging the lives of many patients who otherwise were deemed hopeless by mainstream oncology. In a handful of remarkable cases, complete cures were achieved. As word of Dr. Burzynski's results spread, so too came the need to develop synthetic analogs of these peptides to keep up with demand. Dr. Burzynski dubbed his synthetic peptides, "antineoplastons" (ANPs), derived from the word "neoplasm," the term for a cancerous tumor. Anti-neoplasm. Anti-cancer.[10]

Based on extensive analyses of blood samples from his patients — using techniques he pioneered — Dr. Burzynski determined that ANPs influence roughly one hundred of the genes involved in tumor cell growth — helping to switch off oncogenes and activate tumor suppressor genes. ANPs were also nontoxic, posing no harm to healthy cells. Word spread.

In 1977, Dr. Burzynski opened his clinic to treat terminally ill cancer patients — people who either chose to refuse the debilitating consequences of traditional cancer therapies, or people who had tried everything conventional medicine had to offer and had no place else to turn. Many of these patients had positive results, finding genuine reprieve from intractable cancers when mainstream medicine had told them all hope was lost.

CELESTE!

On the evening of March 28, 2016 — while Wendy and I were still trying to digest all this information — Neil and Evie were sequestered upstairs in his room for a virtual visit with Celeste Sabbaugh from Argentina. Of course, Wendy and I were intensely interested in this conversation as well, so our attention was somewhat divided. The kids visited with Celeste for thirty-five to forty minutes, and they heard her story firsthand:

---

10 *The Burzynski Breakthrough*, by Thomas D. Elias, 1997

Celeste was twenty-four years old and in college studying economics when she began having symptoms somewhat similar to Neil's. She went to several doctors, who could find nothing wrong with her. In March of 2011, she was finally diagnosed with DIPG.

As with all DIPG patients, her prognosis was grim, and her doctors recommended a strong course of radiation along with an oral chemo called temozolomide — pretty much the "standard of care" prescription. With no other options apparent, she agreed. Celeste tolerated the radiation well enough, and it reduced the tumor by half, but taking the chemo on top of radiation was too much. She felt increasingly tired; her muscles weakened; her appetite faded; and she had dizziness, nausea, depression, trouble sleeping, and hair loss — the typical side effects from such a harsh course of treatment. To help stabilize her condition, she needed many blood and platelet transfusions.

Celeste's side effects were so debilitating she spent most of her time in the hospital. All the while, her oncologist kept increasing her dose of chemo. In August of 2011, Celeste asked about her prognosis and was told she might live another two years — an extremely ambitious projection based on statistics, but bleak to her mind if her condition was to be so depleted. That was when she declared "enough is enough." If she wasn't going to survive and recover, why should she go through such suffering? She stopped all treatment and went home.

Despite her decision, Celeste's family refused to give up, and they made an appointment for her to visit M.D. Anderson in Houston, Texas, one of the premier cancer treatment centers in the US. In November of 2011, Celeste and her father flew to Houston to meet the oncologist who would look at her case. Celeste recalls feeling a renewed sense of hope, but after the oncologist reviewed her MRI and medical records, she was told there was nothing M.D. Anderson could do for her. "Go home and enjoy the time you have left."

So, home to Argentina she went, convinced there was nothing to do, no more treatments to try. Those were the worst days of Celeste's life. She recalls waking up each day surprised to be alive. Her family, however, was unwilling to surrender, and while searching for options, they found one more possibility — a clinic back in Houston, of all places — that was using an experimental therapy with some reported success for DIPG patients. These reports were, in FDA parlance, "anecdotal," the sort of evidence that relies heavily on personal testimony; thus, its value is downplayed or dismissed in the formal world of conventional medicine. However, when one is drowning in despair, anecdotal evidence shines like a lighthouse appearing from out of the gloom in the darkest of nights on the roughest of seas.

Celeste's father "overnighted" her records to the Burzynski Clinic, and soon thereafter, they were traveling again, although Celeste said she did so to please her father more than anything else. It was February of 2012 when they arrived at the Burzynski Clinic — "where hope exists," according to the clinic's motto.

Dr. Burzynski made no guaranties, but he felt Celeste could be helped by antineoplaston therapy. First, however, she would have to ask the FDA for permission under "compassionate use." Fortunately, she received approval without too much delay, so Celeste had a catheter surgically implanted, by which daily infusions of antineoplastons (ANPs) would be given.

During her time in Houston, the Burzynski Clinic's staff treated Celeste with great care and respect, and they trained Celeste's father on how to prepare and administer the nontoxic ANPs. He also received training on how to change the dressing on her catheter-wound until it healed (a task Celeste's mother would assume). As soon as Celeste's father was certified, they flew home to Argentina with the equipment and enough ANPs to last several weeks.

Thus, Celeste's parents became her nurses, and Celeste received her daily infusions of ANPs prepared by her father. He was one of her guardian angels. The other was her little dog, Amando, who stayed by her side through thick and thin, and this was no easy time. Celeste felt tired and sleepy all the time. On top of that, she was still barely able to walk, and being connected to a pump for most of each day — even if it was portable — was daunting. Nonetheless, Celeste's hope was being slowly renewed, and once again, she graced her family with the smile they so dearly loved.

Over the next year and a half of taking ANPs, Celeste slowly began to feel better. Throughout this time, she and her dad communicated with the Burzynski Clinic on a daily basis, reporting her status and getting instructions on dosing adjustments. Celeste also had a sympathetic doctor in Argentina who monitored her health and ordered periodic MRIs to gauge her progress.

As time passed, Celeste's MRIs showed stable disease. For a girl who was supposed to be dead, this was no small thing. Finally, her ANP therapy was tapered down and eliminated. As soon as she was untethered from the ANP pump, she started spreading her wings and living a full life. Her neurologist viewed her MRI and told her she could lead a normal life. She was officially in remission, and at the time of this writing, Celeste had a child of her own.

That's the gist of the story Celeste told to Neil and Evie, (the same story available on the "Burzynski Patient Group" website).

Neil was literally floating on air after his conversation. "She's amazing," he beamed. "As far as she's concerned, the Burzynski Clinic saved her life!"

"Like Jessica Ressel," I smiled at his enthusiasm.

"Sort of," Neil tipped his head quizzically, "but she tried standard therapy first. Jessica went straight to Burzynski, as I recall."

"Yeh," I nodded, "I think that's right."

"Celeste didn't have a cake walk," Neil continued. "Some days she felt terrible, had no energy to do anything, but when she started noticing small improvements her hope blossomed."

"If you believe in what you are doing," Wendy smiled, "that has healing power by itself."

"Positivity," Neil nodded. "I'm down with that!"

"What did you think? " I asked Evie.

"I'm glad I found her," she answered. "Her story is amazing. She coached Neil to be optimistic: 'If she could do it, so can he! Be fearless, and never give up hope!' But I'd like to know more about the Burzynski Clinic in general and their clinical trial in particular."

"We'll get more information," I promised her.

Neil beamed. "She kept saying, *'If I can beat DIPG, so can you!'* She told me to call her anytime."

"FAN-TASTIC," Wendy smiled, wiping the corners of her eyes.

"I'd like to visit Dr. Burzynski as soon as possible," Neil concluded.

"You still need to qualify for his clinical trial," I cautioned.

Neil raised an incredulous eyebrow.

"We'll get a consult, regardless," I assured him.

"That's more like it," he cuffed my shoulder.

Having no reason to take Celeste at anything less than her word, we were swept up in the excitement of the moment. From where we were sitting, promising studies were just that — promising — while Dr. Burzynski's antineoplastons had already worked miracles, albeit "anecdotal." ANPs might not work for everyone, but they had worked for many who were otherwise doomed, with DIPG patients obviously being of particular interest. And Neil had just spoken to a long-term survivor! Even if ANP therapy was a long shot, it was looking like it might be his best shot. We were more determined than ever to visit Houston and meet Dr. Burzynski.

HINDSIGHT

For all intents and purposes, the kids' conversation with Celeste put an end to the wrangling with Mary. In all fairness, however, she was not wrong about Sloan Kettering. As of 2020, enrolled patients have apparently enjoyed a median survival of just over two years, with one patient living six years! That is absolutely FAN-TASTIC! Unfortunately, at the time of Neil's diagnosis, these results must have been closely guarded, because none of the doctors with whom we spoke discussed them, and they certainly would have. Even had we known, there was Jessica Ressel, Celeste Sabbaugh, Tori Moreno, and a handful of others in Dr. Burzynski's favor. Some of these survivors have children of their own! Why mainstream medicine is determined to dismiss these survivors is distressing beyond words, but no amount of official quibbling can dim such miracles when they're witnessed in-person by someone whose life hangs in the balance.

15

IMMUNOTHERAPY OR ANPS

"Focus is what gives life direction;
determination is what helps one stay the course." NF

While we were eager to visit the Burzynski Clinic, with Neil's trial eligibility still uncertain, we wanted to keep exploring the immunotherapy trial at the University of Louisville, so I was pleased to hear back from Nurse Comings:

> **To: Dean**
> **From: jennifer**
> **Subject: RE: Immunotherapy trial - University of Louisville**
> **Date: March 29, 2016**
>
> Hello Dean,
>
> Thank you for the Easter wishes!
>
> I'm sorry to hear of Neil's diagnosis and what he and your family are going through right now. I have been linked in a few email conversations between you, Dr. Plant and Dr. Kieran in the last week. Before I responded to an email, I wanted to get a few questions answered by Dr. Lucas and Dr. Elster.
>
> I understand you were inquiring about the possibility

of eligibility and inclusion into the trial without having standard of care treatment first. I double checked the possibility with Dr. Elster. This is an FDA requirement for the study. Being that this is a phase 1 clinical trial, a patient must meet the eligibility requirement of having standard of care therapy and either be refractory to treatment or relapsed before treatment can begin.

But because of his diagnosis of DIPG he would be eligible to have his cells collected and the vaccine made and stored for use if needed.

Below is a brief overview of the study. I'm happy to go into further detail, or answer any questions you may have! I would also be happy to discuss anything over the phone, as sometimes it's easier to answer questions in a conversation.

This is a phase 1 clinical trial, meaning this is the first phase of the study. We do not have clinical data at this point on the effectiveness of the treatment in this patient population.

Cells are collected through a central line that is placed on the day of collection.

This is an all day visit. The central line is placed in the groin and the line is then pulled on the same day, prior to discharge. Some patients require some type of anti-anxiety medications to take the edge off while the line is being inserted, others require sedation (our little ones) and some of our older patients have not required anything but the local anesthetic

Once cells are collected, it takes about 6-8weeks to generate a vaccine ready for use.

Then the treatment phase starts. Scans are needed within 1 week to determine disease status (doesn't have to be 'No evidence of disease,' but a large tumor burden with metastatic disease is not optimal in enrolling into the trial)

Week 1 is chemo (decitabine) days 1-5 given

Week 2 Day 1 is vaccine and hiltonol (2 injections in the arm)
Day 4 is hiltonol (injection in the arm) and counts/physical exam
Days 1-5 GMCSF is given (given by parents mon-friday)

Week 3 Day 1 is vaccine and hiltonol (2 injections in the arm)
Day 4 is hiltonol (injection in the arm) and counts/physical exam
Days 1-5 GMCSF is given (given by parents mon-friday)

Week 4 Rest week (counts and physical exam are checked once this week)

Week 5 Rest week (counts and physical exam are checked once this week)

This is repeated again for cycle 2. On week 5 of cycle 2, scans are repeated to see if the patient's disease status has changed, stayed the same or progressed. Depending on results cycles are repeated for 2 more times, for 4 cycles total. Each cycle lasts about 35 days.

Please let me know any questions that you have
Regards,
Jen,RN BSN
Research Nurse Coordinator
Kosair Charities Pediatric Clinical Research Unit

So, there it was. As exciting as it sounded — formulating a custom immune system vaccine — radiation was mandated by the FDA. While disappointing, in the spirit of refusing to take no for an answer, I would keep trying to finagle a way in for Neil. Thankfully, at the same time that Louisville began looking more like a long shot, prospects for participation in the Burzynski Clinic's trial took a positive turn.

To: Dean
From: "Sheryll"
Subject: RE: Treatment at the Burzynski Clinic
Date: March 29, 2016 reply from Sheryll

Hi,

Dr. Burzynski stated the medicine will be available in 3 weeks. He advises you and your son to come here around April 12 so we can see him and have the scans done in Houston. Dr. Burzynski feels your son will qualify, since there is one criteria that may not require an enhancement, providing we do a PET/CT brain. The consult and medicine and doctor's visit will be free of charge if he is entered into the clinical trial. We can also discuss other options in the event your son does not meet the criteria.

If this works for you, let me know and set a date so I can put you on Dr. Burzynski's schedule

Take care
Sheryll

That was promising, especially on the heels of the kids' conversation with Celeste, but I could half-imagine the Burzynski skeptics hollering, "Scam! He won't qualify! It's a bait and switch!" Thankfully, we were beyond reach of such trolling. On the other hand, Dr. Kieran's wave-off carried weight, but his story of that failed overture still left the door cracked.

Raffaele, too, had voiced caution, but at the end of the day, he would tell us to trust our instincts.

"Hey Neil," I hollered up to his room. "We're a definite 'go' from Houston!"

"FAN-TASTIC!" he yelled back. "When?"

"I haven't given up completely on Louisville," I replied. "That needs a little more time, but it looks like the second week of April for Houston."

"Let's get'r done," Neil drawled, inspiring a smile. We were going to Houston for a consult. Before that, however, we wanted to "consult" with Charles if he could make time:

To: Charles
From: Dean
Subject: Re: Panobinostat-histone deacetylase (HDAC) inhibitors slowed DIPG cell growth; see last article
Date: March 29, 2016

The articles you sent are very informative, but we need to make a decision soon. It's all such a complex guessing game. Would you have time to talk in person? Thank you for all you have done to help!

God Bless,
Dean

As happened so frequently, as this email went out, a new pair of emails arrived from "Dr. Mary" within hours of each other: *"I think Harvard would be very careful and do a very targeted biopsy with imaging guidance. The more I read the more I think you all need to know exactly what's in that tumor. Guys, I'm a pathologist. Seeing is believing. Think on this for me. Love you. I'm working today at Evanston. I'm going to talk to our neuropathologist and get his thoughts."*

Then: *"I talked to our neuropathologist. He called a colleague at Brigham who says the reason they probably want a biopsy/tissue diagnosis is because they want to determine possible molecular genetic targets. These may affect prognosis and potential new drugs' predicted efficacy. He said they would likely take biopsy in less critical area such as near or in the cerebellum as to cause least possible adverse sequelae.*

I encourage you to trust your Dr Kieran. I have really never met a single physician in my years of practice that I didn't think always had his/her patients best interests foremost in their mind."

Mary was expressing similar thoughts to those of Dr. Arrillaga, Dr. Cahill, and Dr. Kieran. If any had suggested that the biopsy process was, in fact, likely to match Neil's tumor to a therapy that could have a real impact on his DIPG, Neil would have been more enthusiastic. However, everything we had read and been told suggested the process offered no better results than "standard care." In that instance, the benefit of biopsy was collecting samples for research.

Neil had said it before, and he would say it again: "I support research, but I won't take that path unless I'm convinced there's no better option for my own personal survival."

With time growing short, the immunotherapy trial still seemed to beckon with that sort of potential, but it would take real finagling to get in. On the other hand, just speaking with Celeste had been a huge lift for the Burzynski Clinic. If he went to the Burzynski Clinic, Neil knew he would not have to take radiation. That freedom was very important. I replied to Sheryll: *"Some logistical questions: Assuming we are there by April 11th, how long should we plan to stay? If treatment would potentially start shortly thereafter, I'm wondering if we should just plan to come down and 'camp out.' Neil is doing reasonably well. We're doing all we can to keep him fit enough to travel and take treatment, but he does get tired more easily than he did a month ago; he's having increasing trouble with his eyes; and he's fairly strong but his motor-skills are increasingly challenged. I'm just trying to sort possibilities into a rational plan. Any thoughts or suggestions you might have on what we should plan for would be greatly appreciated.*

Another question: Regarding the PET/CT scan – should we get it done here and bring the results, or wait and do it there when we visit? It might be preferable from an insurance standpoint to do it here, but if there is an advantage to waiting until we are there, we can accommodate that as well. Please advise."

She responded: *"Definitely plan to stay here for at least 3 weeks. The plan is to initially screen your son to enroll in the study. With the protocol requirements, an MRI should be within 14 days prior to starting or else we will have to repeat it. PET/CT scan can be done there if you wish, but keep it close to a few days prior to your arrival here.*

A central catheter placement to a major vein in his chest will be scheduled once he meets the requirements. The catheter surgery will be done at a local hospital by a surgeon who routinely performs this procedure. The catheter is how the antineoplastons will be administered.

In the clinical study, the treatment and services at our clinic will be free, but other expenses such as lodging, transportation, scans, blood tests and catheter placement will be paid either through your insurance or self pay if insurance does not cover it. No compensations will be given to the patients enrolled in the study. You should plan ahead with expenses as well.

I have not heard a confirmed date yet on when the ANPs will be available, but they stated it should be by the 2nd or early 3rd week of April. I'll keep you informed."

COMPASSION CENTER

In the midst of our finish line frenzy, Wendy went to Dr. Slattery's office to pick up a referral letter for Neil to get a medical marijuana card, then she and Neil took a drive into Providence to visit the RI Department of Health. After submitting his referral letter and completing the application, Neil received his card within half an hour. As his caregiver, Wendy received a card too.

The next step was to visit the Slater Compassion Center, one of three state-run "compassion" centers at the time. Wendy and Neil were greeted with professional courtesy and given a tour of the facility — from growing rooms to the "candy store." The center sold dried cannabis flowers, concentrates, and edibles. The compassion program also provided free products to extremely ill patients. Because it was Neil's first visit and his prognosis was terminal, they gave him samples of CBD capsules, CBD/THC bud-blends, and some drop-delivery syringes filled with "Phoenix Tears."

On the ride home, Neil and Wendy debated how to use this new "weapon." Unfortunately, finding the right balance of CBD and THC would be no better than guesswork. There are no real guidelines, just anecdotal stories. Neil and Wendy were truly venturing into the realm of "experimental alternative medicine." Could adding medical marijuana to Neil's nutrition protocols help slow the growth of his DIPG? Could it help slay the monster in his head or at least buy him more time? Could it make matters worse? This would be an ongoing debate between them, but at least it would help Neil feel more comfortable.

EXPENSES — SNAPSHOT

Sheryll had twice mentioned that if Neil were accepted into the clinical trial, the Burzynski Clinic would cover the costs of clinic visits, in-house tests, and ANP medication. That would be a huge burden off our plate! Neil's school insurance would likely help too. Could we handle the rest? Before this nightmare began, Wendy and I had been preparing to buy a house in South Carolina; we had deposit money set aside. Neil also had money given to him by his Grandparents over the years, which he gladly offered to the cause. With these reserves, we figured we could manage for at least a year — assuming Neil was accepted into the clinical trial. Otherwise, we would have to dig deeper, but that was secondary to helping him find the right path to start out.

VALIDATION

In the midst of ruminating upon all the information we were juggling — which made hours seem sometimes like days — Charles replied to my request for a visit in person: *"I can potentially come over if you want. It might be easier as this stuff is complicated. I am available tonight. It would be tougher tomorrow, Friday and Saturday. Sunday is a possibility. But if it's easier for you, tonight's the best night. Anytime."*

"The sooner the better," I replied, and he came over that evening.

We greeted Charles at the door, exchanging hugs, and Neil was anxious to tell him about Celeste.

"I spoke with a DIPG survivor who went to the Burzynski Clinic!"

"That's fantastic!" Charles grinned.

Neil beamed approval at Charles' choice of words, and on that SLTP note, we sat in the living room while Neil told Celeste's story, his enthusiasm increasing each moment. "It's almost three years since she went to Burzynski, and her life is pretty much back to normal!"

"And she was treated with antineoplastons?" Charles asked.

"Yup," Neil nodded.

"Hold on, hold on," I interrupted. "How about we step back to put everything in perspective and work our way back to Burzynski."

Neil waved me ahead, if a little begrudgingly.

"Let's review what we've learned," I said, "to make sure we don't miss something crucial." With that, first up was 'standard care.'"

"I'm not interested in radiation," Neil punctuated the discussion. "And not much in chemo, for that matter."

"Cut, burn, and poison," Charles shrugged. "It's what they've been doing for fifty years."

"At least," I agreed.

"Although they've gotten better at modulating doses," Charles observed in all fairness. "Narrowing the beam, controlling the power with greater finesse."

"But it still goes through healthy tissue," Neil shook his head. "That causes damage. And with DIPG, the tumor is so intertwined with healthy cells, the whole ball gets whacked!"

"Even if the side effects have been minimized," I shook my head, "radiation increases the odds of getting another cancer later on."

"Chemo is hardly better," Wendy squinched her nose. "Whatever goes in a vein goes everywhere else in the body, not just to the tumor."

"Obviously the side effects are difficult," Charles nodded.

"Dean's mom, Neil's Grandma — the kids called her 'Maga' — had some nasty side effects from chemo," Wendy agreed, briefly describing Maga's experience.

"Then there's the biopsy-and-tumor-typing procedure," I continued down our list.

"Jump shots," Neil guffawed.

"What?" Charles looked quizzically at him.

"It's what the neurosurgeon said when I asked about potential side effects," Neil explained. "'The chances of death are fairly remote,' he told us. 'But let's say, if you play basketball, it could throw off your jump shot.' Made me cringe a little," Neil finished.

"Well," I steered back toward the subject. "The idea of the biopsy is to match the tumor against any drugs known to impact its particular gene mutations."

"Some of the studies you sent suggest intriguing possibilities," Neil observed. "But that promise has yet to translate into clinical success."

"And there's still the issue of whether the chemo can cross the blood-brain barrier," Wendy jumped back in.

"That's what 'convection-enhanced delivery' is about," I nodded. "Drilling a 'keyhole' in the skull and delivering chemo direct to the tumor."

Neil shook his head. "Didn't Raffaele express some doubts about that — at least for DIPG — because healthy cells are so intertwined? Once again, the whole ball gets whacked!"

"Chemo and radiation are both indiscriminate," Charles observed. "They hit healthy cells too. Of course there's a continuum," he added. "Less radiation is less toxic. Some chemos are less toxic than others. But at the end of the day, they're both used to 'whack' the cancer. And healthy cells get whacked too."

"Which brings us to the research links you sent," I said.

"The main theme is epigenetics," Charles nodded. "Influencing gene expression to combat cancer — many diseases for that matter. There's been a lot of research in this area," he continued, "and it looks like they've discovered an existing drug, 'panobinostat' — 'a drug designed to change the way cells regulate genes' — which can inhibit DIPG cell growth in lab animals."

"Yes," Neil nodded. "That's one of the ones I meant. It was nice see Dr. Kieran's name in there!"

"Unfortunately," I raised my hand, "the clinical trials have thus far not been successful. Dr. Kieran made that observation in the study-paper from July 2015, and he effectively reiterated the same thing when we met with him a week ago."

"Hmmm," Charles sighed. "I get epigenetics. The concept is intuitively 'functional.' But I agree, it's discouraging to see that this research has yet to bear fruit in the clinical trials."

"There's always a chance," Wendy echoed Dr. Arrillaga, and Charles nodded.

"But what they've done so far is pretty narrowly focused," I observed. "They're targeting a small number of genes when it looks like dozens if not hundreds could be involved in DIPG."

Charles nodded.

"It's discouraging," Neil shrugged.

"But there's always a chance Neil could be the breakthrough," Wendy said, playing advocate again.

"Always a chance," Neil sighed. "But based on what I've seen so far, I'm not sure I want to bet my life on it."

And that was the "bottom line." It was Neil's life on the line. No two ways about it.

"It's a lot to go through," Charles nodded. "A biopsy procedure, standard care, and then chemo. The only real certainty is that science will get some more samples to study."

Neil harrumphed.

"But there's another possibility we're looking at," I reviewed our communications with the folks in Louisville. "But it looks like he would be required to do radiation."

"Which I really don't want," Neil repeated. "It should be my choice."

"I'm asking if there's any way to get around that requirement," I said.

"The prospect of an individualized vaccine — of training a person's immune system to fight cancer — is tantalizing," Charles agreed, "but remember, what they're doing is even newer than the biopsy/tumor-typing process. Correct me if I'm wrong, but Louisville is a 'phase one' clinical trial. There's zero data on efficacy."

"Correct," I nodded.

"Which brings us to Burzynski," Neil came back around to where he had started. "There's no arguing about Celeste. She's a DIPG survivor. After M.D. Anderson turned her away."

"What Burzynski is doing," I offered, "treating people with peptides, it's an epigenetic therapy to my mind, don't you think?"

"Yes," Charles nodded. "But less like a hammer. More like a massage."

"That's an interesting way to put it," Wendy smiled.

Charles pondered thoughtfully for a moment. "Well, there have been some reported side effects from antineoplastons, but from what I've read, they are rare and reversible."

"So, I'm going to Houston," Neil pumped a fist.

"I think that's a good idea," Charles agreed. "It seems to me you've got your ducks lined up pretty well. It's worth a consult."

Thank you, Charles! His visit was a great affirmation: we had been putting the time available to good use — not perfect, but good. Given Neil's priorities and the information we had, our choice narrowed down to the immunotherapy trial in Louisville (if we could work around the radiation requirement) or the Burzynski Clinic. While the biopsy/tumor-typing process might be the leading edge of standard care — especially when coupled with convection-enhanced delivery — results on a par with just doing radiation could not compete with survivors, especially when Neil had just spoken with Celeste.

FINAL PUSH TO DECISION

We breathed a collective and satisfied sigh after talking with Charles. We could stop juggling so many balls. While we still had Neil's daily regimen to manage — as well as his experimenting with medical marijuana — as far as pursuing active treatment was concerned, just the two balls remained: our instincts were directed toward Houston, but our brass ring hopes were still pinned on Louisville. Even though we had "telegraphed" our decision to forgo treatment at Dana-Farber or Mass General, Ashley Plant was still gracious enough to help expedite our overtures with Louisville, which prompted this email from Nurse Comings:

To: "Plant, Ashley"
From: Jennifer Comings
Subject: RE: Immunotherapy trial
Date: March 30, 2016
CC: Dean

Thank you Ashley for your email.

If Dean would like to request Neil's current medical summary and recent images/reports be sent to us, I can pass them along for review and consideration to enroll and collect cells to manufacture the vaccine. If anything is going to be sent, my contact details are in my signature line. It can be emailed, mailed or faxed! If someone will just let me know if something is being sent, I will keep my eye out for it.

Thank you very much for your response!
Regards,
Jen Comings RN BSN

* * *

To: Jennifer
From: "Plant, Ashley"
Subject: Re: Immunotherapy trial
Date: March 30, 2016

CC: Dean

Great. Thanks. I can ask our coordinators to send the information once Dean gives us the final go ahead. If Neil is getting an MRI Thursday maybe we can wait until then and send that as well.

Ashley S. Plant, MD Fellow, Pediatric Hematology/Oncology DANA Farber Cancer Institute Children's Hospital

* * *

To: "Plant, Ashley"
From: Jennifer Comings
Subject: RE: Immunotherapy trial
Date: March 30, 2016

Thank you! I think it would be best to wait until the MRI on Thursday and send the information at that time.

Jen

While this exchange took place on Neil's behalf, Evie wanted to get more information from the Burzynski Clinic:

To: "Sheryll S. Acelar"
From: Dean
Subject: Clinical trial...
Date: March 30, 2016

Sheryll,

My daughter wants to learn more about your clinical trial:

> "I would be interested to read up on the specific antineoplastons being tested, range of dosage

> levels, and basic clinical trial procedures. Its important to get as much information as possible to have questions ready when Neil goes to Houston."

Any information or links you can send would be greatly appreciated. I'm sorry to bombard you with so many questions, but as you can imagine this is a critical time for us, and we want to be as prepared as is humanly possible. I look forward to hearing from you soon.

Thank you again,
Dean F.

Sheryll replied: *"I can send you an article about the clinical trial and previous studies – hard copies – but I cannot provide you the specific protocol of the study."* Then Sheryll sent another brief note: *"Hi again. Dr. Burzynski gave me several articles to overnight to you."*

I replied to Evie: *"They can send hard-copy articles, but no specific protocol data."*

She answered: *"Okay, have them send whatever materials they can."*

While Sheryll and Dr. Burzynski seemed a bit guarded, given the decades of harassment he had suffered, some reticence did not seem unreasonable. She would overnight the articles, so we would have them soon enough. I replied to her: *"Thank you. We are looking forward to seeing what you send. We are still exploring whether to fly or drive, but as of now we are planning to be there no later than the 12th. Also, let me know whether we should arrange to get the PET/CT scan done up here or just wait. It's almost one month since Neil's diagnosis, and while he seems to be doing reasonably well, we are certainly eager to see what changes the tumor has undergone."* Yes, it was coming up on one month since Neil had been diagnosed. The milestone loomed like a deadline: the time to decide was at hand; we had to make a final effort with Louisville, leading to a flurry of emails between myself, Dr. Plant, and Nurse Comings:

To: Jennifer Comings
From: Dean
Subject: RE: Immunotherapy trial
Date: March 30, 2016
CC: Drs. Kieran and Plant

Dear Jennifer,

Thank you for your thorough response. I have a couple of comments which I am happy to share with Dr. Kieran and Dr. Plant.

First, regarding optimal conditions for enrolling, your email states, "a large tumor burden with metastatic disease is not optimal for enrolling into the trial." I would obviously defer to Dr. Kieran, but I think Eugene's (Neil's) tumor would be considered fairly large, and it's doubtful whether radiation could shrink it sufficiently to alter this characterization. Though uncommon, there is also a chance of metastasis in his spine. (He will be getting a spinal MRI on Thursday.) Thus it appears to me Neil might not make an optimal candidate.

Second, in the case of DIPG – where his prognosis without intervention is roughly three months from diagnosis, and the prognosis with "standard care" perhaps doubles that estimate – it strains common sense to consider "standard care" as anything more than an extended hospice prescription; there is no ray of hope, just prolonging despair. While some people – perhaps most – might wish to struggle for every possible second, the quality of those seconds is more important than how many we get. To us and to Neil, the benefit of "standard care" is outweighed by the cost, especially when there may be alternatives – like your trial – which reason argues would offer a better chance of success if "standard care" could be avoided: "Immunotherapy" screams for just that – therapy for the immune system, not an assault by radiation. This seems like such simple logic. Have I missed something?

If we agree on this premise, I would happy to write a formal appeal to the FDA – submitted as an open letter to whatever publications or web sites you might choose. I would be happy to do so, not so much for my son's potential benefit – that time may slip by too quickly – but for the benefit of your research and for anyone whose quest to obtain the treatment he or she wants has been confounded by a suffocation of regulations. In cases where the prognosis is as bleak as that of DIPG, participation in an experimental clinical trial should not be gated by any FDA-mandated precursor treatment. This becomes all the more true when "standard care" would threaten to compromise the very biological system the trial is attempting to stimulate.

Thank you very much for your time.

God Bless,
Dean Fachon

* * *

To: Dean
From: "Plant, Ashley"
Subject: Re: Immunotherapy trial
Date: March 30, 2016
CC: Jennifer Comings

Hello Dean (and Jennifer),

We can work on getting Neil's next MRI sent to the Louisville team for their assessment on the tumor burden/size and whether it is appropriate for the study, but from my standpoint, that should not hold up enrollment. In regards to radiation, my take is that radiation be an attempt to halt growth of the tumor long enough to manufacture the vaccine. We do not typically think of radiation therapy as drastically altering the immune system in the same way high doses of chemotherapy or steroids do. For this reason, standard therapy makes sense to me, not only because it is "standard," but because it can keep the tumor at a more manageable size prior to vaccine manufacturing. Immunotherapy is thought to work best with the smallest amount of disease possible.

I understand this is a complicated and frustrating process and the regulations can appear burdensome. Most regulations are meant to optimize safety of the patient in settings of "experimental therapies," but in this situation I understand why it appears burdensome. Please take some more time to think about radiation and enrollment on this study and we will wait to hear from the Louisville study group on moving forward.

Dr. Plant Ashley S. Plant, MD Fellow, Pediatric Hematology/Oncology
DANA Farber Cancer Institute

* * *

To: Dean
From: Jennifer
Subject: RE: Immunotherapy trial
Date: March 30, 2016

Hello Dean,

I understand your thoughts on the eligibility criteria for the inclusion with the study, but since this is a phase 1 clinical trial I do not know if there is any possibility of waiving that inclusion. I will be happy to pass your email on to Dr. Lucas and Dr. Elster for review and discuss this in our meeting.

Before we bring anyone into the trial for consent and cell collection, Dr. Lucas and Dr. Elster review images and reports prior to the journey here to determine if they are a potential candidate. I request a current medical summary from the treating physician to be sent with the patient's current disease status, and the most recent images for Dr. Lucas and Dr Elster to review and determine whether or not the patient would be eligible. So if this is something you and Neil think may be a possibility, I would be happy to pass anything on if you would like to request these to be sent to me.

Even if submitting an FDA appeal is a possibility, as you said, it may not be a potential benefit for your son, as I think you know that endeavors like these are not always a quick turnaround. As I stated earlier, I will pass your emails and bring it to discussion in our next meeting.

In the meantime if you have any questions, please contact me.
Regards,
Jen Comings RN BSN

* * *

To: "Plant, Ashley"
From: Dean
Subject: Re: Immunotherapy trial

Date: March 31, 2016
CC: jennifer.comings

Dear Ashley,

We began this journey at MGH. That's where the brain and spine imaging was done, and where the repeat spine-MRI will be done today. DANA Farber does have Eugene's (Neil's) brain MRI and the MGH records that go with it, along with Dr. Kieran's notes. It might be best to send those ahead to get an initial evaluation, as the tumor size (3.6 x 5.7 x 5.1 cm) may well put Neil at the very margin of acceptability, if not out altogether. It would be good to get that feedback as soon as possible, then we can forward additional tests if Dr. Lucas feels the trial is a promising route for Neil. Meanwhile, we are evaluating other treatments – "alternative" treatments – that show significant promise (if anecdotal), so please do not fear that we feel we are down to our last best hope.

Thank you, and God Bless,
Dean

PS. Does Neil need to sign any sort of authorization? Hopefully these communications are sufficient, but if a release form is needed, please send a .pdf of the form and we will have him sign it and send you a scan ASAP.

MEETING NEIL'S BIG

The time finally arrived to bring Neil back to Mass General for a do-over of his spinal MRI. We thought this should have been done before any biopsy discussions, but at least it would now add an important missing piece to Neil's puzzle. For this second spinal MRI, we were sent to an imaging center located in an older building we had not been to before.

Finding the center took some wandering — much like finding the records department. Once there, Neil reported to the receptionist, and we took a seat. The waiting room — tiny and windowless — was a curious change from looking over the city from ten floors up.

While the three of us were waiting, Charles Cormier popped his head into the room. Charles was Neil's "Big" (as in "Big Brother") from the fraternity he was pledging, the Eta Zeta Chapter of Beta Theta Pi.

"Wow," Neil exclaimed. "You made it! It's great to see you!"

"Likewise," Charles shook Neil's hand and hugged him warmly, then Neil introduced us.

"We're psyched to have Neil as a pledge," Charles told us.

We were delighted to hear it, but not wanting to take up Neil's precious time with his friend, Wendy and I excused ourselves to go find some coffee. By the time we returned, Neil was "in the tube," and Charles was waiting for us.

"It was so nice to meet you," he said.

"And you," we told him. "It's wonderful of you to come all the way here to be with Neil. That tells us a lot about you and your house, and it means everything to him!"

Charles smiled. "We're all pulling for him. If anyone can beat this, Neil can. He has amazing positivity."

We talked several more minutes about his plans for the future. Charles was unhurried and gracious, but then, it was finally time for him to head back to campus. He shook our hands warmly and gave us hugs too. It was an emotional moment.

"Please call if there is ever anything we can do," he said, giving Wendy his number. This was the first of many times Neil's fraternity brothers would stand by him.

DOCUMENTATION

When we got home from MGH, an overnight package from the Burzynski Clinic was waiting. It contained several articles published in *Neuro-Oncology* and a study published in the *Child's Nervous System* journal. The articles reviewed individual pediatric patients who suffered from brainstem gliomas, including DIPG. The study compared forty such patients, all treated with antineoplastons. The study also specified which antineoplastons were used, the median dosages given, and before-and-after brain scans of patients with exceptional outcomes.

Of the patients in the study, seventeen suffered from DIPG. All had been previously treated with "standard care," and their tumors were recurring. (This is called recurrent pediatric DIPG, or RPDIPG.) According to mainstream oncologists, there was nothing more to be done for these patients except prepare for an imminent end. After receiving antineoplastons, six of these patients lived progression-free for an additional six months, five survived at least one year, two survived two years, and one patient was alive and well fifteen years later.

These documents spanned from the late 1990s into the early 2000s, and they reinforced what we had come to expect: Dr. Burzynski had no magic bullet — no cure-all for cancer — but he had something no other therapy we knew of could point to — a precious handful of long-term DIPG survivors, now including Celeste. Could any other doctor we'd met point to similar results? I would ask, point blank.

I called Evie to discuss the package, and she was eager to take a closer look. In addition to the documents from the Burzynski Clinic, there were more emails to attend to, but thankfully, the number of was beginning to shrink.

To: "Sheryll S. Acelar"
From: Dean
Subject: RE: Treatment at the Burzynski Clinic
Date: March 31, 2016

Hi Sheryll,
Thank you for the articles and the guidance. As there are clearly some timing issues regarding scans and testing, it feels like we should wait to do them once we are there.

Does that sound best from your perspective? Our plan is to be there on or before April 11th unless there is a delay with the ANPs. We have yet to decide between flying or renting a mini-van for the trip, and we are still evaluating housing arrangements.

Talk soon, and God Bless,
Dean

Then, I heard from Dr. Plant regarding my request to start transferring records:

To: Dean
From: "Plant, Ashley"
Subject: Re: Immunotherapy trial
Date: March 31, 2016

Okay, sounds good. I'll start working on this.

Ashley S. Plant, MD
Fellow, Hematology/Oncology

And Sheryll quickly replied: *"Neil's next MRI should be done here. The screening process takes awhile before any treatment can begin. However, the PET/CT scan can be done up there if it helps you with cost. Our receptionist is on vacation today, but contact her on Monday if you have any questions about accommodations."*

AT THE WIRE
APRIL 2016

Nearly a month had gone by since Neil's diagnosis, and he was doing well all considered — better than when he'd come home. Healthy food, moving bowels, plenty of sleep, and lots of hugs from family and friends make a difference. Don't let any doctor tell you otherwise. But we knew Neil had to start one form of treatment or another. It was time to start pushing back on the monster in his head.

I replied to Sheryll's last email: *"I will try to arrange the PET/CT scan for next week in time to bring the results with us."*

She answered: *"Thank you. We will see you soon. If I hear any updates I will let you know."*

LAST MINUTE COACHING

On April 2, we received an email from Evie, providing a summary of the Kentucky Trial: *"I did some supporting research and wrote up a summary of the Kentucky trial – an attempt to explain each of the elements and why they are supposed to work. It might be a little easier to read and understand than the clinical trial website. Hopefully it will be helpful!:"*

KENTUCKY TRIAL

Radiation + Decatibine + Cancer Vaccine + Hiltinol

Overview:

This is a four-pronged approach designed to target different aspects of tumor growth. Radiation shrinks the tumor and generally works best on the higher-grade tumor cells (lower grade cells are less affected). Decatibine is a chemotherapy agent with anti-cancer properties, but its main purpose in this trial is to cause the cancer cells to produce more identifying proteins, helping the immune system to target them. The vaccine itself is made with the patient's blood cells that have been exposed to tumor-specific proteins in the lab, and Hiltonol is an experimental drug which supports the function of the blood cells. Hiltonol works best at stabilizing the low-grade tumor cells that are left after radiation therapy, which is part of the reason that radiation is required for the trial.

Trial process:

1. Blood cells harvested pre-radiation
2. Standard radiation treatment
3. Decatibine administered over 5 day period (low dose)
4. Two weekly vaccinations with blood cells that have been exposed to tumor-specific proteins
5. Hiltonol will be injected immediately after the vaccination
6. Cycles will repeat every 5 weeks for two cycles, with the potential for 2 more if the disease is not progressing

Note: <u>Study is only taking 10 participants, total</u>

Decitabine - anticancer drug (chemotherapy)
Demethylating agent — too much methylation (DNA is wound too tightly) can prevent cancer-supressing genes from being expressed.
Antimetabolite – like a Trojan horse, looks normal, but is toxic to cancer cells that incorporate them
Good blood-brain barrier penetration.
In this trial, the purpose of the decatibine is to cause the cancer cells to increase production of their marking proteins; making them easier for the immune system to identify.
Given by: IV infusion
Side effects (all reversible) include:

- common - Low blood count, fatigue, fever, nausea, cough, bowel issues, hyperglycemia
- less common - headache, insomnia, swelling, chills, low nutrients, bruising, rash, dizziness, cardiac

murmur, soar throat, abdominal pain, mouth sores, drowsiness, abnormal liver function, confusion, anxiety, itching, heartburn

Things to do when taking decatibine: drink lots of water, avoid exposure to potential sickness, small frequent meals, avoid sun

Vaccine - made from subject's blood cells (specifically autologous dendritic cells); these cells will be exposed to a combination of tumor-specific proteins.
Hiltonol - helps promote immune action, supports dendritic cells and has avaccine-boosting effect
Past studies: low doses administered to malignant brain tumor patients – showed regression or stabilization of tumor (glioblastoma patients performed less well than the rest of the group)

"Chemotherapy and radiation are generally more effective against rapidly dividing malignant cells, but are less so against low-grade tumor elements. Based on information available to date, agents such as Hiltonol may be more effective in stabilizing certain of these low grade tumor elements and could thus be useful in treatment of low grade tumors or in maintaining remission after more aggressive chemotherapy or radiotherapy."

Can't find much information about side effects...

Questions:

1. What is the likelihood that the tumor proteins being targeted will be active in Neil's tumor?
2. Is a confirmation biopsy definitely required?
3. Side effects of Hiltinol?

A+ Evie! An awesome summary that reinforced and elaborated on the information Nurse Comings had sent on the twenty-ninth. Evie was also correct in inferring we were suffering from information overload. Her "translation" re-invigorated our sense of groundbreaking potential in the Louisville trial — even so, she also highlighted potentially serious side effects. This upped the ante for pressing the argument for allowing Neil to participate — preferably without radiation.

To: Ashley.Plant
From: Dean
Subject: Status update
Date: April 3, 2016
CC: Dr. Kieran, Raffaele

Dear Ashley,

Dr. Kieran is away until the 6th, I believe, so I thought I would run this by you. Eugene (Neil) is doing reasonably well – in some ways improved, in others slight deterioration. We have him on a strict diet and a supplement regimen that seems beneficial, but we also realize that our final decision is close at hand. These are the options which seem most appealing: Louisville (if they deem Neil an acceptable candidate), the Burzynski Clinic, or doubling down on our current regimen by employing medical marijuana (which D/F is no doubt familiar with).

Louisville is attractive because it seems the most "leading-edge" and logical. If there is a good match between the proteins the trial is using to train the patients' immune cells and the most likely DIPG mutations, that would seem to hold real promise. The downside is the radiation and chemo side-effects, but if the trial is having some good results so far, I think Neil would still consider that route.

Next is Dr. Burzynski. Dr. Kieran warned us away from him in no uncertain terms. While we greatly respect Dr. Kieran's opinion, in a situation like this it would seem short-sighted to rule Burzynski out, especially when his patients include some 3-year-and-more survivors of DIPG, one of which Neil "skyped" with a few nights ago.

And finally, the diet/supplement/medical marijuana alternative. While the evidence we've found is all anecdotal, medical marijuana appears to have amazing curative properties, shrinking and in some cases eliminating cancers.

For the record, Neil is not interested in any sort of biopsy procedure. While he is likely to donate tissue should he succumb to this disease, he wants to preserve the best possible chance for a full recovery, and pulling out tiny plugs of brain-stem does not seem conducive. Even though recovery from DIPG is a long shot, if anyone can do it, it would be Neil.

While we wait on Louisville, the Burzynski clinic is Neil's top choice at the moment. However, Dr. Burzynski requires a PET/CT scan prior to admission into his trial. Since it has been just over a month since Neil's diagnosis, could you order such a scan, both to fulfill the clinic's requirement and to check on how things have changed in a month? If we found that nothing appears to have changed significantly, that could auger towards maintaining our current regimen for a while longer...

If you think we have missed anything else we should

be considering, please say so. Regardless of which path we take, we hope D/F would consider monitoring Neil's progress independently. That's it in a nutshell. You have been tremendously helpful, and I look forward to hearing your thoughts.

God Bless,
Dean F.

* * *

To: Dean
From: Raffaele
Subject: Re: Status update
Date: April 3, 2016
CC: Ashley.Plant

Dear Dean,

Thank you for the update. I understand Neil and your standpoint on the situation. The following comments are not medical advice, but personal thoughts, as always intended in the best of ways.

One thing I would say is that any examination to be done prior to treatment by one specialist/investigator has to be ordered/scheduled and planned by that provider. If Dr Burzynski needs any exams to start therapy for Neil, he would be the one to plan and order those. Only the treating physician knows why, how and when tests need to be done. As a pediatric oncologist, I would find it difficult to understand the rationale behind a PET/CT for Neil at this time, outside of a clinical trial that specifically asks for it. So I would address the question of ordering the test to be performed directly to the person asking for it.

This same point applies also to follow up. It is best to be followed closely by those who deliver treatment. It is very hard to advise on anything when patients are treated with approaches that are foreign to our practice. I think that only Dr Burzynski ultimately knows what the treatments he uses does to the human body. They might be excellent effects or toxicity, but only his clinic would know what to do. If you go there for treatment, his team should be in charge of the follow up. They are supposed to know what to expect and how to deal with the relevant observations.

Regarding medical marijuana, I have little experience, so I cannot comment. Its use in children is very limited and I have no scientific evidence to support its use outside of symptom-management. It is very effective for nausea and/or anxiety for example.

Warmest wishes, as always,
Raffaele

* * *

To: Raffaele
From: Dean
Subject: Re: Status update
Date: April 3, 2016

Thank you Raffaele! Your points are well taken. We do not know for sure if Neil will take treatment in Houston. If he does, the Burzynski clinic would of course be in charge of monitoring and advising. I was just thinking it would be invaluable to maintain some independent oversight to help interpret results once we return home. Wouldn't you think so? That may prove impractical, but at least the idea is on the table. We're hoping the picture will crystallize in the next few days, and I'll keep you posted. On balance, we are maintaining a positive attitude, largely because of all the well-wishes and prayers from friends near and far!

Thank you again,
Dean

* * *

To: Dean, Raffaele
From: "Plant, Ashley"
Subject: Re: Status update
Date: April 3, 2016

Dear Dean,

I very much agree with Dr. Raffaele's response. A PET/CT is not typically indicated in a case like Neil's, so it's hard for us to order this on behalf of another doctor and also may become an insurance issue for coverage.

In regards to the other treatments by Dr Burzynski, although I respect your interest in alternative approaches, it's hard to recommend these therapies given only anecdotal evidence at best. When there is not robust evidence for a treatment, we are accustomed to only trying these therapies in the setting of a clinical trial to make sure patient safety is number one priority.

I cannot imagine what you and your family are going through and we do want to help in any way we can, but I want to be very honest about what we know and how we think about experimental therapies. My recommendation would still be pursuing radiation while considering clinical trials. Some of the alternative therapies may not be allowed while on a trial because of the unknown interactions, so it's important to mention that up front. Your doctors should know about all therapies so we can do our best to make sure therapies are not going to interact or cause worse side effects in combination. If you decide not to do the trial, I'd still recommend radiation and if you want to try alternative therapies after then that's fine.

I'm sorry to hear Neil is now possibly having more symptoms. Did he decide to take steroids for symptomatic management?

Please keep in touch and let us know how we can be of help.
Ashley
Ashley S. Plant, MD
Fellow, Hematology/Oncology
Boston Children's Hospital/Harvard Medical School
DANA Farber Cancer Institute

ONE MONTH ANNIVERSARY

It was one month to the day since Neil had been diagnosed. He ostensibly had two months to live, although objectively, he did not seem worse for the wear since coming home. Regardless, the time for decision had arrived.

To: "Plant, Ashley"
From: Dean
Subject: Re: Status update
Date: April 4, 2016
CC: Dr. Kieran, Raffaele

Dear Ashley,

Thank you for your concern about Neil's condition. He has not worsened enough to want the steroids, although he still holds them in reserve. As mentioned, in some aspects his condition has improved. He is having a slightly easier time swallowing, and he is able to use the bathroom more easily. His gait is more or less the same, but his eyes are a bit more fixed and his speech a bit slurred, especially when he is tired. His spirits are nothing short of amazing.

Regarding the PET/CT scan, I think the need pertains to getting a better-understanding of the tumor's metabolism – the granularity between "enhancing" vs "non-enhancing." If so, logic suggests that information could be valuable. If we go to Houston, the test can be done there, but the timing is such that it would be nice to get a comparative look as soon as possible. As regards independent monitoring, since we would return home after a month to continue under remote supervision, having a local advocate would be helpful to objectively assess the treatment's effectiveness. If DANA Farber cannot not act in that capacity, I understand.

We are still very interested to learn if the Louisville trial would accept Neil. (Unfortunately, we have not gotten results from his repeat spinal MRI of last Thursday, but if something were seriously amiss I think we'd have heard.) If Louisville would accept Neil, and if your expert consensus believes the proteins being used to train the patient's immune cells are a strong match to known DIPG mutations, that would offer a compelling argument. Has

Dr. Lucas given any indication? Is there any word on how effective this trial has been to date?

We have made no final decision on treatment, but knowing the status of Neil's tumor would be helpful, as a stable appearance would suggest we are already on a good course – under the guidance of a Naturopathic Oncologist – so it might be worthwhile to continue. Bottom line: We are still uncertain about the most hopeful course of action, but "standard" treatment offers no hope beyond a short-term pause, which pretty much sets it aside unless done in conjunction with something that holds genuine promise. That leaves us searching for promise. While anecdotal evidence is not scientific, it can be very compelling when delivered by an actual DIPG survivor. **Do you know of any 3-year DIPG survivors Neil can reach out to?**

Thank you, and God Bless,
Dean

* * *

To: Dean
From: "Plant, Ashley"
Subject: Re: Status update
Date: April 4, 2016

Hello again Dean,

I'm glad his symptoms have slightly improved, that's great. He sounds like a very strong person with a lot of resilience. I will allow Dr. Kieran to weigh in on how he feels about follow-up and monitoring going forward since he has seen you both in person before. I believe Dr. Lucas is waiting for the MRI. We were able to send notes to him but since the MRI was done outside our institution I be-

> lieve it has to be sent from MGH. Once he has the scans, Dr. Lucas can then weigh in more definitively about the options for the trial. This trial is very much a phase I trial in which we have very few patients enrolled thus far. This early into the trial, we are unable to say anything about the efficacy of the therapy. I apologize that we aren't able to say much more than that at this point. **I unfortunately do not know of any 3+ year survivors of DIPG.** I am skeptical that the other doctor does as well, and many times it is a misdiagnosis and not true DIPG. Just to put in another plug for standard therapy – "pausing growth" is a benefit here because it can make it more likely that other therapies can be effective because the more minimal the disease the better for things like immunotherapy and maybe even for the alternative therapies you are considering. I know this is a difficult decision and you and Neil have been thinking very hard about this
>
> Thanks again for keeping in touch,
> Dr. Plant Ashley S. Plant

Dr. Plant's response, ever gracious, had a sadly familiar ring to my query about survivors: "misdiagnoses." In Celeste's case, having passed through the renowned halls of M.D. Anderson on her way to the Burzynski Clinic, we were inclined to believe her diagnosis was accurate. Regardless, I wasn't sure what Ashley meant by, "*Dr. Lucas is waiting for the MRI,*" so I replied immediately: *"Waiting for which MRI? The brain or the spinal? D/F has the original brain imaging. Dr. Kieran returned the CD to us, but he also pulled the file up on his computer, so it is on your system. If that hasn't been sent to Dr. Lucas, please do so ASAP – electronically if possible. I can overnight the CD otherwise. If Dr. Lucas is waiting for the repeat spinal, I'm not sure when that will be available. I have a call into MGH, but they operate on voice mail and it's difficult to communicate with anyone over there. Please advise."*

Dr. Plant replied instantly: *"I was told we cannot send uploaded images from other hospitals. I double checked again today and it has to be sent from where it was done. Sorry about this! I believe the brain MRI is most important to get sent. Sorry for the hassle."*

Wait, what? Such formalities at this stage of the game? Liability issues, no doubt, but I had to take a deep breath before answering: *"I had no idea. Last I knew, all that was needed was the authorization we gave you. Now it's almost too late. We have to move on Houston. Please send me the address to forward the CD and I will send it overnight, but we will need to get word back almost immediately – from Dr. Lucas and Dr. Kieran – to justify backing off Houston. This seems a shame, but then maybe it's as it should be. I believe Dr. Burzynski deserves a lot more credit than he has gotten. Let's hope Neil proves that to be the case!*

Dr. Plant replied again, instantly: *"Sorry for the delay! Our staff that works in this doesn't work on weekends, so we just figured this out."*

Oh my goodness. We just lost a few precious days. With no electronic transfer available, we would send the disk via overnight courier; even so, we were still waiting for Neil's second spinal MRI results. It seemed like MGH had lost interest the moment Neil failed to jump at their treatment plan. Regardless, since bad news usually travels fast, we assumed the retake was negative, or we would have heard. That meant no tumor involvement in his spine. While negative findings are usually something to celebrate, for us, it just meant the chance of Neil's tumor being something less lethal than DIPG was ruled out. We continued planning for a visit to Houston. With time suddenly growing short, we decided to fly.

To: "Sheryll S. Acelar"
From: Dean
Subject: Touching base...
Date: April 4, 2016

Sheryll,

We have made reservations to arrive on the 12th. Staying at the Marriott Townplace Suites. Things are coming together. I also wanted to advise Dr. Burzynski of Eugene's (Neil's) current condition; he is probably a 65 on the Karnofsky Scale. I hope he will maintain roughly that level for another week to 10 days. We have him on a diet and supplements (prescribed by a Naturopathic Oncologist) which seems to suit him, so thus far he's avoided any "standard" intervention. At what, if any, point would Dr. Burzynski advise Neil to use the steroids prescribed by MGH (Dexamethasone)?

Thank you, and God Bless,
Dean Fachon

Since we were traveling to Houston for a consult — at minimum — it seemed like a good idea to ask the airline about "special-needs" travelers.

Submitted: 4/4/2016 12:05:21 PM
United Airlines Support
Name: Dean Fachon
Subject: Future Travel

In the near future I will need to transport a cancer patient from Boston to Houston. We may need some assistance in the terminal and boarding. Also, we would be traveling with the patient's medications. Can you help navigate him and his meds through TSA security? I have reserved round-trip tickets; if I need to change the return date, how can that be handled with minimal expense? When making reservations, I was unable to select seating. Can you assist in selecting seats so we are all together?

Thank you,
Dean Fachon

ONE FINAL QUICK "LOOK AROUND"

While waiting for the final pieces of Neil's treatment puzzle to slip into place, Wendy found another article — about epigenetics and cancer — on the National Institute of Health's (NIH) website. In the article, a familiar name was mentioned, Dr. Jane Fountain. She had also been quoted in at least one of the links from Charles. This time, the name clicked. I'd met Dr. Fountain years before, when she was just "Jane." Now that she was with the NIH, perhaps she could offer some additional insights? On that premise, I tried contacting her at the same time we fine-tuned plans for Houston.

To: Dr. Fountain
From: Dean
Subject: Do you recall...
Date: April 4, 2016

Dear Dr. Fountain,

Do you recall the name "Dean Fachon?" Some years ago we met while you were doing your post-doctorate. We only saw each other a few times, so you might not recall. I am writing now because I was directed to the NIH web site to read an article in which you were mentioned:

> "Study points to possible treatment for lethal pediatric brain cancer
>
> NIH-funded preclinical study suggests epigenetic drugs may be used to treat leading cause of pediatric brain cancer death"

I'm doing research because my 19-year old son was diagnosed with DIPG about a month ago. Since then my family and I have been looking at every treatment approach we can possibly find. When I saw your name and your area of expertise, I had to reach out. We are looking for all the guidance we can get. If you do not recall meeting, or if this email is unwelcome, please accept my apology for the intrusion.

All the best, and God Bless,
Dean Fachon

* * *

To: Dean
From: Fountain, Jane
Subject: RE: Do you recall...
Date: April 5, 2016

Hi Dean,

Where did we meet? I need something to jog my memory.

You have already found your way to one of the most exciting advances for DIPG recently, the panobinostat clinical trial.

https://clinicaltrials.gov/ct2/show/NCT02717455?term=DIPG&rank=5

This is an experimental treatment your son could consider. Other trials are listed on the clinicaltrials.gov site. The eligibility criteria are provided for each study so you should be able to quickly tell which ones are possible. Any questions should be directed to your neuro-oncologist or the lead on the trial.

Your son is fairly old for a DIPG diagnosis, so I would encourage getting a 2nd opinion. Understanding the genetics of his tumor might also be key to deciding upon other treatments, so a biopsy could be very informative. However, often in the case of DIPG, this is not possible. Has this procedure been discussed with you both? Is it clear the tumor is inoperable? Have you gotten this opinion from at least two neurosurgeons or neuro-oncologists who have expertise in treating DIPG patients? While your son is in between the adult and pediatric worlds, the expertise for DIPG is going to be on the pediatric side.

There is also a DIPG registry/consortium to support the performance of clinical trials, care for patients, and advance research. I would encourage you to contact this consortium and have them review your son's case. Getting as many expert opinions as possible may prove invaluable in deciding on the best treatment course.

http://dipgregistry.org/patients-families/second-opinion/

There is also a preclinical DIPG consortium of scientists actively engaged in identifying new, effective treatments for DIPG. Dr. Michelle Monje is one of the investigators noted in the panobinostat link below.

http://www.cristianriverafoundation.org/

It's an exciting time for research, with some promising, novel therapeutics moving into trials. Precision medicine is driven by understanding the genetics of the tumor, but most DIPGs have common alterations, so experts may be able to make good educated-guesses on the genetics, even if a biopsy is not possible. What's key is making sure the diagnosis is correct.

If you have any questions, let me know. As you are probably aware, I am not a physician so cannot provide

medical advice. My goal is to steer you to those who can
I wish the best for both you and your son.

Jane
Jane W. Fountain, Ph.D.

What a surprise! I had no real expectation she would ever even read my email, let alone answer. While she could not know it, Dr. Fountain had just outlined much of our search efforts to date. That was reassuring. As for the study she referenced, the *Trial of Panobinostat in Children With Diffuse Intrinsic Pontine Glioma*, while intriguing, it wouldn't commence until late June of 2016. Almost three months away. Was this study so promising it justified waiting? Not with other strong possibilities much closer at hand. Even so, Dr. Fountain's enthusiasm for epigenetics was another plus, if unintentional, for the Burzynski Clinic.

To: Fountain, Jane
From: Dean
Subject: RE: Do you recall...
Date: April 5, 2016

Hello Jane,

Yes, we have a second opinion from Dr. Mark Kieran at DANA Farber. There is little doubt of the diagnosis. A biopsy was suggested, but Neil is not keen absent a real benefit in subsequent treatment. To date, no such benefit has been demonstrated.

The "Panobinostat" trial is certainly interesting, but I don't know that we can wait for 3 months. Of the many trials we have reviewed, there is an immunotherapy trial in Louisville Kentucky that seems promising. We are still trying to determine if Neil would be considered an acceptable candidate.

After this, we keep coming back to the Burzynski Clinic. Though widely decried in mainstream circles, his anecdotal results are very compelling. Neil spoke with a three-year DIPG survivor via Skype a few nights ago. None of our doctors can point to any DIPG survivors of that duration, and they discount such people as most likely having been misdiagnosed. The young woman Neil spoke with had been turned away as incurable by M.D. Anderson, which suggests a correct diagnosis.

I'm not sure exactly where we met, but I'm glad I recognized your name. Thank you for your insight and help!

God Bless,
Dean

* * *

To: Dean
From: Fountain, Jane
Subject: RE: Do you recall...
Date: April 5, 2016

Hi Dean,

I have heard of Dr. Kieran but not the Burzynski Clinic. Anecdotal stories suggest similar outcomes occur for others who don't go to this clinic. Speaking from family experience, my brother-in-law is a pediatric brain tumor survivor. His tumor was deemed inoperable at the age of 8. My in-laws drove from New Mexico home to Stanford. The neurosurgeons said "no" and sent him down the hall to Radiology. This was the mid-60s. My brother-in-law is now 57 years old. One of my colleagues had a child diagnosed with a pilocytic astrocytoma who received treatment at Johns Hopkins University and is alive and well. One of my niece's best friends was diagnosed with a chordoma 2 years ago. She had a very cutting edge endonasal surgical procedure done at U. Pitt. She is in graduate school now. (I fully appreciate that a DIPG is a more difficult tumor to treat than the 3 examples provided above.)

You can ask your neuro-oncologist about the possibility of being treated with panobinostat off-label (compassionate use). It is unknown if this therapeutic will be effective in people but there is science supporting its use. No matter what you decide to do, I would ask for scientific evidence that the agent or procedure has the potential to be beneficial. I would be cautious proceeding with anything "anecdoctal" in nature. I am a scientist, however, and have an obvious bias in this direction. A publication is not all that's important here; it has to be clear the study was performed in a rigorous way, diagnoses were correct, etc, etc.

Overall, I would consider vaccine or other immunotherapy trials. Immunotherapy has been quite successful in other cancers recently.

The Novocure device is also something that might be considered. Has anyone pointed you in this direction? The results have been a bit difficult for some in the community to accept but the scientific premise is viewed as solid. I am not sure if the electrodes can be customized for a DIPG. I would ask questions about this.

http://www.novocure.com/.

The world is a small place. Thank you for reaching out,

Best of luck with deciding how to proceed.
Jane

ANECDOTAL BONUS POINTS AND A LAST-MINUTE LONG SHOT

Despite her disclaimer, Dr. Fountain's personal accounts lent a degree of credence to anecdotal evidence. It seemed odd she hadn't heard of Dr. Burzynski, but then, most of his dustups with the alphabet agencies had been many years ago, and his anecdotal successes had been marginalized. Regardless, it was good to know she was enthusiastic about immunotherapy. As unlikely as the Louisville trial was beginning to look, we would cultivate the possibility until the last possible moment.

But there was also something new Dr. Fountain had mentioned — "Novocure." It was a company using "Tumor Treating Fields" — tuned electromagnetic radiation — to treat cancer. According to their website:

> "Tumor Treating Fields is a cancer therapy that uses electric fields tuned to specific frequencies to disrupt cell division, inhibiting tumor growth and potentially causing cancer cells to die.
>
> By using physics to influence biology, Novocure discovered another way to treat cancer. Tumor Treating Fields utilizes the natural electrical properties of dividing cancer cells."

Any treatment that promised to attack tumor cells while leaving normal cells unharmed was very exciting — the exact sort of treatment Neil was seeking. It was time to launch one more ball into the air, even at this late date.

To: Patientinfo@Novocure
From: Dean Fachon
Suject: DIPG treatment with TTField
Date: April 5, 2016

Hello,

My 19 year old son was recently diagnosed with DIPG. Because of your company's work with Glioblastoma, Dr. Jane Fountain at NIH/NINDS suggested I get in touch. Could your TTField be tuned for DIPG? Are the TTFields typically used stand-alone, or as an adjunct therapy? Are there any clinical trials under way? Where are your TTFields being used? Any further information you can send would be greatly appreciated.

Thank you,
Dean Fachon

NO ARGUMENT

While I juggled this new ball, Wendy and Neil were doing their best to pin down the right way to use medical marijuana. Neil would sit by his bathroom, window open to not stink up the house, puffing away on the various "smokable" blends he'd received at the compassion center. Then, there was "Phoenix Tears." Neil had been instructed to take no more than a single drop the first day, then add an additional drop on each subsequent day. Until how many drops? Who knew? There was one time in particular when Wendy feared Neil would stumble and fall after getting too loopy.

"You need to take it easy, Honey," she tried to coach him. "This is trial and error."

"Thith Thtuff'ith thmack," he chuckled sheepishly.

Finding the right amount of CBD and/or THC to make a "therapeutic dose" was pure guesswork. There were no guidelines, certainly not for treating anything more than a patient's discomfort. The absence of guidelines made this experiment more dubious by the day in my book, but Neil wanted to do it. At the very least, it did help him relax, helped when he had a headache, and helped him escape, if for just a few hours. Who could argue about that with a terminally ill patient? And I had plenty else to keep up with:

To: Dean
From: "Sheryll S. Acelar"
Subject: RE: Touching base...
Date: April 5, 2016

Hi Dean,

Based on the protocol, we do have plans to place him on a steroid such as dexamethasone prior to, or during, the screening process. If the doctor there indicates that he needs to be placed on steroids, we have no objections, nor will it impede him from proceeding to Houston.

I spoke with Dr. Burzynski, and since he would like to make sure Neil does well with the medicine, you may want to plan on staying longer than 3 weeks if you decide to proceed. I will keep you posted on the status of clinical trial preparations.

Sheryll

* * *

To: Jennifer Comings
From: Dean
Subject: RE: Immunotherapy trial
Date: April 5, 2016
CC: Ashley Plant

Jennifer,

I learned late yesterday that DANA Farber has not forwarded Eugene's (Neil's) image files due to their rules about sharing electronic files that were originally taken by another hospital (MGH in this case). While this is now the eleventh+ hour for us to make a decision, we do not want to completely rule out the trial unless the trial rules out Neil, so I have sent the original MGH disk and files via "FedEx overnight." The envelope should arrive there at 8AM tomorrow. Please advise as soon as you have the material and can estimate the time frame for getting back to me with an opinion on Neil's potential candidacy. Hopefully this "heads-up" will help you stage events more efficiently. Thank you for your time and effort.

God Bless,
Dean

* * *

To: Dean
From: Jennifer Comings
Subject: RE: Immunotherapy trial
Date: April 5, 2016

Hello Dean,

I will keep my eye out and let you know. I do have a meeting scheduled with Dr. Lucas tomorrow, so I'm hoping to have the disk so he can review. If not, I will give him the medical summary I received today. I'm aware of the need for reviewing Neil's records as quickly as possible. Dr. Lucas is usually very prompt once the information needed is given to him. My aim is to respond as quickly as possible.

Regards,
Jen

* * *

To: "Sheryll S. Acelar"
From: Dean
Subject: RE: Touching base...
Date: April 5, 2016

Sheryll,

Thank you. The doctor here did not make the steroids a requirement, and Neil has been very reluctant to take them, but a short period of symptom relief might outweigh the risks. For the time being, Neil is using medical marijuana to help with symptom relief. He was given a referral by his local doctor. I am also appending a list of the supplement regimen Neil is on. Please advise if there is anything he should discontinue prior to testing and treatment.

We are booked for a month and can probably extend as long as our finances hold out. I have not been able to arrange the PET/CT scan, so that will have to be done in Houston as well.

Thank you again for all your help.

God Bless,
Dean

> ***Supplement Regimen, each taken at various intervals and some more than once throughout the day:***
> Vitamin D3
> Methyl Protect
> Host Defense
> Critical Colon
> MSM
> Colloidal Silver
> Magnesium
> Iodine
> CoQ10
> Omega 3

Meriva Curcumin
Alpha-Lipoic Acid
Warrior Juice (herbal tincture)
Poke Weed Tincture
Resveratrol
Herbal tea blend
Phosphatidyl Serine
Melatonin
Colon Max

* * *

To: Dean
From: "Sheryll S. Acelar"
Subject: RE: Touching base...
Date: April 5, 2016

Hi Dean,

The supplements are fine, but he cannot use medical marijuana in Houston. It is not legal in Texas. If Neil is enrolled in the trial, he also cannot take Meriva Curcumin. Its properties could impact results. Let me know is you have further questions.

Best, Sheryll

LAST CALL

Late on the morning on April 6, I received a call from Jennifer Comings in Louisville. In addition, she sent the following email, which reviews our discussion:

To: Ashley Plant, Mark Kieran
From: Jennifer Comings

Subject: RE: Immunotherapy trial
Date: April 6, 2016
CC: Dean

Hello Dr. Plant and Dr. Kieran,

I received Neil's medical summary and images this morning. Thank you for the summary. In looking at both the summary that you had sent and the med history and images sent by MGH, there were a few discussions regarding the possibility of Neil's participation in the trial. I did phone Dean after the meeting and discussed this with him.

I told him I would follow up in an email to let you know our conversation and he had asked that I CC him as well. If there are any questions, please contact me or email Dr. Lucas directly.

I did discuss that because this is a phase 1 trial, that unfortunately there is no possibility of a waiver of the inclusion criteria, one must have had SOC therapy before beginning treatment into this trial.

Although the inclusion criteria per protocol allows collection of cells prior to any initiation of SOC treatment, Dr. Lucas felt it would be better to have some sort of treatment initiated to possibly stabilize the tumor (steroids/radiation) before flying Neil here to Louisville for collection.

We discussed the timing of this and that it usually takes 6 weeks to grow the vaccine. I encouraged Dean to please reach out to me if they chose to begin radiation and if a cell collection is something they would want to consider.

He had no further questions at this time, but I let him

know that I'm available to answer anything in regards to the trial if he had any in the future.

Please contact me if you have questions about our discussion.
Thank you!
Jen

That shut the door on Louisville unless Neil changed his mind about radiation. On the other hand, the concern about flying raised a familiar red flag. To hear it again was a bit disconcerting at this stage in the game. It had been weeks since Dr. Panis had cleared Neil for flying, and while he seemed to be doing okay, a lot could have changed. Dr. Lucas was evidently concerned that changes in cabin pressure could cause Neil to have a seizure. Wendy did some quick research and found some support for this concern. I needed to ask Neil's doctors again.

In the same breath, the Novocure device presented a new possibility, which I was trying to explore as quickly as possible.

To: Jane Fountain
From: Dean
Subject: RE: Do you recall...
Date: April 6, 2016
CC: Evie

Dear Jane,

The Novocure TTField device is very intriguing. Are you familiar with Royal Raymond Rife? TTFields sound similar to his "Mortal Oscillatory Resonance or MOR" technology. (Interestingly enough, Royal Rife was persecuted for his brilliant work.) If the TTField results are "a bit difficult for some in the community to accept," I infer that to mean better than some might have hoped for. Can you send any links to results? Since the device is FDA-cleared for treating Glioblastoma, I sent Novocure an inquiry about DIPG. Thank you for that lead!

Yes, it's a small world, even so it's often quite large in its indifference. Sometimes too it seems simple, and then overwhelmingly complex. It's a world of opposites attached. We make our way as best we can. I'm glad I recognized your name, and I thank you for having the compassion to respond! We will do our best in the days ahead.

Thank you, and God Bless,
Dean

* * *

To: Dean
From: Jane Fountain
Subject: RE: Do you recall...
Date: April 6, 2016

Hi Dean,

The Novocure device has gone through Phase III testing. Some in the field were initially skeptical. I believe the results should be available through a PubMed or Google search. I don't know for sure, but they may have interest in testing on other types of brain tumor. I just don't know if the location of the tumor would make it difficult to direct the fields. I think they've also been working to reduce the size of the battery pack to make it more transportable and less noticeable. At minimum, there is evidence it is efficacious for GBM.

Best,
Jane

I copied Evie so she could research "TTFields" as well. She got back to me quickly: *"Novocure looks very interesting...would you like me to send them an inquiry? They have contact information for clinical trials on their website."*

I replied: *"I did already. We like the sound of it too..."*

And then Novocure replied to my query:

To: Dean
From: Patient Info, Novocure
Subject: RE: DIPG treatment with TTField
Date: Wed, 6 Apr 2016

Dear Dean,

As you requested, we are providing you with information about OptuneTM (Tumor Treating Fields). There have been no clinical trials conducted to date in DIPG tumors. TTFields are used to treat tumors in the supratentorial region of the brain (upper brain).

Optune is a noninvasive regional therapy that targets dividing cancer cells in the brain and generally does not harm healthy cells. Optune works by creating alternating, "wave-like" electric fields called Tumor Treating Fields (TTFields). TTFields travel across the upper part of the brain in different directions to help slow or stop recurrent glioblastoma cancer cells from dividing.

Optune is delivered through 4 transducer arrays that are placed directly on the scalp to target the tumor. The transducer array placement is determined based on each patient's MRI results to maximize the therapy's effect on the tumor.

Indications for Use

The U.S. Food and Drug Administration (FDA) has approved Optune for use as a treatment for adult patients (22 years of age or older) with histologically-confirmed glioblastoma multiforme (GBM).

Optune with temozolomide is indicated for the treatment of adult patients with newly diagnosed, supratentorial glioblastoma following maximal debulking surgery and completion of radiation therapy together with concomitant standard of care chemotherapy.

For the treatment of recurrent GBM, Optune is indicated following histologically-or radiologically-confirmed recurrence in the supratentorial region of the brain after receiving chemotherapy. The device is intended to be used as a monotherapy, and is intended as an alternative to standard medical therapy for GBM after surgical and radiation options have been exhausted.

The most common (™10%) adverse events involving Optune in combination with temozolomide were low blood platelet count, nausea, constipation, vomiting, fatigue, scalp irritation from device use, headache, convulsions, and depression.

The most common (™10%) adverse events seen when using Optune alone were scalp irritation from device use and headache.

Only a physician properly trained and certified in the use of the device may prescribe the therapy. A list of certified treatment centers/physicians located in the United States can be found here: http://www.Optune.com/

We hope this information is helpful, and best of luck.

Thank you for your interest in Optune.
Novocure

One ball up, then down just as quickly. And the moment of decision was pounding at the door. While going to Houston was effectively certain, there was still a last minute chance of pivoting to Louisville if Neil changed his mind about radiation. Immunotherapy seemed like a breakthrough opportunity, despite the "standard care" drawbacks. Would Neil change his mind? And whichever direction he chose, how would he get there if flying was out? The logistics were daunting, and the window of opportunity was closing. We didn't panic, but we flailed a little — at least I did.

To: Ashley Plant, Mark Kieran
From: Dean
Subject: Safe to travel?
Date: April 6, 2016
CC: Raffaele

Hello Ashley and Mark,

I just spoke with Jen Comings about the Louisville trial. While they would not rule out Eugene's participation, they would want him to undergo radiation in advance of even doing the cell collection because Dr. Lucas has some concern as to whether or not it is safe for Neil to fly. He feels there could be a risk of seizure due to changes in cabin pressure. This concern is based on an image taken over a month ago. Should another image be taken to ascertain if the risk has increased substantially? Whether we go to Houston or Louisville, if this is a serious concern, it shakes up our options. Please advise.

Yours,
Dean Fachon

* * *

To: "Sheryll S. Acelar"
From: Dean

Subject: Urgent issue
Date: April 6, 2016

Sheryll,

As mentioned previously, we are in touch with a group in Louisville Kentucky that is conducting an immunotherapy trial. We had almost ruled out that option due to a snafu of information-exchange between hospitals, and due to the trial's radiation requirement, but we made one final inquiry about visiting Louisville. After seeing Neil's records they replied with a caution: Based on the size of his tumor, they are concerned about flying – that changes in cabin pressure could cause him to have a seizure. This impression is based on the images taken a month ago. What is your/Dr. Burzynski's assessment of the potential risk? We are "all systems go" to fly to Houston next Tuesday, but if there is a significant risk then we need to change plans. We can drive if we must, but doing so would change our arrival time and prolong Neil's wait for intervention. Please advise.

Thank you,
Dean F.

* * *

To: Dean
From: "Sheryll S. Acelar"
Subject: FW: Urgent issue
Date: April 6, 2016

Hi Dean,

Dr. Burzynski cannot decide without examining the patient, but if it's a big risk his advise is to drive.

I hope this helps
Sheryll

* * *

To: Jennifer Comings
From: Dean
Subject: Follow-up question regarding Eugene's possible participation...
Date: April 6, 2016

Hi Jen,

We are pinging Neil's doctors about flying. Please thank Dr. Lucas for bringing it to our attention! We are now back in a quandary. In addition to pursuing the Louisville trial, we were set to fly to Houston for a visit at Burzynski Clinic. Now we're figuring out logistics if we have to drive. As for Louisville, as much as Neil wants to avoid radiation, he is still intrigued by the novelty of the immunotherapy approach. However, if he wanted to join, the time lag is troubling. Waiting twelve+ weeks is a long time for a DIPG patient. How about this possibility: We could drive to Louisville in roughly 14 hours. You could get the lymphocytes and start training them while Neil is returned home for radiation. Both the radiation and cell prep would be finished at about the same time. Then it would be a matter of waiting whatever time must elapse between the end of radiation and the trial's commencement. If this seems potentially workable, let me know so we can factor that into our last minute deliberations.

Yours,
Dean F.

* * *

To: Dean Fachon, Ashley Plant, Jennifer Comings
From: "Kieran, Mark W.,M.D.,Ph.D."
Subject: RE: Safe to travel?
Date: April 6, 2016

Dean,

I have no idea what the concern is for flying. We allow all of our patients to fly (in fact we send many of the kids on Make-a-wish trips to places all over the world). The risk of seizures is small but real in any patient with a brain tumor. This risk is not influenced by flying except in cases where there is severe fluid buildup and pressure within the brain. You are absolutely fine to travel. Ashley had also asked about continued follow-up here at DFCI if you partake in alternative treatments. This is also fine. While we can't be giving those treatments, our responsibility is to make sure Neil is as well as he can be, and we will always do everything we can.

Mark

Thank you, Dr. Mark Kieran! He knew we were on the cusp of choosing a path he could not approve, yet his candor and compassion were utterly gracious — a true gentleman to whom we will always be grateful.

FINAL "POW WOW"

"Hey Neil," I hollered upstairs, "let's you, mom and I have a quick pow wow."

"I'll be down in a moment," he hollered back.

"Sit right where you are," Wendy stepped into the office and motioned me to follow her upstairs. "We'll be up."

"Give me second," Neil answered, and a minute later, he called down,

"Okay." He was sitting on his bed, the aroma of marijuana still wafting from the bathroom.

"Are you good to talk?" I wondered.

"Jus'a whitto buzz," he bobbed his head and held up a hand, thumb, and finger about half an inch apart.

"Yeh right!"

"C'mon Dad," he sat up straight. "JK, JK. I'm good."

I shook my head. "Got me again."

"So what's up?" Wendy asked.

"Dr. Kieran says it's fine to fly," I told them. "The risk is when there's fluid and pressure in the brain."

"No one mentioned anything like that in my scans," Neil observed.

"Dr. Kieran would certainly know," Wendy agreed.

"So we can," I said. "The question is where to?"

"Louisville still requires radiation," Wendy frowned a little.

"But immunotherapy could be a major breakthrough treatment," I had to admit.

"Could be," Wendy agreed, "but there's no track record. Nothing for DIPG."

Neil nodded thoughtfully. "That's why it's a 'phase one' clinical trial. They're making their best guess at this point."

"Yup," I shrugged.

"You know I'm not keen on radiation," Neil reiterated for the umpteenth time.

"We know," Wendy and I nodded.

"Dr. Burzynski has been successful," Neil continued. "I don't buy all the negative hype. Just look at Celeste," and he gestured in frustration with his hands. "Let's not lose our nerve at the last minute. Let's stick with that plan."

Later that day, I heard back from Nurse Comings:

To: Dean

From: Jennifer Comings

Subject: RE: Follow-up question regarding Eugene's possible participation...
Date: March 7, 2016

Hello Dean,

I anticipated your question from you yesterday, so I did propose this in our meeting yesterday. Dr. Lucas still felt very strongly that even though our protocol allows for collection of cells before the initiation of treatment, in Neil's case he felt it would be in his best interest if you are going to enroll in the trial to have some sort of tumor stabilization before traveling here (even if by car), and going through the procedure of having cells collected.

I know that this proposes a time lag that you are trying to avoid, but this was his assessment.

Unfortunately it is a process to get someone here for a cell collection. It usually is not an overnight turnaround. We have to get prior insurance authorization; I must coordinate with another department to arrange for the collection of cells; and a surgeon must place the line. To line all this up may take a couple of weeks.

You all have a lot to consider at this point, and I'm trying to be as prompt as I can to get all of the information to you and answer any questions so that you all may make a decision quickly. I'm happy to answer any and all questions!

Please let me know if there are any other questions.

Regards,
Jen Comings RN BSN

And that put the final "nix" on Louisville. We were going to Houston.

Period. I replied to Jennifer: *"Thank you. All considered, the trial is not the right way for us now, but we wish you and Dr. Lucas tremendous success! Maybe we'll have a chance to talk again."*

She answered: *"Thank you Dean. I wish you and your family the best in whatever decision you all make as I can only imagine how difficult it is to make the one that you all feel is the best for your son. Please feel free to contact me again if you do have any more questions."*

Then I sent a quick note to Dr. Kieran, 'CC'ing' Dr. Plant and of course Raffaele: *"Thank you for your indispensable candor and continued concern on Neil's behalf! As much as you would rather not hear it, he wants to go to Houston. Let's hope for another anecdotal success-story to help gum up the works. That's what we pray for, but we know there is no guaranty. We will keep you all in the loop either way."*

BURZYNSKI

What seemed like an eternity ago, Raffaele had said, *"At the end of the day, I can only encourage Neil and you to form your own opinions and decide what is best for him."* We had been through a gauntlet, looking at as many therapies as possible in what little time we thought Neil could spare. In his words, *"Of all the options available, antineoplastons seemed by far the least toxic, while giving my body a fighting chance for a future. For me this was safety."*

The Burzynski Clinic was the last ball in the air, and only time would tell if this decision was wise. I sent a quick note to Sheryll: *"We have the green light to fly from Dr. Kieran at DANA Farber. Our schedule is unchanged. Thank goodness. Talk soon. See you soon."*

Sheryll replied: *"Dr. Burzynski has informed me the Antineoplaston medicine will be available by April 21. We have a 2 week screening process prior to starting the therapy. We will perform the necessary tests and if Neil meets the requirements we will set up the catheter-placement appointment. The clinical trial requires a lot of paperwork, so we should take care of this as soon as possible. We will schedule your first visit for Wednesday, April 13, 2016 at 9:30am. See you all soon!"*

FINAL INPUTS

Neil had one last appointment with Dr. Noé before we planned to take off. We sent her a letter in advance, including all the information Dr. Burzynski had sent us:

> *Dear Dr. Noé,*
>
> *If you can, please review the enclosed documents – reports and a study of patients who took the treatment Neil is committed to trying. We have tickets reserved for this coming Tuesday to fly to Houston. Whatever impressions you have of Burzynski's therapy, we would like to discuss them.*
>
> *Neil has been taking your prescribed supplement regimen and Mary's tinctures (and doing quite well all considered), and he recently received his "medical marijuana" card and began using MM, but he will not be able to continue when we go, and he may be asked to stop taking at least some of the supplement/tincture regimen if he is enrolled in the clinical trial. He will instead be asked to take a steroid for at least a little while.*
>
> *I'm sure there will be lots to talk about when we see you, but we especially wanted to get the Burzynski information into your hands so you would have time to evaluate.*
>
> *Thank you, and God Bless,*
> *Dean, Wendy and Neil Fachon*

Since Neil had now been to Dr. Noé's office a few times for craniosacral therapy, he was well-known by her staff and warmly greeted. We sat in the familiar waiting room, and a few minutes later, Dr. Noé greeted and took us back to her office. She had reviewed the material we sent.

"As I mentioned before, I've met Dr. Burzynski," she nodded. "I've already seen much of this information," she continued, handing back the documents we had sent. "To me, his approach is logical and groundbreaking. You are wise to go see him."

"I'm glad you think so," Neil smiled.

After giving him a thorough exam, Dr. Noé noted some weight loss and admonished us to feed him more. "Hold his weight! He needs more protein."

Wendy was doing her best but promised to try harder. Dr. Noé had a few more suggestions, then she told us to call anytime if we needed her help. She escorted us back to the reception area where she wished Neil good luck and gave him a hug. With that, we made our announcement to our family and friends:

To: Family and Friends list
From: Dean
Subject: Update from EG
Date: April 7, 2016

Dearest Family and Friends,

It has been awhile since our last installment. It has been a constant roller coaster around here. We had our options narrowed down to a choice between the Burzynski clinic or a clinical trial in Louisville Kentucky that is exploring immunotherapy...

...While immunotherapy is very promising, the timeframe we have is too short, and this trial is too new. They have no way of knowing how effective the vaccine will be...This approach is fairly narrow, but it may well be strong. Will it be strong enough to thwart the tumor in its entirety? Who knows? Burzynski's approach, although lacking a sharp point, is much broader, and it has the advantage of a positive track record. Neil also spoke with a 3-year survivor who underwent treatment at the Burzynski clinic. When we asked Dr. Plant at DANA Farber to refer us to a 3-year DIPG survivor, she said there are none that she knows of. So we are booked for Houston.

Keep us in your thoughts and prayers.

Lots of Love, and God Bless,
Dean

And we received countless replies, all of which resonated in our hearts, much like this:

To: Wendy Fachon, Dean Fachon Dean
From: Charles
Subject: Re: Update from EG
Date: April 8, 2016

Hello Dean, Wendy, Evie and Neil,

Thank you so much for keeping me in the loop. I know this is daunting and exhausting. Take one day at a time. I am really excited for you! That might be a strange thing to say, but I feel there is so much hope and promise with Dr. Burzynski's approach. When do you leave for Houston? I am also curious to know if Neil has spoken to other survivors? Keep on praying and I will too!

Hugs to all,
Charles

16

"GO" FOR HOUSTON

"Imagine yourself conquering life and beating your fears. The act of imagining can help to make it reality." NF

With Neil's decision behind us, things flowed easily and with optimism, but we still had plenty of logistics to attend to — like arranging for someone to keep watch on the house. Thankfully, we are blessed with wonderful neighbors, so there was no shortage of help being offered. Cindy and Ted, along with our next-door neighbors — Tim and Sherri, and Carl and Donna — would keep eyes on the house, doing things like watering plants, checking the furnace, making sure the power was on, clearing any tree limbs that might fall in a windstorm, and just making sure things were secure. We would have our mail forwarded to Houston, but there was always the chance a package could show up, so someone would also check the doors. By splitting responsibilities, no one felt overburdened.

With worries about the house put to bed, we could focus on packing. That sounds easy enough, but packing for any length of time always seems to become an unsettled rush. How cold will it be? Should we bring rain gear? What books do we want? Where are the chargers for the computers and the cell phones? What supplements and medications should we bring? Each of these questions and plenty of others took careful thought. We made multiple lists. Of course, we could also buy things in Houston. Indeed, we would buy many things in Houston because we would be staying in a suite with a kitchen. We could do our own cooking, but we hoped to avoid buying too much else besides kitchen supplies.

Neil also had his special gear for eye exercises and his digestive wellbeing. This would all need careful packing. We debated bringing his juicing equipment, but it would have been very bulky and heavy on top of everything else. If any place would have organic juice bars, we reasoned, it would be Houston, so the juicing equipment stayed home.

CALL FOR BACKUP

Of course, Neil also wanted to bring his medical marijuana.

"We can't bring that," I said. "It's illegal in Texas."

"For medical purposes," Neil scoffed. "Come on! We can double-wrap it in ziplock bags and tuck it in the luggage."

"I don't think so," I shook my head, but he wasn't convinced.

Because second-mom Cindy had been instrumental in getting Neil "hooked up" in the first place, Wendy called her for "backup." After Wendy explained the situation, Cindy came right over. "Hey you," she hollered upstairs. "C'mon down here!"

A few moments later Neil shuffled into the kitchen, trailing that certain aroma. "Hi Mrs. G!" he beamed and gave Cindy a big hug.

"What's up buttercup," she smiled, delighted to see him looking so happy. "You ready?"

"And raring," Neil nodded.

"Yeh," she cocked an eyebrow. "You smell ready!"

Neil chuckled sheepishly.

"What's this your mom tells me?" Cindy continued. "You want to bring that stuff with you?"

"I do," he nodded. "It's helpful."

"I'm sure it is," Cindy sympathized, "but you can't bring that on the plane."

"But," he started.

"No buts! Do you want to get arrested?"

Neil scowled and opened his mouth, but Cindy cut him off. "Don't make me go up there and flush that sh*t down the toilet!"

Neil burst out laughing uncontrollably, as did Cindy and Wendy.

"I guess there's no point in arguing," Neil chuckled, slowly regaining composure.

"None at all," Cindy pursed her lips and shook her head, wiping tears from her eyes.

Touché, Cindy!

RE-ENTRY LOGISTICS

If everything went as smoothly in Houston as we hoped, we would return home and continue Neil's treatment ourselves. Preparing for that would take planning. While Dr. Kieran offered to help monitor Neil's condition, we wanted to find someone closer to home, someone who could take a more active role in Neil's treatment. We hoped Dr. Heinrich Elinzano, the chief neuro-oncologist at Rhode Island Hospital, would be willing. Wendy touched base with his office administrator, and she asked for Neil's latest records. All we had available were copies we had made to a thumb drive, so Wendy drove into Providence to drop it off. Before she even got home, Dr. Elinzano's office had called and left a message: "We cannot open the files on the thumb drive."

To: Stephanie at Lifespan
From: Wendy Fachon
Subject: Eugene Fachon's MRI files for Dr. Elinzano
Date: April 8, 2016

Dear Stephanie,

We'll ask that the MRI disk we sent to Kentucky be sent on to you. We have the go-ahead for flying from DANA Farber, so we are heading to Houston on Tuesday. The Burzynski Clinic will begin Eugene's (Neil's) evaluation/tests Wednesday morning.

The clinic will do another brain MRI as well as a spine MRI and PET scan. We still have not heard back from MGH on the results of the spinal MRI done there over 10 days ago, although we will have Neil check his portal again tomorrow. What we need is a doctor here at home to join "Team Neil" as we embark on this journey. We were uncomfortable at MGH. DANA Farber will monitor but cannot be directly involved. We are hoping Dr. Elinzano can help fill the gap for when we return.

Please call me with any concerns or questions.

Thank you!
Wendy Fachon

I contacted Jennifer Comings to request she send Neil's MRI CD directly to Dr. Elinzano. She replied immediately: *"Yes Dean, I will do this Monday morning."*

Now, that was supportive!

TOO LITTLE, TOO LATE

As final plans took shape, Evie found an online resource with some very interesting testimony from adults who had been diagnosed with DIPG. Neil was in the gray area between pediatric and adult oncology, but we had not heard much at all about adults who'd been diagnosed with DIPG.

To: Wendy Fachon
From: Evie Fachon
Subject: DIPG in Adults
Date: March 8, 2016

I found a message thread full of adults who have been

> diagnosed with DIPG, spanning 2011-2015. Worth a read: https://csn.cancer.org/node/233406

While very few adults get diagnosed with DIPG, some had found their way to this blog, and they shared their experience with radiation. It was much better than we had come to expect. Some patients had lived well beyond their prognosis — living years. From their descriptions, however, it seemed like their tumor burdens had been significantly less than Neil's when they started. One described an area of one centimeter by one centimeter. Neil's tumor was the size of a golf ball teed up at the base of his skull. There was almost no room left to grow. Even so, had we seen these comments sooner, Neil might have given radiation more consideration, but the die was cast.

17

NEVER GIVE UP

"So my question is, what are my threats. How do you block them, and how do you create counter-threats?" NF

On the afternoon of Saturday, April 9, a pair of old friends, Mike and Kristine, stopped by to wish Neil good luck. Mike was holding a brown paper shopping bag under his arm.

"Where's Neil?"

"In the study," I told him as Neil popped his head around the corner.

"Hay-lohh," he greeted his visitors with a slightly lopsided grin.

"Hay now," Mike clapped Neil's hand. "How you doin'?"

"Can't complain," Neil said warmly. "Can't complain."

"That's the spirit," Mike smiled. "I've got somethin' for you. Can we sit someplace?"

"Use the study," I suggested, and Neil led the way.

Mike sat in a lounge chair overlooking a large chess table that was handmade by Neil's Great-Grandfather Gene. Neil plunked down on the sofa alongside as Mike reached into his bag and took out what looked like a high school yearbook. "Let me show you this," he said, using the chair's arm to prop open the book. It was a yearbook of sorts — of Mike's training and graduation from Army Ranger School. As soon as Neil realized what he was looking at, he took off the eye patch to see up close.

Mike began turning pages and narrating — from his arrival at boot camp to live fire training, and from survival training to graduation. Mike's pride of accomplishment was evident, as too were the tears that crept into eyes. "A lot of these guys were killed later on — in overseas combat," he frowned for a moment.

To say Ranger School was grueling would be a gross understatement. Only the toughest apply, and most wash out. At one point, near the end of his training, Mike had become very ill and almost had to drop out, but he stuck it out.

"I was sick as a dog," he pursed his lips, "on top of no sleep for days, but I wouldn't quit," and he shook his head no way. Then, Mike reached into his bag and pulled out something that jingled. "You know what these are," he asked, handing Neil a short ball-chain from which dangled a pair of stamped metal tags.

"Dog tags," Neil answered.

"Sort of," Mike chuckled. "They're 'toe tags,' the spare set they give you in case you get killed or blown up, and they can't find your dog tags. This is what they put on your big toe to mark your body." Neil was speechless as Mike continued. "These went with me everywhere, through some very nasty sh*t you don't want to know about," he nodded, "and I brought them back." He handed Neil the tags and reached into the bag once again, extracting an old "Boonie hat." I'd seen Mike wear it many times — another token from his career overseas. He handed the hat to Neil too. "I want you to have these for good luck," Mike said simply.

Neil was flummoxed. "Holy mackerel!" He held the tags and donned the hat carefully, taking a few deep breaths to absorb the heft of these tokens — the significance of all they had silently witnessed with the man sitting next to him. "Thank you," he said almost reverently. Not knowing what else to say, he motioned to the chess board in the middle of the table. "Want a game?"

Mike accepted with glee. "I'm gonna get you back for the last time we played," he blustered, and so a hardened war veteran and survivor of scrapes we can't even imagine would do ritual battle with a young man given three months to live.

Neil got up from the sofa and settled into the overstuffed chair opposite Mike. On the table was a large hardwood chessboard where two armies of pieces — one maple and the other ebony — stood at ready attention. These beautiful pieces, from the House of Staunton, were a gift to Neil when his rating broke 2000 — making him a "chess expert" — several years earlier. Neil offered white, but Mike wanted black.

They made a few opening pawn moves when Neil said, "I'm just gonna keep playin' standard," basically offering to "kibitz" as he brought out his queen's knight.

"Alright, now you're..." Mike said, hesitating, with his fingers dancing over the board but touching nothing, as if probing Neil for his thoughts.

"Trying to get control of the center," Neil explained. "Because if you control the center, you have more control over how the game will develop."

"Alright," Mike nodded. "How many saddles do you have on that horse? He's coming to get me!" And he snorted a laugh as he advanced a central pawn one space.

"Um hmmm," Neil hummed.

"That bad?" Mike asked. "You're scaring me."

Neil laughed, a goofy chortle he tried to stifle. He knows his condition makes him laugh inappropriately, and he does not want to offend Mike.

"Don't be quiet on me now," Mike reassured him.

"Om jus' tinkin," Neil choked back another chuckle and cleared his throat, "I'm just thinking."

Moments passed.

"Alright, that's long enough," Mike loudly laughed, coaxing Neil to laugh with him.

Neil moved out the light-squared bishop.

"Okay," Mike rubbed his chin. "Alright. Hmmm. You make me feel all warm and fuzzy!"

Neil made a goofy laugh. "Hmm," he hummed. "I try. I try."

While they played, Wendy, Kristine, and I made a peanut gallery at the doorway.

Mike inhaled a chuckle and moved a knight off the back rank. "Was that good?"

Neil gave him a thumbs up. "Looked good to me."

"That's why I'm scared," Mike quipped, drawing giggles from the peanut gallery.

Neil chuckled and then got serious for a moment. "Don't worry about this; don't worry about me judging you for any moves you make. It's... Playing chess is really about what's going on in your own mind, not your opponents. I had a friend, Lexie, who came over, and I was teaching her about chess, and she was saying how she thinks it's such a psychological game, and I'm like, 'It's funny you say that. Because I couldn't find it less psychological.' I mean, it's really just about the position on the board. Doesn't matter who my opponent is, I'm playing the position. But when you're not quite sure of the moves you're making, then it's definitely a little more psychological because you're thinking, 'Oh Boy! I'm playing this knight move here. What's he gonna think, what's he gonna see that I'm not seein?'"

"Yeah," Mike agreed, suddenly pointing at me, "We do that! Me and you."

"Exactly," Neil nodded. "You second-guess yourself when all the information is right in front of you on the board, not in your opponent's mind."

"You know what I do with him," Mike said with impish glee. "We'll be playing, we'll be all focused, and I'll start telling a story." While he was speaking, Mike was moving his hands like a magician to weave a distraction.

Neil blurted a belly laugh, and Mike grinned from ear to ear.

"That's definitely trying some psychological tactics," Neil smiled.

"Alright," Mike continued. "So it's your move, right?"

"Yup, it's my move now," and Neil focused back on the board while Mike took a long swig of his beer. "Okay," Neil narrates his decision. "Play simple," and he castles, king side.

"Yup, alright," and Mike quickly pushed his queen's bishop out to A6 on the right edge of the board.

"Hmmmm," Neil pondered. "So what makes you play it here instead of the long diagonal?"

"Alright," Mike explained, "the reason I did this is because it puts you in line here," pointing to Neil's knight, "and I can take it. And if you move it, I can take your castle."

"Okay, okay," Neil nodded.

"But that's not good?"

"Umm," Neil gestured noncommittally. "In general, when people have already pulled this pawn out," and he pointed to the pawn on B6, "they bring the bishop over here," and he pointed to B7. "Right now, your bishop is out on the edge, kind of out of the way."

"But I figured he's protected by this," Mike pointed to the B8 knight.

"Well yeah," Neil nodded. "What I'm thinkin' right now is if I take, and you take back..." and while discussing this "variation," he was moving the pieces to illustrate, completely changing the board.

"Yup," Mike followed along.

"Now you ideally want to be developing your knights towards the center," Neil said, "which is what I'm trying to do.... Whereas, if you make this exchange, your knight ends up on the outside of the board. Now once you move a piece you want to be thinking, 'Okay, where can I go with this guy next? What is he doing in this area?' He should at the very least be applying some sort of pressure to your opponent, even if it's just passive pressure..."

"Towards the center of the board," Mike said, but with no certainty.

"Something like that," Neil nodded. "Whereas, in this exchange, what can you do with him next, if that knight was the only thing you could move?"

"I could go here," Mike said, putting his finger on C5, "to move in on you, but I gain absolutely nothing because your queen would have me trapped."

"Yeah."

"And I can't take that pawn because of your castle," Mike continued, "and from what else I see, I can't go there, again because of your queen, and I can't go there because of your pawn."

"Okay," Neil agreed. "So?"

"The only thing I can do is move back, basically," Mike concluded.

Neil nodded. "The idea I'm getting at is your knight will be isolated, like a man on the battlefield has gone AWOL," Neil gestured with his hands. "He's just run off in the distance, not performing his duty at post."

"I should've done that a long time ago," Mike guffawed. "Drinking margaritas under a palm tree somewhere!"

"See you later," Neil laughed, grabbing Mike's knight and galloping off the edge of the board. "Oooh, run away..." Then, he put it back and continued, "but if that's the way you want to go, by all means, send your knight riding away!"

"There you go. I can't afford the horse food!" Mike snorted. "Not to mention Rhode Island tax!"

Mike was in typical form, entertaining everyone, but especially the kid with the brain tumor, taking his mind off that problem completely.

Turning his attention back to the board, Mike murmured, "You're great, Neil."

"The general idea, Neil said, looking back at the board, too, "is if something like this exchange happens," and he continued moving the pieces to illustrate, "now I'm threatening your knight, and you don't have a good advance, so might you end up retreating — wasting effort."

"Gotcha."

"So what typically happens in an early situation like this," Neil continued, putting the knight back and moving Mike's bishop to B7 to illustrate a different line. "In a situation like this, with the bishop out here," he said, gliding his hand over the long diagonal through the center of the board, "this is what the bishop would control."

"Right." Mike nodded.

"It will be a nice diagonal for the whole game," Neil continued. "With that move, without even being threatened, the bishop will apply nice pressure in very key areas, and if something steps into that line," Neil snapped fingers, "it's ready to take out the threat."

Mike smirked and pointed over Neil's left shoulder at Sable, a small stuffed German shepherd on the side table behind him — a memento from my youth. "Is she whispering in your ear?"

Playing along, Neil leaned towards Sable. "What's that?" he asked, his ear next to her snout.

Mike used the moment to slip his second queen on the board — the reserve queen used for promoting a pawn that makes it all the way to your opponent's back rank.

As if replying to something Sable said, Neil whispered, "We'll talk to him about that in a little bit," then he looks back at the board.

Mike taps the new queen, snickering. "You gotta stay alert."

"I saw that," Neil chuckled and taunted Mike right back, "You wanna do that? Keep her."

"NO," Mike held his hands up and removed the piece, "Just break it to me easy!"

Neil smiled and gave a sage nod, gesturing over the middle of the board, "So yeah, my general suggestion is just keep..."

"Control of the center," Mike completed the sentence.

"Especially at the beginning of the game," Neil agreed. "You wanna control the center, and just in general, move pieces with an eye towards the next move they could make. So with this errant knight," he returned to the piece that started the digression, "I would bring it to D7 so it covers these squares." He pointed them out and demonstrated how this cover would allow the adjacent pawns to advance, "to apply more pressure in the center later on."

"Nice," Mike murmured. "So it's your move now, right?"

"Yup," Neil said and moved all the pieces back where they were.

"What," Mike sat up with a questioning look. "Are you starting over?"

"No, no," Neil shook his head. "Just putting things back where they were. Unless you want to start over."

"Oh, I see," Mike was dubious. "Okay, alright," he pondered. "Wait, you just... You remembered all that?!"

"Yup."

"Holy crap," Mike sat back. "He's unbelievable.... So now, based on all that," Mike wondered out loud as Neil pushed a pawn.

"So now," Neil explained, "I'm not going to take the bishop."

"And I'm doing that," Mike says, retreating the bishop.

"So you're going back. Okay." Neil rubbed his chin and stared intently at the board, then he advanced a pawn onto Mike's side of the board.

"Okay," Mike said, rubbing his chin as well. He reached for a piece then pulled his hand back to his forehead. "Oh I see," he murmured, looking at Neil. "He's starting on me."

They both chuckled.

"Oh no," Mike feigned distress, then he hovered his hand. "Alright," he said, capturing Neil's advanced pawn with one of his own.

Neil quickly took back with his knight, advancing more power onto Mike's side of the board.

"Oh boy," Mike murmured, leaning over the board and thinking. "So it's my move now?"

"It's your move," Neil nodded.

"I was afraid you'd say that."

"You don't want him moving twice in a row," I chuckled from my vantage point.

"Is that why you like to play black," Neil asked. "So you can wait?"

"No," Mike was a bit flustered. "I just knew I was going to get my butt handed to me. I wanted to make the second move to see what your first move would be, was the real reason."

Neil nodded with a chuckle. "Gotcha."

"Now," Mike said and raised a hand, paused a few seconds, then continued, "I'm going to do it." And he takes Neil's D4 pawn. "Is that what you were trying to lure me to do?"

"I don't know," Neil choked back a giggle.

"What would you have done?" Mike asked.

"What's that?"

"You wouldn't have done that? No?"

"Hmmm," Neil looked at the board and then at Mike. "Well, I haven't really calculated my full plan yet."

"Oh boy," Mike looked to us for commiseration.

"But uh," Neil chuckled, "this looks fun, so," he picked up his knight, takes Mike's F7 pawn and attacks Mike's rook in the bargain. "So I'm gonna do this."

"Owe," Mike winced. "I thought you liked me dude! Well that sucks!" And he laughed, slapping his thighs, then he thought for a while before moving his rook to G7, out of harm's way but also sacrificing some of the rook's leverage.

Neil pressed his attack by advancing his queen to a diagonal, which doubled up protection on the knight while taking a pawn and attacking Mike's king in the process.

"Holy crap," Mike sounded less chipper. "This guy don't mess around. Jeepers creepers. Man you've got that thing pretty well protected, eh?"

"Yup," Neil agreed. "Why didn't you just take the knight? Could've taken it with your king."

"You mean earlier," Mike asked.

"Yeah," Neil nodded, "instead of moving the rook."

"Because you intimidate me?"

We laughed hard, the lot of us. That was comedy! Mike is intimidated by nothing.

"Yeah, no," Mike wagged his head with chagrin in the light of hindsight.

"You wanna go back a couple of moves," Wendy piped up from the peanut gallery.

"No, no," Mike scoffed. "I'm good. I'm learning. It's not every day I get to play the best," he added, continuing to ponder. "Alright," he finally reached for a piece, but then stopped, shaking his head. "I don't see anything else I can do, do you? To get out of that?"

"Well," Neil commiserated, "you only have one move you can do right now."

"And I don't even see it," Mike admitted.

"You can block," I suggested.

"Well yeah," Mike nodded reluctantly, moving his king's knight to block Neil's queen.

"That's the only move you can do," Neil concurred. "If you want to keep playing."

"Just shortening my..."

"Execution," Kristine finished her husband's thought with a giggle.

Now, Neil took a long look at the board, hand on his chin and tipping his head back and forth ever so slightly as he ran various moves through his mind.

Mike thumped his foot nervously. "I can see smoke coming from your eyes."

"See," Neil shared some of his own battle experience, "you can get into a tournament and do this for an hour straight, just thinking about one move."

"I've seen you do that," I boasted a little. "I've seen you play full-length games back-to-back — eight hours straight — and win both."

After a couple of minutes, Neil finally moved his queen's bishop, severely hampering any chance Mike might have had at a counterattack.

"Um Um Um Um Ummm," Mike ruminated, then he reached for a piece but withdrew his just as quickly. "I see that one! Son of a gun."

Now "smoke" was coming from Mike's ears as he moved a bishop to attack Neil's bishop, then withdrew it. "That's kind'a dumb," he spoke softly. "Right?"

"Uhh," Neil spoke softly too, "from my perspective, I would have to say yes."

Then, they both broke out laughing, and Mike looked at us. "Oh that's funny! But he's honest." Half a minute went by, then he moved his G pawn.

Neil reached out and touched Mike's queen. "What about her?"

"What?" Mike asks.

Neil wiggles a pawn, which can take Mikes' queen.

"Oh! Why did I not see that?" Mike shrugged, sitting back in his chair. "It is what it is."

"Go back a move and do something different," Wendy suggests again.

Neil coaxed him too. "Where would you move your queen?" he said as he slid Mike's pawn back where it was.

Mike started thinking out loud while gesturing over the board. "I could put it here to pressure your queen, but then you'd just kill me with your knight, so I can't do that. And then I could go over here, but you kill me with this knight. And I could go over here, but you can still get me with the knight, and then I thought about going over here, which would probably be my most lucrative move. Correct or incorrect?"

"I would say that's a good analysis, soldier," Neil smiled warmly.

So, Mike brought his queen back to protect his king and get out of harm's way.

"He's infiltrated your side of the board," Wendy sympathized.

"Yeah he has," Kristine gently nodded.

"I'm just playing like..." and Mike squinched his nose and gestured like he was juggling turds before taking another tug on his beer.

After a minute or so, Neil moved his queen straight back one square.

Mike's hand went to his face. "Umm Umm Um Um Ummm," and out came that knight again.

Neil immediately retreated his queen on a diagonal.

"Was that a good one that I just did," Mike asks him.

Neil agreed with a small nod as he stared at the board, then he looks up. "I don't know, was it?"

"Hey now!" Mike did a double take at his position. "Oh my lord. Now I see what you're doing."

"What am I doing?"

"You want to punch through," Mike said, tapping a square on the board.

Neil chuckled softly and shrugged with his hands. "Maybe, maybe not."

"And you said this game is not psychological?!"

We all laughed.

"How about, I don't want to find out," Mike smirked with good humor as he continued to contemplate. He reaches for a piece. "Not cool," and withdrew his hand to his cheek. "Alright," he started, "that's not bad, but I don't know. I see that," and he hummed. At last, he took hand his from his cheek, tapped the table, and moved his knight, attacking Neil's bishop. "Bad?"

"No, I wouldn't say so," Neil shook his head.

Mike chuckled softly, and Neil laughed again, then he took his time inspecting the board before moving his bishop right next to Mike's queen-side knight.

Mike quickly pushed a pawn to attack Neil's vulnerable bishop, and Neil immediately advanced his queen all the way to the sixth rank on the G-file. The resulting threat to Mike's king forced him to move it before he could take Neil's bishop. (That's the nature of chess, setting up hidden threats in advance and unveiling them to throw off your opponent's plans.) When Mike's move introduced no unexpected variations, Neil just made the move he had planned a few moves ahead of time.

After a minute's pause, Mike grabbed his king's knight and whinnied. Smirking, he moved the knight back to defend against Neil's queen.

Neil smiled and choked back a laugh, maybe with just a touch of predatory glee. "What made you do that?"

"Oh wait," Mike realized his blunder. "What did make me do that? Good Lord! It is what it is. I see. Nope, I really screwed that one up. Oh my Lord."

"Maybe," Neil commiserated. "Take another second on that one. On that move."

"Are you sure?" Mike asked.

"Absolutely," Neil nodded. "Think about it a little more."

"It was here, right?" Mike asked as he returned his piece to its former position.

"Yup," Neil nodded.

"Yeah, that was dumb," Mike mumbled. "Way dumb. But I'm kind of screwed though, and he hummed softly. "Wow, I see where you're going with this program. I can't really do much to stop it from happening," he said finally, rubbing his chin.

"Well, I think you can," Neil replied softly.

"Walk him through it a little bit," I coaxed.

"Well," Neil leaned forward, "what am I threatening?"

"You're gonna get this right now," Mike said, tapping a piece on the far side of the board.

"Well, if I take it, what do you do?" Neil asked, and he started moving pieces to demonstrate.

"Pardon me," Mike said as once more he was whisked to the "classroom."

"If I take this, what do you do?" Neil repeated, holding his queen over the piece he could take.

"Cry," Mike smirked.

"You say, 'Thank you very much,' and take my queen," Neil told him. "Even exchange," and he removed his queen from the board.

"Right," Mike nodded. "I guess it's not over."

"But you wanna," Neil started to say, but then dissolved into laughter. He just looked Mike right in the eyes and chuckle-talked as he put the pieces back in the positions they were. "So, right now, taking this guy is not a question for me because I'd lose my queen, which I don't want to do. So what am I threatening?" As Mike pondered, Neil continued, "If you move your knight here, then, uh, I guess I'm not threatening," and he smiled.

"Yeah, yeah," Mike said. "I see it now."

Neil chokes down a laugh, not wanting to be rude.

"I understand," Mike nodded. "Don't worry about it. But what happens now is you'll move this and put me in check."

"Okay," Neil agreed. "So, what's my threat if I do that?"

"My king. The king himself," Mike said.

"It's just putting you in check," Neil agreed. "There's worse things that can happen."

"Correct," Mike nodded, and pointed to various squares on the board as he ran through his options. "The smartest thing I would think of is probably this," he said, sliding his king out of check while giving Neil a questioning look.

"Don't look at me," Neil shrugged, still holding down chuckles.

"Alright," Mike stopped fishing. "Let's see what you do with this," and he sticks with the king move.

"That's the only move that keeps you alive," Neil nods.

"That is?"

"Yup," Neil confirmed and goes back to inspecting the board.

Mike looked at us, made an exaggerated wipe of his forehead, and grinned, then took another pull on his beer. "When you come back from Houston," he tells Neil, "I'm going to show you how to drive an eighteen-wheeler."

Neil chuckled.

"And you get five hours to figure out the rest," Mike snorted, and Neil chuckled with him.

"Your dad came with me," Mike recalled. "Twice, right?"

"At least twice," I nodded. "I think maybe three times."

"And you know what I do on a CB radio," Mike grinned manically, winding up for a pitch.

"Oh my goodness," I laughed at the memory of the back-and-forth between the truckers. "That was some funny stuff! I couldn't understand half of it. I'm sitting there thinking, 'What the heck did they just say?'"

"Oh yeah," Neil smiled, trying to stay focused on the board.

"It's because of the slang we use," Mike slapped his thighs with glee at the chance to unwind. "'Captured four wheels, plain wheel wrappers' and..." Then, he noticed Neil made a move. "Did you just move?"

"I did indeed," Neil drawled sardonically, not taking the bait and pointing at the bishop, which was formerly alongside Mike's queen-side knight. "Right here."

Mike wouldn't have it and tried a new trick. "My German shepherd has four of those," he chuckled as he grabbed two bishops and held them to his chest like a pair of nipples.

At that point, we all "lost it," and Mike rolled with it.

"You should have seen me when I was younger," he aped, repositioning the bishops to his forehead, like horns, and impersonating Kristine's voice:

> "'Honey, did you stop at the bar?'"
> "'Nooooo!'"

Next, he held a bishop to the tip of his nose, "Pinocchio!" He was relentless. Then, letting the laughter subside, Mike clapped his hands. "Alright, let's get back to looking at the board."

"Let's get serious here," Kristine wiped her eyes with a chuckle.

"He's trying to distract you Neil," Wendy wiped her eyes too.

"Umm hmm," Neil chuckled. Try as he might to focus, he couldn't wipe the grin off his face.

"Ask your dad, I'm really good at it," Mike grinned again, then he finally looked back at the board.

Neil stifled another goofy laugh. "Alright...Alright."

"You wanna break it to me easy," Mike said, "I can tell." He looked at the board and thrummed his fingers on the table. Almost a minute went by before he picked up his queen. "Would I be dumb to do this," he asked as he moved her. "It doesn't really accomplish anything, but..."

"Well," Neil resumed his prodding too. "Why would you play that move?"

"Umm," Mike said. "Try to keep this under suppressing fire," he said, gesturing to Neil's queen. "I know you could kill it anyway with the pawn. Kinda makes it kinda dumb, huh?"

"Well," Neil began, "right now you kinda have to think, 'What are my threats, and how do I start to get counterthreats,' because you've kinda been on the defensive all game."

"Yup."

"So you wanna think about ways you can you do that," Neil said as he picked up Mike's queen. "And to me, this move," he moved Mike's queen one way, "or this move," then another, "would instantly put my knight under pressure, forcing me to back up a little bit. So that's a good place to start. From there, you wanna think about getting more of your pieces into the game."

"I'd say by probably trying to open this up," Mike gestured towards a pawn.

"Yes," Neil agreed, likewise gesturing as he continued his critique, "'cause right now this bishop is closed off; this knight is on the rim with no way back; and your rooks are kinda out of the game."

"Right," Mike nods.

"Okay," Neil continued, getting tired and slurring a little, "so now you're thinking, I'm in a bad position. How do I coordinate my pieces to work together again?"

"Alright," Mike agreed. "I'll go with this method," and he advanced the pawn. "That alright?"

"Opening up for the bishop," Neil nodded, "sure."

"That's good, right," Mike asked again, smiling as he took another swig of his beer.

"It's a move," Neil replied coyly. "I'm not going to say it's the best move, but it's a move," he chuckled, teasing a little, then he resumed his inspection of the board, left hand to chin, right hand on his knee.

Mike cleared his throat, but no jokes were forthcoming.

Half a minute of silence, then there was a flurry of moves: Neil slid his queen's rook to D1, taking more control of that file. Mike quickly moved his rook to E8, attacking Neil's knight. Neil withdrew his knight to a location that threatened Mike's queen. Mike moved his queen to a new square and held his finger on the tip of her crown, taking a moment to see how the position looked before committing.

"Dumb, or good?" Mike asked, removing his finger.

Neil quickly moved his bishop and said almost immediately, "Well, that actually doesn't help me." He squinted his left eye briefly to exclude double vision. "No, it doesn't. Oops. Too late."

"Go ahead," Mike offered.

"What's that?"

"You can take it back," Mike offered.

"No," Neil says, "I mean you haven't taken any moves back."

"Ha," Mike smiled broadly. "I think I might have."

"I'll figure something out on the fly," Neil smiled.

"Oh I'm sure," Mike smirked back, and they chuckled softly together. Then, Mike resumed his inspection of the board, trying to decide how to take advantage of this new opportunity. He hummed and started to reach for a piece, but then quickly pulled back, "not so fast" written on his face, then he sighed and took Neil's vulnerable knight. "Dumb? Smart?" he asked.

"Smart," Neil nodded. "That was me pulling a 'dumb,'" he smiled and looked Mike right in the eyes.

Mike grinned ear to ear, making big dimples and hand gestures as if batting something back and forth. "He's playing 'Tom and Jerry' with me."

Neil snorted, then he moved his king's rook alongside his queen's rook, inviting a trade of rooks.

Mike rubbed his chin for several moments, then he cleared his throat. "Aye-yi-yi-yi-yi-yi!" He slid his rook one square to the right and mumbled to himself, "That's f*ckin stupid. Oops, excuse my language, stupid," he laughed. "Am I right about it being stupid? I mean you're just gonna come down," he gestured "hopeless" with his hands, "and take that."

"Probably not the brightest move," Neil mumbled, squinting at Mike's side of the board.

"Huh?"

Neil cleared his throat, "It's probably not the brightest move."

"Right," Mike mumbled as he tried to imagine Neil's potential responses, "'cause then that puts me in check. But then I could kill with that, but now your queen can come in..." and Mike grimaced.

"Once again," Neil said, also speaking with his hands, "my question is, what are my threats right now?" And he reached over the board and lifted his bishop, revealing an attack on Mike's queen from one of Neil's rooks. "If I move this bishop anywhere, your queen is under threat. So I've got a lot of options with this bishop right now," and he slid it back and forth to illustrate, "which puts your queen under threat in addition to whatever I attack with the bishop. So if you move your rook," and he slid Mike's rook, "I can just take you first."

"And I just opened up the door for you to come in," Mike shook his head.

"Yes," Neil agreed, "and you're not figuring that I've revealed a threat on your queen," he said. "You're not addressing the root problem right now."

Mike leaves the rook where it is.

"I may not move the bishop," Neil continued. "I haven't really decided. But until you've addressed the root problem, the move you were planning is the best."

"Hmmm," Mike barely mustered a sound, feeling stymied.

"What's that called?" I asked. "A revealed check?"

Neil squinted at me. "A revealed attack. If it were his king, that would be a revealed check."

Mike looked at me too. "You got yourself a smart individual over here, cap'n," then he straightened up. "Where were you, years ago?" he asked Neil.

"Years ago," Neil looked up with a grin. "Well, let me tell ya," he puffed up like he was about to make up his own joke.

"Let me tells you a story," Kristine laughed.

"Let me tell you a story," Mike jumped on the opening. "When I was driving my stroller..."

"Your eighteen-wheel stroller," I added a twist.

"My CB radio went out," Mike did not skip a beat, "and I tell you what, I threw my pacifier right out the window!"

That tickled Neil's funny bone so hard he burst out with a belly-laugh he couldn't contain in the least. The look on his face was priceless.

"When I came out'a my momma," Mike continued, "I looked at the doctuh n' said 'Get me a beer!'"

What a line!

It took several moments for everyone to catch their breath, tears rolling down our cheeks. When the laughter finally subsided, Mike smirked, "I'm not right, by the way. In the head." Then, he leaned towards Neil and reached his hand across the table. "It's like this."

"Say again?" Neil asked.

"It's like this," Mike repeated. "Take my hand."

Neil reached out and grasped Mike's hand.

"Never give up," Mike said somberly.

Neil chuckled, not meaning to, and choked it back.

"Got me," Mike asked, a bit of flint in his eyes.

"Okay," Neil nodded.

"That's what you do on the battlefield," Mike told him.

"Yup," is all Neil could manage, taken completely aback by this sudden shift.

"Never give up," Mike repeated, then he released Neil's hand, and it was back to the races. "I've got some sh*t to do with you when you get back. I'm gonna kick your ass!"

Neil laughed, but he was still trying to absorb what just happened.

"Alright," Mike continued, punctuating his message with a slap on the table that jiggled the board, then he drilled his eyes back down on the pieces. "You're tough, man. You are one smart individual," he spoke softly as he tapped the table. "I've got to hand it to you. I've never seen anybody as smart as you."

"Oh c'mon," Neil fended off the compliment.

"Oh no," Mike replied. "Dude, I've seen you play at my house. I know you're playing 'cat & mouse,'" he laughed. "You're being nice to the company." After a few more moments of looking at the board, Mike groaned, "I suck at this game."

Neil chuckled softly in commiseration. He'd been there too.

Then, louder, Mike said, "You got a gift!" And after a few more seconds, he moved that knight, which had been sitting off on the side of the board the whole time.

"Gettin' the knight back in the game," Neil smiled, then he pushed a pawn forward, putting more pressure on Mike's already pressure-packed position.

"Man, he's tough," Mike scowled at the board and groaned again, his queen completely embattled. "You got something against black women," he teased unflinchingly. "Man oh man oh man, you're killin' me," he shrugged, reached for a piece, then pulled his hand back. "Nope." He looked up at Neil, put his hand to his mouth and sighed. "Man, this sucks," expressing the frustration most chess players try to hide. Mike finally reached for his queen, moved it, moved it back to where it was, then moved it again, his finger poised on its crown. "Good or dumb?"

Neil smiled and resumed playing possum, "I dunno."

"I hate it when he does that," Mike grimaced playfully, releasing the queen. "He makes my liver quiver!"

Neil waited a moment, squinted at the board, then captured a knight with his bishop.

Mike chuckled, resumed his hand-to-chin gaze at the board, and hummed. A few moments later he looked up. "Did I ever tell you how much I suck at this game?!"

He and Neil snorted in unison.

"Ohhhh sh*****t," Mike dragged the words out under his breath. The end was drawing near, but he took Neil's bishop nonetheless.

An even exchange, except Neil reached immediately to take Mike's bishop with his queen, then he leaned back, squinting his uncovered left eye.

Mike moved his queen one diagonal square, and Neil reached quickly again to push his queen all the way to the eighth rank — the side closest to Mike — which put his king in check and attacked his rook at the same time — a classic fork.

Mike reached quickly to move his king, and then realized he'd been trapped. "Ohhhh!" He smirked at Neil and wagged his finger "naughty boy."

Neil inhaled an awkward laugh, nodded, and smiled warmly, reveling in the camaraderie.

Mike moved his king to the only safe square, and Neil reached over and swept Mike's rook off the board. The end of the game was at hand.

"Yeah," Mike acquiesced. "I knew that was coming."

Neil smiled, appreciating Mike's grace.

"Oh my," Mike declared as he reached for a piece. Then, he pulled back, saying, "And then you kill that. I'd say my ending is here, huh? Pretty much. In two moves?"

Neil nodded gently. "The cookie crumbles pretty quick, yeah," he agreed, his eyes brimming with respect for Mike's humor, courage, and humility.

Mike looked at me with a big smile. "Son of a gun, he's smart, I'll tell you what," and he laughed. "Nice!" Then, he reached across the board to "high-five" Neil. "You're the best. Unbelievable. Wow!" Then, Mike added, "I went wrong like four moves ago. Well, the whole game, really."

"The whole game was an interesting prospect," Neil nodded, prepared to debrief, which is what usually happens after a tournament game, in the "Skittle's room."

"But I was on defense the entire game, from start to finish," Mike marvels.

"That's often all black can do," Neil tried to allay Mike's chagrin.

"But I couldn't get in there," Mike pointed to Neil's castled king, "because your king is well protected."

"M'yup," Neil nodded.

"And you've got," Mike gestured over Neil's defensive line of pawns. "I would've had to forfeit maybe two pieces to get in there!"

"M'Yup," Neil agreed again. "You couldn't force your way in there. That game was more about getting control of the center, getting your pieces working together."

"Even with that scenario," Mike stated, "you have to get to the corner at some point to attack a castled king."

"What's that?"

"How could I keep everything in the center?" Mike asked.

"Well," Neil demurred. "You don't necessarily keep your pieces in the center. It would get pretty crowded. But you wanna make sure they're on active squares where they can..." and he gestured over the center of the board.

"Control the center," Mike nodded.

"Generally, yeah," Neil nodded back. "Have some control of the center."

"But I didn't have a chance to even break through there," Mike pointed, "because of the way you..."

"Yeah," Neil nodded. "No, you never had a chance to attack my king. Sometimes that happens. You can't always be on the offensive. Sometimes you are just going to play defense. But if you're stuck on the defensive, you wanna," and he thumped the table and slurred a little. "You definitely wanna make sure that queen doesn't get around the back. Secure the corners."

"I see that now," Mike smiled appreciatively.

Mike and Neil had one last good chuckle, then Wendy announced that dinner was ready. In the last forty-five minutes, Neil had laughed more than he had in the previous four weeks combined.

As they got up from the table, Mike looked at Neil with a sober expression and extended his hand once again, "Thank you, Sir!"

Wearing Mike's Boonie hat and holding his toe tags, Neil grasped Mike's hand warmly. "Thank you, Sir! Thank you very much!"

"You know why I gave you those, right,? Mike quizzed him.

"I have some guesses," Neil answered.

"'Cause I want you to hand'm back to me when you're better. Never give up!"

As the "boys" finished up at the chess board, Evie and Alex arrived to join us for dinner. The table banter was much more subdued, and when we all finished, Mike and Kristine took their leave.

"Remember what we talked about," Mike hugged Neil.

"How could I ever forget," Neil beamed back, the Boonie hat still perched on his head.

"Rematch when you're back," Mike added.

"You go it," Neil smiled.

After Mike and Kristine departed, Neil asked Evie and Alex if they'd like to play some *Mario Kart* on the old Game Cube.

"You need, you ask," Evie winked, and the three of them holed up on the porch to get a good dose of togetherness before we departed for Houston. For the next hour or two, hoots erupted intermittently from the porch — the indelible sounds of a home being lived in. When it came time for Evie and Alex to leave, we gathered in the kitchen to say our goodbyes.

"I'm gonna miss you," Neil told his sister, his trusted companion through so much of his life, eyes watering.

"Oh Buddy," she smiled and gave him a big hug. "I'm gonna miss you too!"

"But you'll come down for his birthday," Wendy said.

"Of course," Evie assured us. "I wouldn't miss it."

"Make it so," Neil winked and hugged his sister and Alex in a three-way farewell.

18

HOUSTON APPROACH

"Commitment, passion and belief is the foundation of action." NF

APRIL 10, 2016

With two days to go, we focused on final preparations for an extended stay in Houston — clinical trial or not. Such was the clinic's focus as well:

> **To: Dean**
> **From: "Sheryll S. Acelar"**
> **Subject: Re: Urgent issue**
> **Date: April 10, 2016**
>
> Hi Dean,
>
> I want to confirm your date of arrival to Houston. Since the ANPs will not be available until April 21, we will have time to do the following while you are here with Neil:
>
> 1. To do a complete and accurate history, physical examination and neurological examination performed by Dr. Burzynski
> 2. Initiate Neil on steroids such as dexamethasone prior to getting his MRI brain and spine and PET/CT brain.

He must be on a fixed dose for at least 5 days prior to the scans

3. Acquire baseline labs, Chest xray and ECG.
4. Start the initial training for preparation of medicine which will be guided by an infusion nurse
5. Read the consent form thoroughly, go over any questions and sign
6. Discuss finding a doctor at home who will help your son. The doctor will need to sign a form to become part of the study – a sub-investigator – if Neil enters the trial.

We will discuss all additional details, and we are hoping Neil qualifies for the clinical study. If he does not for some reason – if we find anything from the blood test, clinical condition or scans that disqualify him, then Dr. Burzynski will discuss other possible options. If options other than the trial are pursued, you will be responsible for the costs.

We hope to see you soon.
Best,
Sheryll

We knew we would need a local doctor to help once we returned home. Now, we learned that if Neil gets enrolled in the trial, this doctor would also need to become part of the study — a "sub-investigator." For the moment, we took it in stride, assuming this piece of the puzzle would fall into place.

I replied to Sheryll: *"We are arriving on the 12th at 7:52PM, UA flight 372. Staying at Marriott TownePlace Suites. We have dexamethasone but Neil has not taken it yet. Would 2 MG be a sufficient dose? We can start him tomorrow if you can let me know early enough. The rest sounds logical and we look forward to seeing you and hopefully starting treatment. One other question: For roughly how long do you expect Neil will have to take steroids? He is not a big fan of the idea."*

Sheryll answered: "*Dr. Burzynski says he would like to see Neil before he starts taking the dexamethasone. Dr. Burzynski will discuss the length of time and steroid dose at that time.*"

As serendipity would have it, at the same time we were preparing for our journey, a new video series about alternative cancer treatments was published — "The Truth About Cancer." Created by Ty Bollinger, the series promised a deep dive into cancer treatments — mainstream and alternative — the latter being the path we certainly felt we were on. We looked forward to watching the series when time would permit, but for the moment, we took its arrival as "good karma." Save for a complete remission of Neil's illness, our spirits could not have been better.

APRIL 11, 2016

Most of our bags were packed, and we went through our checklists again and again, trying to imagine everything we might need.

"Whatever we've forgotten, we can buy in Houston," Wendy smiled. "Just so long as you have all your gear," she told Neil.

"Yup," Neil agreed. "All packed."

"I think we're set," I clapped my hands. "Unbelievable."

Neil gave a "thumbs-up." All that was left was dropping a spare set of house keys off with Cindy. Wendy gave her a call.

"C'mon down anytime," Cindy answered. "We're here."

Wendy walked down to the Grady's to deliver the keys.

"We've got this," Cindy promised. "Everything will be fine. You focus on taking care of business!"

"We'll do our best," Wendy nodded.

"How are you getting to the airport?" Cindy asked as she gave Wendy a farewell hug.

"We're taking a limo," Wendy told her.

"Uh huh," Cindy grunted, a skeptical look briefly crossing her face, then she smiled. "Good luck my friend! We're here if you need anything. You call us!"

"We will," Wendy promised as she stepped out the front door. "Thank you." She blew Cindy a kiss, then she turned and walked home.

"We are blessed with good friends," Wendy said as she hung up her jacket in the back hall.

"We sure are," I agreed, then we took one more "last look" at our checklists.

A little while later, the phone rang. It was Anne Palumbo. "I'm driving you to the airport tomorrow," she told Wendy, having learned of our "limo" plans from Cindy.

"That's not necessary," Wendy thanked Anne gratefully. "We have a limo lined up."

"Well un-line it up," Anne insisted. "Of course I'm driving you! I want to see my Neil off."

Anne was like Cindy — any friend of her kids was one of her kids. Neil had known her son Mark since kindergarten, when he, Neil, and Andrew all took Taekwondo lessons together. So, we had a ride to look forward to.

"Couldn't be better," Neil chuckled when he heard the news.

DEPARTURE
APRIL 12, 2016

No more juggling emails, no more balancing one course of action against another. We were committed: Neil was two thumbs way up; the plants were watered; our friends were briefed; we were packed, and our bags were piled in the kitchen, ready to shuttle out the back door. It was a formidable pile. For the first time in my life, I could foresee needing porters for help at the airport.

Anne drove a big SUV, tailor-made for lugging kids and equipment to Taekwondo tournaments, even if those days were long past. Now, the vehicle was cleared out just for us. Our luggage completely filled the rear compartment, then we piled into the seats. On the ride to the airport, we reminisced about Taekwondo and school memories, and Anne asked Neil about college and girlfriends. Every so often she would glance in her mirror at Neil. "You got this," she told him.

The traffic was light until we neared downtown Boston, then the usual brake lights began to appear. Anne checked her phone for a traffic report. Nothing unusual coming up, but we had planned an extra hour just in case. Traffic at the airport was dense. Cars were pulling up two-deep at the curb, but Anne would have none of it. She carefully, but aggressively, nosed her way right up to the curb, and as luck would have it, we were next to a curbside check-in. We piled out and unloaded the SUV.

"You've got this," Anne repeated and hugged Neil a long time. "You're all in my prayers every night. Keep me posted, and let me know if there's ANYTHING I can do!" Then, she gave Neil another hug. "I'm picking you up when you come home," she promised.

"I look forward to it," Neil grinned, a grateful tear in the corner of his un-patched eye. We watched as Anne nudged her way back into traffic, beeping goodbye, then she disappeared.

Turning to the attendant at the check-in kiosk, we started the second leg of our journey. Curbside check-in was remarkably easy. With our bags neatly tagged, stacked, and in the airport's custody, we had only our carry-on bags to manage. This made it much easier to navigate through the throng of foot traffic. We located the nearest TSA officer to explain our situation. Having contacted TSA ahead of time, they were expecting us. The officer whisked us to the head of the security line and offered to get a golf cart to take us to our gate. We had already been sitting on the drive, and we would be sitting for the next several hours. Neil was in good spirits and happy to walk, so we thanked the officer and set off on foot.

Flanked by his parents, Neil ambled toward the gate. With our flight not departing until 4:33 p.m., we had well over an hour to wait, so we stopped at Hudson News to look at the magazines and buy some gum to help keep our ears clear during takeoff and landing. Neil also wanted a neck pillow — one of those horseshoe-shaped pillows you put around your neck with the thickest part under your chin, so the padding supports your head if you nod off. This was vaguely reminiscent of Neil's "Ninja" days playing soccer. We got him a "premium" pillow to support his head and neck as much as possible.

The waiting area was almost empty as we looked for seats near the gate. Of the few people there, a couple slightly older than Wendy and I had noticed Neil's eye patch and irregular gait and asked politely if we needed any assistance.

"No, but thank you," Wendy smiled and sat next to them. Neil and I plopped down as Wendy struck up a conversation with our "neighbors." Upon learning of Neil's situation, the woman confided that she and her husband had suffered a similar experience. It's a small world where cancer is concerned, and the conversation helped pass the time quickly. Soon, the flight was announced, and the agent at the ticket counter motioned us to board first. Between that and the business-class seats we tucked into, our "sailing" was going as smoothly as possible.

The flight to George Bush Intercontinental Airport was uneventful. Looking at Neil, one might think we were taking him to visit a college. He had taken off his eye patch, popped in his earbuds, and was snoozing, his pillow doing exactly what it was designed to do. Wendy and I browsed the flight magazines and passed the time quietly.

ARRIVAL

Daylight was beginning to wane as we approached Houston, and a patchwork of lights began to wink into life. We touched down at 7:52 p.m., deplaned with well-wishes from the crew, and made our way to the baggage claim area. By then, it was dusk, and travel weariness was settling in. We enlisted a porter to help collect our baggage and load it onto an airport golf cart, then he drove us through the airport to the rental car check-in.

The rental area was nearly empty, but the customers that were there were lined up at the same rental company I'd reserved with, so we patiently waited. Wendy held our place in line while Neil and I "used the facilities," then she took her turn. At last, we were first in line, and I was greeted with a smile by the desk clerk. My reservation popped up, my identification and credit cards were accepted, and we ran through the obligatory checklist — insurance and filling the gas tank — then the clerk asked if we wanted GPS or a "speed pass."

"I don't think so," I shook my head. "We brought a GPS. But what's a 'speed pass?'"

"Some of our highways have high-speed travel lanes," she explained, "to bypass local traffic."

"Can we get around without one?" I asked

"It's mostly for rush hour," the clerk observed. "You should be fine otherwise."

"In that case," I smiled, "we're all set."

With the details sorted out, the clerk printed our contract, gave us a map, explained how to exit the airport complex, and directed us outside and up some stairs to the area where we could pick from the available compact cars.

"Just show your contract to the attendant on our way out," the clerk smiled and bid us goodnight.

We felt like overdressed camels — me with two bags in each hand and a bag over my shoulder; Neil with his backpack over his shoulder, his computer case in one hand, and towing a large two-wheeler with the other; and Wendy loaded down with the rest. It was dark, and the night air was balmy by the time we managed to lug our things out to pick our "new car." There were several compact Toyotas and Nissans to choose from.

"Which one do you want?" I asked Neil.

"Let's take this one," he pointed to a white Corolla. "She looks pretty smart."

I popped open the trunk and started loading her up. The trunk wasn't quite big enough, so one bag had to take the seat next to Neil.

"No big deal," he smiled. "I'm not planning on laying down. I wanna see this place!"

The car started right up, then it took me a few minutes to adjust the seat and mirrors, to figure out where all the important buttons and knobs were located, and to get our little GPS (an old "TomTom ONE") plugged in and booted up. We gave it a few minutes to triangulate, but it just couldn't lock onto a signal while we were inside the garage. Fortunately, there wasn't much traffic departing from the rental area, so once outside, we pulled over to let the GPS figure out it wasn't in Rhode Island anymore, then we commenced the third leg of our journey.

I'd been to Texas once before — to Houston and Galveston — when I worked as a "doodlebugger" on an oil exploration boat in the gulf, but that was thirty years earlier. Things had changed "just a little" since then. I was a newcomer just like Wendy and Neil, and while it may be a cliché, our first impression of Texas was, "This place is HUGE!" Ribbons of light ran everywhere — a giant network of taillights and headlights merging and splitting onto multiple access roads and up onto highways, some of them with so many lanes it was like seeing double. And there were power lines everywhere. Some ran parallel to the roadways, others crisscrossed in a labyrinth extending as far as we could see. And all of it was capped in the hazy glow of ambient light trapped under a gathering haze. We struggled just to follow the path our little GPS drew through this maze, a lone turtle amongst hares.

More than once, we nearly wandered off route as we headed south, skirting around downtown Houston, then turning west on Route 10. What a highway! Six lanes each way, traversing cloverleaf interchanges with on-ramps and off-ramps stacked like layers in a cake. Each side of the highway had two-lane feeder roads, and almost the entire paved expanse was flanked by glass-faced office buildings, many brightly outlined in neon lights, some red, some white, and one lit up blue. A few also had spotlights pointing up at giant American flags — like thirty feet by fifty feet — waving gently. It was like driving through a giant video game.

Just after 10:00 p.m., we arrived at Towne Place Suites on Katy Freeway and were graciously welcomed by the night duty manager. With the last of our energy, we loaded our luggage onto a cart. I parked the car, then we trundled to the elevator, went to the second floor, and walked to the end of the hallway where the long-term suites were located — on the quiet side of the hotel. Wendy swiped a keycard and opened the door, and we got our first look at what would be "home" for the next few weeks. The suite had two bedrooms and a large common area combining a living/dining room with a fully equipped kitchen. There was a dining table at which four people could sit, a large over-stuffed chair with a footstool that doubled as a coffee/game table, a fold out couch, and a TV atop a credenza. Each bedroom had a TV as well, along with sitting chairs and dressers. The larger room had a king-sized bed and a writing desk too. The décor's color theme was burnt orange — not exactly our taste, but a sight for tired traveler's eyes.

Wendy and I took the larger bedroom, and Neil took the room with a queen-sized bed. The fold out couch would be perfect for Evie when she visited. The suite also had several windows we could open to provide good cross ventilation. Everything was clean and tidy, even sterile, but that would change as soon as we unpacked and settled in. In all, the suite looked like it would suit our needs nicely. We unpacked enough to retrieve what we needed to turn in, sent word we had arrived safely at our final destination, then we tucked into bed feeling buoyed by a successful journey and the prospect of meeting Dr. Burzynski the following day.

THE BURZYNSKI CLINIC
APRIL 13, 2016

We slept well our first night — a comforting beginning — and upon waking we got our first good look outside. Our bedroom windows looked directly at a twenty foot earthen levee with a drainage ditch running along its base. The levee surrounds George Bush Park, a seven thousand eight hundred acre nature sanctuary through which the Buffalo Bayou runs. The park also serves as a catch basin to hold stormwater runoff, hence the levee. We could occasionally see someone walking or biking along the top of the levee, so there was a path for pedestrians. Running parallel to the levee was Grisby Road, the access road upon which our hotel and several other businesses were located. Across this road, we noticed a small path which crossed the drainage ditch and went up to the top of the levee. Nature walks beckoned.

We hadn't brought anything to eat besides snacks, but the hotel had a breakfast buffet we could graze. Unfortunately, there wasn't much for Neil except fruit, but he was happy with that until we could get our bearings and find the right food for lunch. Our excitement grew throughout breakfast: the Burzynski Clinic was just eight miles east on Route 10, the last leg of this part of Neil's journey.

It was the tail end of rush hour traffic when we got in the car, so we gave ourselves extra time. The hotel's parking lot abutted the feeder road to Route 10, so from the moment we turned out of the lot, we were on full alert. Merging onto Route 10 required timing and a heavy foot, but big city traffic is just that, and we got used to it. Driving to the clinic was another dose of Texas-huge. In daylight, the expanse of lanes seemed wide enough to land a pair of jumbo jets side by side.

The Burzynski Clinic was on the opposite side of Route 10, so we had to drive beyond the clinic and take a U-turn, then we proceeded slowly to avoid overshooting the address. We found the clinic soon enough, a glass-encased three story office building, fairly typical for the outskirts of Houston. The clinic is set well back from the access road, and the first thing we noticed as we pulled into the parking lot were Bougainvillea hedges in full bloom. The hedges surrounded the lot and lent a festive air to the moment. At last, it felt like we were where we needed to be.

"I'm pretty excited," I said as I pulled into a space close to the main entrance.

"I've got goosebumps," Wendy admitted.

"Me too," Neil smiled with a gleam in his eyes.

The air was supercharged with optimism as I held open the front door and we entered the lobby, a large open area with three-story ceilings and filled with light, plants, various places to sit and a glass-encased elevator in the center. We would later discover a cozy café down the corridor on the opposite side of the elevator, and beyond that, an indoor botanical courtyard. A security guard sat at a desk to one side of the lobby. He greeted us pleasantly and directed us to the second floor. "The entrance to the clinic is directly opposite the elevator doors," he told us, and we stepped aboard the elevator as if it were a rocket gantry.

"Here we go," I said in hushed anticipation.

"We're really here," Wendy nodded.

"Blastoff!" Neil pressed the second-floor button and pumped his fist in triumph as the doors closed.

We lifted off slowly, and when the doors opened, we were greeted by a faint aroma — nothing objectionable — but an aroma reminiscent of urine.

"The 'piss doctor,'" I winked at Neil, and he chuckled.

"People sure like to pick on things they don't accept," he observed.

"Or what they don't want others to look at too closely," I added.

"Okay," Wendy chided, "let's not be cynical right now."

The clinic's entrance was twenty feet in front of us. Neil stepped eagerly into the lead and opened the entry door for us. Upon entering the waiting area, we were immediately reminded of the waiting area at Dana-Farber — except for the silence. We were the only visitors there. These were difficult times for Dr. Burzynski. He was in the midst of yet another confrontation with the Texas Medical Board. Nonetheless, the waiting area was very welcoming, with a large area to the left of the receptionist's counter devoted to children. This area was playfully decorated and had a collection of children's books, a variety of toys, and some games. The right side of the room was for adults, with leather sofas and chairs, side tables with lamps, and a coffee table with a few magazines.

Neil walked confidently up to the receptionist's counter. "I'm Eugene Fachon," he announced.

The receptionist had piercing, kind eyes. "It's good to see you," she replied with a warmth you might expect more from an Aunt. "We've been expecting you. I'm Irena." Then, she smiled at us, "He's so handsome!"

We chuckled softly and smiled back. "A pleasure to meet you!"

Irena had a Polish accent, an accent with which we would become very familiar. After she officially signed Neil in, she motioned for us to make ourselves comfortable. "I'll call Sheryll. It will just be a few minutes."

Irena's kind demeanor set us completely at ease as we took in our surroundings in greater detail. The walls were covered with framed pictures of patients, many accompanied by letters — some in crayon — thanking Dr. Burzynski and the clinic for doing what their own doctors had told them could not be done.

"Wow," Neil shook his head and smiled as broadly as his smile would stretch. "Just wow!"

After admiring some of the pictures, Neil sat down where he felt most at home, in the children's area, and soon thereafter, a petite and vivacious young woman stepped through a nearby side door. She had Filipino features and wore a traditional white lab coat.

"Hello Eugene," she said cheerfully with a hint of a Latin American accent. "I'm Sheryll Acelar," and she extended her hand. "I'm the coordinator for the clinical trial."

"I'm very pleased to meet you," Neil smiled. "My friends call me Neil."

We exchanged greetings all around, briefly discussing our trip and reactions to Houston. It was nice to put a face on the woman with whom so many emails had been exchanged. Sheryll then motioned us through the door into the clinic's inner sanctum. To the left was a nurses' station and a corridor lined with doors, the first standing open to a small conference room. To the right, we caught a glimpse of exam rooms. Sheryll took us left to the conference room.

"Make yourselves comfortable," she said, motioning to the chairs. "Would you like anything? A juice or bottled water?"

"Water would be good," we agreed, and she brought several bottles.

"Dr. Burzynski will be with you shortly," she said and departed, closing the door.

The room was simple, furnished with a dark wooden conference table surrounded by six cushy armchairs upholstered in leather. Three of the walls were adorned with tasteful artwork. The fourth wall, opposite the door, had a large picture window.

"Check this out," Neil nodded at the window.

The picture window overlooked an indoor courtyard that stretched the full width of the building. A glass ceiling let in natural light, and the space was filled with tropical trees, plantings, and a walkway lined with benches — the indoor arboretum.

"How cool is that?" Neil smiled with his eyes.

"That looks very soothing," Wendy nodded. "A space for seeking serenity."

We arrayed ourselves around the table, leaving the seat nearest the door for Dr. Burzynski. Laying in the middle of the table was a photo album that invited perusal. It was filled with photos like the ones in the waiting area — some of Dr. Burzynski with his patients and some just of his patients, including 'then and now' photos of long-term survivors, their baby faces bloated from steroids in one shot and their adult faces normal and smiling warmly in the next. Some of these survivors had kids of their own.

All the photos told a story, not of hyped-up promises, but of grounding in genuine hope. This was the indelible counterpoint to Dr. Burzynski's alleged reputation. The naysayers might claim these people were brainwashed, but more than any video we had watched, any articles we had read, or any person Neil had spoken with, these tokens of love, appreciation, and respect reassured us the Burzynski Clinic was the right place for Neil to be.

TWINKLING EYES

About five minutes later, Sheryll returned carrying a large sheaf of papers that she placed on the table. Dr. Burzynski followed closely behind, a stout man with a full head of reddish-brown hair combed back and a neat mustache. He smiled broadly, a twinkle in his blue eyes that was spritely. The room was immediately brighter. Sheryll left and closed the door.

"Hello," Dr. Burzynski greeted us with his strong Polish accent, shaking hands with Wendy and I, then focusing his full attention on Neil. "So, you are Eugene Fachon."

"Yes sir," Neil managed as he picked his jaw up from the table.

"And you elect to forgo standard treatment," Dr. Burzynski nodded approvingly.

"Cut, burn, and poison," Neil frowned. "Not really interested."

"The only real promise we found is alternative medicine, and your clinic stands on top," I added.

"This is not alternative medicine," Dr. Burzynski shook his head no. "It's science-based, with empirical evidence over many years. It should be 'standard of care,' but we see a lot of resistance."

"We know," I raised my palms in apology.

"So," Dr. Burzynski switched gears. "The name 'Fachon' is very interesting. It means 'we are angry' in French, but we hope you will be happy here," he smiled. "Is your family from France?"

"Eugene's Great-Grandfather emigrated from Pforzheim, Germany just after World War I," I replied to this surprise question.

"Ahh," Dr. Burzynski wondered out loud. "Huguenots? They were persecuted by French Kings, Louis XIV and XV. Many were slaughtered for their beliefs, but some refugees escaped into Germany."

"Yes," I nodded, taken completely off guard by this friendly digression. "I think my Grandfather mentioned a Huguenot connection going way back. His father, Eugene's Great-Great-Grandfather, was a stained glass window maker who traced his ancestry to a gamekeeper who lived in the Black Forest — a gamekeeper who was murdered by poachers, actually."

Dr. Burzynski had a keen interest in history and smiled. "My family saw trouble too, during World War II and later, when Soviet Union took over Poland." He let that hang in the air for a brief moment, then he got down to business. "So, I have looked at your scans and records. I'm very sorry you have this condition," he said, looking at Neil and shaking his head. "DIPG is a difficult cancer, the worst of childhood brain tumors," he confided. "But you are not typical case. You are much older than usual, but I think we can help. We've had good success with it before."

We all nodded appreciatively, and I gestured towards the photo album. "That's why we're here."

"Please," Neil added, "tell us about antineoplastons. ANPs. How they work."

HOW DO ANTINEOPLASTONS WORK?

"Of course," Dr. Burzynski loosely folded his hands on the table, but they would not sit still for long. "With cancer, there are changes in gene expression." He raised a hand to count off his fingers. "Mutations, amplifications, suppressions, translocations, and more. Fortunately, we have natural tumor suppressor genes to protect against cancer. Unfortunately, toxic influence can turn tumor suppressor genes into oncogenes, cancer-causing genes. Conditions which cause mutations usually happen during patient's life — from toxic exposures, a variety of things," he shrugged. "In small percentage of cases, mutations may be hereditary. These are most difficult. But for most others, epigenetic treatment may turn off activity of the mutated or misbehaving genes, and the cancer cell dies. If all cancer cells die, the mutated gene is gone. The root of the cancer is gone." He looked at us inquiringly. Were we with him so far?

"Got it," we nodded.

"Many DIPG patients have certain mutations in common," Dr. Burzynski continued, "but we think there are about two hundred mutations altogether, and which mutations occur can vary between patients. Even within a single patient, mutations can shift throughout course of disease. DIPG is quite tricky. Based on laboratory data, antineoplastons can influence over one hundred common gene mutations." At this point, he held up his hands, spread open and palms facing outwards, thumbs almost touching. "This side is ANPs — Atengenal and Astugenal," and he wiggled the fingers of his right hand. "This is malfunctioning and mutated genes in DIPG," and he wiggled his left. "If there is no overlap between mutations and antineoplastons, there is no response." Then, he began to slowly overlap his right hand behind the left. "The more overlap between antineoplastons and malfunctioning genes, the greater chance of response," and he finished by closing his right hand over his left in a doubled up fist. "With full or significant overlap, we may get complete response."

In my mind, I pictured Venn diagrams:

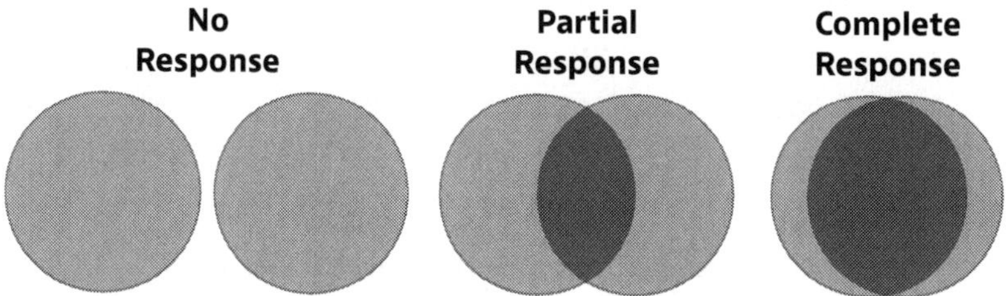

Note: When Evie had requested information on the protocol for the clinical trial, Dr. Burzynski sent copies of articles — published in _Neuro-Oncology_[11] — concerning a variety of patients with DIPG, as well as other brain tumors. He also sent a peer-reviewed history of seventeen patients with recurrent DIPG. Based on this information and what we had gleaned independently from documentaries, articles, blogs, and books, we inferred Neil's chances of a complete response might be roughly two out of ten; and his chance of a partial response, which could significantly extend his life, was perhaps four out of ten.

"When you say 'complete response,'" Wendy asked, "you mean..."

"The tumor dissolves," Dr. Burzynski nodded. "What may be left is scar tissue."

"That would be the goal," Neil beamed at Dr. Burzynski. "When do we start?"

INFORMED CONSENT

"Well, here we have paperwork for the clinical trial," Dr. Burzynski smiled and gestured to the sheaf of papers Sheryll left on the table. The cover page was entitled:

---

11 The articles referred to were first published by Duke University Press. Oxford University Press has since taken over the publication, and Dr. Burzynski's articles have been archived there.

Subject Consent for a Patient Age 3 - 21 With Newly Diagnosed Disease
Who Has Refused Radiation Therapy, to take part in:
"A Phase 2 Study of Atengenal (A-10) and Astugenal (AS2-1)
in Diffuse, Intrinsic Pontine Glioma (DIPG)."

"This document explains the clinical trial," Dr. Burzynski nodded. "Please take your time and review it thoroughly." Then, Dr. Burzynski got up. "Let Sheryll know when you are ready, and I will return to answer any questions." With that, he departed and closed the door.

"Ooof!" Neil hooted softly. "Someone pinch me."

We all chuckled, awash in a sense of relief, excitement, and most of all, hope. Wendy and I moved our chairs to flank Neil as he pulled the paperwork to him, and we all began reading.

The document listed the tests required to qualify for the study — blood tests, urine tests, a detailed neurological exam, as well as MRI and PET scans. The document also outlined the tests and procedures to be routinely performed during the study — tests to monitor the safety and efficacy of the treatment.

The study itself would be a one-hundred-four-week program — two years! To accommodate the administering of ANPs, a vascular access catheter would need to be surgically placed in a vein below Neil's left collar bone. Infusions would need to be given through this catheter six times a day using a programmable electronic pump. The protocol would require weekly lab tests, monthly physical exams, and MRIs taken every eight weeks. The patient was asked to keep a journal describing side effects and changes in physical symptoms, and there was a section pertaining to the patient's right to withdraw from the study. In addition, the document discussed the risks and side effects associated with the protocol. The three most likely side effects from ANPs were fatigue, hypernatremia, and hypokalemia:

- Hypernatremia is defined as high sodium levels in the blood. Hypernatremia occurs in approximately five out of every ten patients and can be severe in three out of ten cases. "Severe hypernatremia (marked elevation of sodium level in the blood) has been implicated in the deaths of 3/1000 patients." Proper sodium levels are maintained through consuming water and proper diet.
- Hypokalemia is defined as low potassium levels in the blood. Healthy potassium levels are maintained through diet and the use of potassium supplements.

The document concluded with financial obligations. The ANP medication and ongoing support from the Burzynski Clinic would be free of charge to enrolled patients. The patient's health insurance and/or the patient himself would be responsible for surgical costs, pharmacy costs, equipment costs, bloodwork, and radiology. Furthermore, the Burzynski Clinic would be indemnified against any harm to the patient, and the clinic would have no obligation to compensate for any failure of the treatment. Participation in the trial would be completely voluntary, and there were no guarantees.

We jotted down a few questions as we read, but for the most part, the document was clear and self-explanatory. When we were ready, I let Sheryll know, and Dr. Burzynski returned soon thereafter.

"So," he said with a serious expression, "what questions do you have?"

"I'd like to know a little more about side effects," Neil asked. "The sodium and potassium-related side effects. How often do they occur, and how severe are they?"

"In general, they are not severe," Dr. Burzynski began, "as long as we monitor blood levels and adjust water intake and supplements. In beginning, there may be some nausea. It may take a few days to adjust, but nothing like radiation or chemotherapy." Then, he elaborated. "Of course, FDA will say otherwise. They point at a case of severe hypernatremia to claim ANPs are toxic. This was a sad case, of course, but there were other fac-

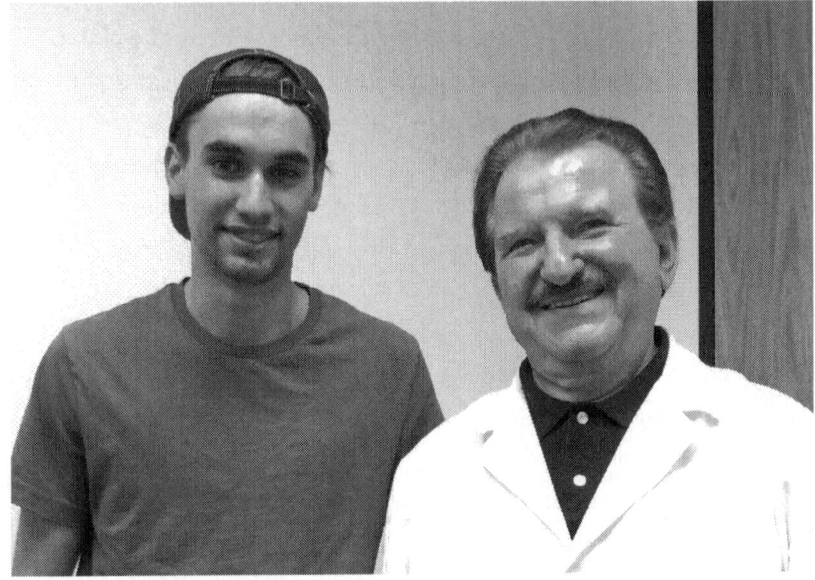

tors. Otherwise, we have very few issues with side effects we can't manage. Overall, they are mild, controllable, and reversible."

If we had any further questions, they were minor and lost in the shuffle. Anything important would come up again in due course. Suffice it to say, Neil was eager to start. "Let's do this!"

He signed the document, along with a standard HIPAA authorization form, and Dr. Burzynski signed too. Both signatures were witnessed, and at roughly 11:00 a.m. on April 13, 2016, Neil became the first candidate-enrollee in Clinical Trial BRI-BT-55.

At this point, Dr. Burzynski wanted Neil to start taking dexamethasone, three milligrams per day. He would need to be on the steroid for five full days before getting the baseline MRI and PET scans. Neil had the unused pills from the MGH prescription, so he was all set for the moment.

"I will see you again later today," Dr. Burzynski said, and a moment later, Sheryll returned.

"We'll need you to get some bloodwork today," she told Neil. "I've set up an appointment at the lab for two o'clock. After that, we'll need you back here at three for your physical examination."

Before leaving, we asked Sheryll and Irena for recommendations on where to find lunch suitable for Neil. This was a common question, apparently, and both suggested Newk's Eatery nearby.

"And what about grocery shopping?" Wendy asked. "We need to stock our kitchen with some fresh organic food."

They advised going to the H-E-B, and Sheryll gave us directions. We thanked them and promised Sheryll we would be back no later than 3:00 p.m.

It was just before noon when we descended back to the main lobby. As we stepped out from the clinic into the bright midday sun, it felt like we should have been carrying weights to keep from floating.

"That was like meeting a rock star," Neil shook his head in mild disbelief.

"No kidding," Wendy smiled.

"It's strange meeting someone you've only seen on TV," I nodded. "They seem bigger than life, but they're real."

"And now you're his patient," Wendy smiled.

"I couldn't be more pleased," Neil agreed.

And that meant a lot!

We could hardly believe how far we had come, that Neil's imminent death sentence had a genuine chance, even if small, of being commuted. He was one step closer to starting the clinical trial — unless the scans and tests contradicted his eligibility. If that happened, we were fully prepared to consult with Dr. Burzynski on alternatives.

LUNCH BREAK

Neil was famished, so Newk's was our next stop. It was close to the clinic, so we got in the car and meandered through a couple of parking lots to park by the restaurant's door. Newk's menu board was posted next to the entry, and it detailed a wide selection of fresh salads and homestyle soups. Everything looked good, and it took a few minutes to decide, then we stepped up to the counter and placed our order. After paying the cashier, she gave us a number placard. "Pick any table and just leave this where the waitstaff can see it."

The dining area was large and had the decor of an industrial mill building, with exposed ducts hanging from the ceiling, brick walls, and a large glassed-in kitchen to one side. We selected a booth in the corner, and our meals were delivered shortly thereafter. Upon taking first bites, we quickly agreed we would be eating at Newk's more than once. Besides that, we spoke little. Neil had some catching up to do as far as eating was concerned.

When we departed the restaurant, Neil noticed a building diagonally across the parking lot that looked interesting, iFLY Indoor Skydiving. "That looks cool," he said.

"We'll check it out some time," I promised.

We had enough time to go back to our hotel for a brief rest before heading to the blood lab, Quest Diagnostics, located halfway between the hotel and the clinic and right off the highway on a feeder road. The lot was full when we arrived, cars parked cheek-by-jowl, but — as Wendy puts it — 'the parking angels were watching out for us.' We found a spot right next to the entrance. It took some time for the receptionist to collect Neil's information, then we sat down to wait. After ten minutes, he was called, and a few minutes later, we were out the door. "Easy peasy," Neil smiled. A busy location, but convenient.

From there, we went back to the clinic. Neil was ushered into an exam room, where the nurse took height and weight measurements to get a baseline, then he was hooked up for an EKG. Shortly thereafter, Dr. Burzynski arrived to give Neil a complete neurological evaluation reminiscent of the exams given him by Dr. Panis and Dr. Kieran. Dr. Burzynski also commented that he felt Neil ranked about seventy on the Karnofsky scale.

Once Neil's examination was complete, we thanked Dr. Burzynski, and he departed. Sheryll escorted us back to the waiting area and outlined the action plan: Neil would take the steroids for five days, and Sheryl would schedule the necessary scans in the days immediately following. If Neil passed all the requirements for the trial, she would schedule the surgery to place a catheter, and soon thereafter, Neil would commence treatment.

"So enjoy yourselves," she smiled. "There's plenty to do around Houston."

"First we need to get a bit more settled in," Wendy replied. "Right now, we need to go shopping. Our kitchen is bare."

"That sounds like a plan," Sheryll agreed. "Please don't hesitate to call if you need anything or have more questions."

We promised we would and shook hands all around.

"See you again soon," Neil grinned brightly.

Excerpts from Dr. Burzynski report, April 13, 2016:

On April 13, 2016, the patient, father and mother presented to the Burzynski Clinic at 10:00AM in consultation room 5 for a screening visit. Prior to procedures being performed, the informed consent was given to the patient and his parents to read. Ample time was given for them to read the informed consent. The Principal Investigator was available to answer all questions to their satisfaction. The patient proceeded to sign the informed consent. The Principal Investigator signed the informed consent. Vital signs were then taken, baseline height and weight measured, and Principal Investigator Dr. Stanislaw Burzynski performed physical and neurological examinations.

Chief Complaint: The patient is a 19-year-old Caucasian male from RI, who presented accompanied by his father and mother, complaining of ataxia, diplopia, dysarthria, intermittent mild headaches, confusion, dizziness, difficulty swallowing liquids, flatulence, constipation, muscle stiffness, shortness of breath with exertion and mood changes. He is able to care for himself but is unable to carry on normal activity or active work.

History of Present Illness: Mr. Fachon was in his usual state of health until January 2016 when he developed difficulty initiating urination and defecation and complained of a lack of coordination, such as when getting out of bed he felt that his arms and legs were affected. He also complained of difficulty writing as well as difficulty swallowing liquids, resulting in choking. At the end of January he noted periodic slurred speech. His parents noted some dysarthria. The patient reported a history of concussions that occurred in August, September, and October 2015. The above symptoms progressively worsened. His headaches worsened and radiated to his neck and the top right side of his head.

On March 2, 2016, he consulted Walter Panis, M.D., who recommended an MRI of his head. On March 3, 2016, the MRI of the head, with and without contrast showed an expansile T2/FLAIR hyperintense 3.6 x 5.7 x 5.1 cm (AP by transverse craniocaudal) lesion that demonstrated alternatively decreased and heterogeneous T1 signal and no significant enhancement. The lesion encased both vertebral arteries and nearly completely circumferentially surrounded the basilar artery with an exophytic component. Findings were consistent with diffuse intrinsic pontine glioma (DIPG).

The patient was referred to neurologist Isabel Arrillaga-Romney, M.D. at Mass General Hospital, who discussed radiation therapy and the risks and benefits of biopsy and referred him to neurosurgeon Daniel Cahill, M.D. An MRI of the spine was recommended for further evaluation of difficulties with urination and defecation, and treatment of dexamethasone 3 mg p.o. daily for diplopia and balance difficulties was advised. A second opinion was obtained at another medial facility [DANA Farber] to explore clinical trial options. The patient refused recommendations and presented to our clinic to explore our clinical trial, according to protocol BT-55.

NEUROLOGICAL EXAMINATION

Alert and oriented x3.
Cranial nerve III defect: left eye ptosis
Cranial nerve V defect: partial palsy
Cranial nerve VI defect: left esotropia
Ataxia gait
Decreased motor strength, 3/5 in all extremities
Karnofsky Performance Status: 70

ASSESSMENT:

Diffuse intrinsic pontine glioma

TREATMENT PLAN:

Dr. S.R. Burzynski recommended: Beginning today, he will be screened under Protocol BT-55 clinical trial, study of Atengenal and Astugenal in Diffuse Intrinsic Pontine Glioma. He will be screened under Cohort 3, which is patients ages 3 to 21 years old with newly diagnosed diffuse intrinsic pontine glioma who (or whose parents/guardians) have refused radiation. The Principal Investigator started the patient on dexamethasone 3 mg once daily for the purpose of following the protocol BT-55.

SUPER SIZE

As soon as we got back in the car, Wendy programmed the GPS with the address for the H-E-B supermarket. Super-duper-market was more like it. The parking lot was a sea of cars, and from where we had to park, the walk to the store was easily two hundred yards.

"You guys go ahead," Neil yawned. "I'm good here."

"Okay," we agreed. "Just keep your phone handy and the doors locked."

Neil "hung out" in the car, tucked into his neck pillow, earbuds plugged in, and his cell phone at the ready, while Wendy I went to shop in a market that seemed more like a labyrinth — half a dozen supermarkets stitched together. We grabbed an oversized shopping cart and started in the produce section, Wendy's number one priority. Fortunately, it was near the entrance, and even better, the H-E-B had a large selection of organic fruits and vegetables.

"This is perfect," Wendy said, and she started loading the cart with kiwis, carrots, green beans, limes, lemons, russet potatoes, onions, celery, kale, spinach, cabbage, avocados and more. Around the corner from produce was a meat department as big as typical grocery store back home. We picked up some all-natural cold cuts and a package of organic chicken, but our list included a lot more stuff — things like spring water, organic juices, spices, olive oil, salad dressing, yogurt, hummus, gluten-free crackers, healthy snack foods, and so on. Given the extraordinary expanse we needed to cover, we split up. I took half the list, and Wendy the other.

"You keep that cart," I told her. "I'll grab another."

In no time at all, we lost track of each other as we walked up and down aisles that seemed as long as football fields, trying to familiarize ourselves with the store's layout. Ten minutes later, my cell phone rang.

"Where are you?" Wendy asked in a small, frightened voice. "I'm lost."

"Head to the checkout area and go to the left side of the building," I suggested. "I'll find you there."

It took about five minutes and a fair amount of wandering around to locate each other, and Wendy was almost in tears. "I feel like a little girl at a carnival who can't find her dad," she admitted.

We consolidated carts and stuck together for the rest of our spree, spending well over three hundred dollars. As we exited the store, it took a few moments to reorient in the afternoon glare of the parking lot. Here too, it was easy to get lost — to lose our car amongst the several hundreds of others. After getting our bearings, we pushed our cart down an aisle, only to discover two hundred yards later that we'd made a mistake. Our car was not there. Fortunately, we were close enough that a few moments of scanning pinned it down, but we'd need to pay more attention in the future.

When we reached the car, Neil was nodding off to his music. We headed for "home," and Neil took his very first three milligram dose of dexamethasone as soon as we got there. Another milestone, although it felt a bit like capitulation to mainstream orthodoxy.

"I don't want to take this any more than I have to," Neil said.

* * *

While the H-E-B's scale would take getting used to, its broad selection of fresh organic foods would make it our go-to market. Indeed, I returned there later that day to pick up some forgotten essentials. By the time I got back to the hotel, Wendy had already prepared a home-cooked chicken curry that filled the suite with a marvelous aroma. There was a lovely mixed green salad to go with it. In the process of "working the kitchen," Wendy also discovered a few more items she wanted.

"Make a list," I suggested, and she held up a piece of paper with several items neatly printed.

Soon thereafter, we were seated for our first home-cooked meal in Houston, and it was delicious. Neil devoured two big helpings.

"Dr. Noé would be pleased," I smiled.

I helped Wendy clean up after dinner, then we all sat together to watch some TV. Nothing much grabbed our attention, and Neil started yawning, which proved infectious, so that was the signal to turn in early, exhausted but happy. Sleep came swiftly and lasted all night. Restorative — the best thing for healing.

19

COUNTDOWN PREPARATIONS

"Live in the present, but for the future." NF

THURSDAY, APRIL 14, 2016

After morning ablutions and breakfast, Wendy heated the coffee for Neil's self-administered enema. We set everything up in our cramped little bathroom, then he went in and closed the door. Twenty minutes later he emerged with a content smile, having accomplished what he needed to do. As mundane as it sounds, regular bowel movements are essential to good health, so we needed to keep him going (pun intended).

While we had been busy, so too had the Burzynski Clinic. On the morning of April 14, the clinic's sister organization, the Burzynski Research Institute, issued a press release:

> **Burzynski Research Institute, Inc. Announces the Launch of a New Clinical Trial in Diffuse Intrinsic Brainstem Glioma**
> April 14, 2016 11:31 AM Eastern Daylight Time
>
> HOUSTON--(BUSINESS WIRE)--Burzynski Research Institute, Inc. (BRI) announced today that it has begun patient enrollment into an FDA-reviewed and IRB-approved, open-label, single-arm phase 2 study of Antineoplastons A10 and AS2-1 in patients > 3 months of age with

a diffuse intrinsic brainstem glioma (DIPG). Study subjects will be placed in one of five treatment groups based on their age and whether or not they have received prior treatment for DIPG. The primary study endpoint is a decrease in the size of the tumor, either a partial response (≥ 50% decrease in the size of the tumor) or a complete response (disappearance of the tumor).

"The response and survival of children with recurrent intrinsic pontine glioma based on a phase II study of Antineoplastons A10 and AS2-1 in patients with brainstem glioma"

DIPG is primarily a disease of childhood, with the majority of patients being between 5 and 10 years of age. However, infants and adults can also be affected. It is the most common brainstem tumor in children, representing 75-80% of childhood brainstem tumors, and affecting an estimated 300 children in the U.S. each year. The prognosis for children with DIPG is significantly worse than that of other primary brainstem tumors. The standard of care for patients with newly-diagnosed DIPG is radiation therapy (RT), which appears to control tumor growth for a short period of time, prolonging survival by approximately 3 months. Within 3-8 months after completion of RT, most patients with DIPG will show progression of their disease. No chemotherapeutic agent has ever demonstrated a significant improvement in outcome beyond that achieved by RT alone. An original BRI paper, "The response and survival of children with recurrent intrinsic pontine glioma based on a phase II study of Antineoplastons A10 and AS2-1 in patients with brainstem glioma" was published in Child's

Nervous System in December 2014, Volume 30, Issue 12, pages 2051-2061 (DOI 10.1007/s00381-014-2401-z).[12]

Now, we had four days to play with, so for our second day in Houston, we planned to just take things easy and get acquainted with our local surroundings. To begin with, we'd head back to the store to pick up a few items, then we planned to find a vendor of fresh-pressed organic vegetable juice. We assumed Houston would have organic juice bars, and we weren't wrong, but neither were we as right as we'd hoped. Flipping through the phone book, we found a few possibilities, but none near the hotel, and our foray to the closest candidate was less than successful. Their juice was pre-pressed and packaged in twelve ounce plastic bottles with no dates. Ideally, we needed juice made to order, within minutes of when Neil would consume it. We picked up a few bottles nonetheless — better than nothing — and admitted we'd have to broaden our search.

"I should've brought the juicing equipment," I lamented.

"We'll find something," Wendy was optimistic.

After our initial juice foray, we stopped at Walmart. (No, not for juice!) Although our kitchen was stocked with pots, plates, utensils, and so on, Wendy wanted a glass roasting pan, a better frying pan, a bottle opener, a paring knife, and a few other utensils for the kitchen. Just those two errands ate up the morning, so we meandered back towards Newk's Eatery. On the way, we passed a small park that looked inviting, so Wendy started a list of "things to do." Little discoveries like that, coupled with our growing familiarity of the general area, helped us start feeling settled in.

After lunch at Newk's, we returned to the hotel to take some downtime, then during mid-afternoon, we made use of the warm sun to walk across the road in back of the hotel and up to the top of the levee overlooking Bush Park. There was a path already worn in the grass leading down to the levee's perimeter drainage ditch — dry at the moment — and up the embankment. When we got to the top, we discovered a paved bike/

12 http://www.businesswire.com/news/home/20160414006163/en/Burzynski-Research-Institute-Announces-Launch-Clinical-Trial

walking path stretching as far as we could see to the west. Half a mile to the east, the path curved to the right, following the levee's eastern boundary. The interior floor of the park was a lush forest of large succulent plants and mature trees — a lot like the vegetation in Florida. Between where we stood and the forest was a low swampy area, dotted with birds. We walked a few hundred yards west until Neil was ready to turn back. In time, we hoped to go further.

Before dinner that evening, Neil spent half an hour doing his eye exercises. He felt it was helping to slow the progression of his double vision, allowing him to forgo his eye patch sometimes. Over dinner, we planned a trip to Galveston for the following day. That evening, we sent emails to family and friends, reporting on everything that had happened to date, and Wendy touched base with Dr. Noé.

MEMORY LANE
FRIDAY, APRIL 15, 2016

The ride to Old Town in Galveston took roughly an hour, ending at the Gulf of Mexico. We turned left and followed the shoreline to Fort San Jacinto Historic Point. The Gulf was breathless and warm in the hazy sun — almost a mill pond. A handful of oil rigs stood at varying distances all the way to the horizon. The only thing stirring the waters were the oil tankers traversing in and out.

"I was just a little older than you when I worked on an oil exploration boat," I told Neil. "We used to steam in and out right past this point."

"That must have been pretty interesting," Neil smiled.

"It was a fun time," I nodded. "We'd go out for two or three weeks at a time, searching for 'salt domes' that indicated the likely presence of oil underneath," I explained. "One time we had to high tail it back just in front of a hurricane. The boat rocked so much that night, I thought she would lay right over and sink."

Neil shook his head, trying to imagine it.

"You would have laughed," I added. "Earlier in the day, when the waves started getting too big to keep working, we had to reel in the mile-long cable array we were towing. The waves washed up the fantail and took us right off our feet more than once!"

"Sounds a bit dicey," Neil raised an amused if incredulous eyebrow.

"Totally serious," I nodded. "But nothing like what we're in now," I added ruefully, tussling his hair with a shake of my head.

"Oh, I think we're doin' okay," he smiled kindly, looking intently into my eyes.

We hung out quietly for half an hour or so, watching tankers disappear into the haze. Whenever I'm near the sea, it tugs at my heart. By the look in Neil's eyes, he felt it too.

"How about some lunch," Wendy finally suggested, looking at her watch.

We passed a restaurant coming in, Miller's Seawall Grill. It looked like fun and we stopped. Their menu listed a variety of classic gulf-shrimp dishes with hush puppies on the side. It was a major break from Neil's normal diet, but he deserved it. He enjoyed the fried shrimp so much he had seconds. And for dessert, we indulged in key lime pie.

"Well that should do it," Wendy smiled as Neil swallowed his last bite of pie. "Talk about cheating!"

"That was worth it," he grinned.

We drove back through Old Town and took a detour to see the inner bay. Unfortunately, there was not much to see, just commercial buildings and warehouses, but behind and looming high above the buildings were the towers of oil rigs — in for service or laid up. In a few spots, we could spy between buildings to the wharves where a variety of vessels were tied up, some very similar to the boat I once worked aboard. Then, we headed for "home."

After returning to the hotel and relaxing a bit, Neil and I went for a workout in the small hotel gym. It had an elliptical, a treadmill, and some free weights. Neil used the elliptical and spent some time with the free weights. He wrapped up with some balance exercises, then we grabbed some waters and sat next to the hotel's small outdoor pool.

"Not quite right for playing catch," I lamented.

"But fine for a dip," Neil smiled.

Soon thereafter, Wendy called us upstairs for a dinner medley of stir-fried veggies and baked lemon chicken. Neil once again ate his fill.

"Delicious," he pronounced. "Thank you Mom."

"You've eaten well today," Wendy smiled.

"Thank you both," Neil nodded gratefully.

After dinner, we discussed plans for the next day — run some errands and go back to that little park we'd discovered the day before — then we tried to watch some TV. Unfortunately, the hotel's cable network was programmed to run commercials way too often. Very frustrating.

"A DVD player would be nice," I frowned. "We could just watch what we want."

"I don't think we need a DVD player," Neil shook his head. "I'm pretty sure I can hook my computer up to the TV. All we need is an HDMI cable, then we can watch DVDs."

"Clever," I patted his shoulder, so we augmented our plans for the following day. We would also stop at Best Buy to get an HDMI cable. With that, Neil ducked into his room to do eye exercises and make some calls to his friends; I cleaned up the kitchen; and Wendy sent a quick email to Neil's "other moms."

SATURDAY, APRIL 16, 2016

With a few days under our belts, we were getting into a routine. After a leisurely start to our day, we took a ride down Route 6 to find an HDMI cable. On the way to Best Buy we saw a "hobby store" that was the size of a supermarket — a normal supermarket — but BIG for hobby store!

"That looks like it has to be fun," Neil observed. "We'll have to check that out!"

"Absolutely," I agreed. "Not today, but put it on the list."

Wendy just laughed at her boys.

Neil found the cable he needed at Best Buy, and we picked up two movies, *Heart of the Sea* and *Revenant*. On the way back to the hotel, we also stopped at Barnes & Noble. Wendy wanted a large map of Houston.

After she found what she wanted, we passed a Target, and Wendy wanted to check there for a few more kitchen items, then it was time to return home for lunch.

After lunch and some downtime, Wendy suggested, "Let's check out that little park."

"Sounds fine to me," Neil agreed, so we set out once again in our car.

After turning south on Route 6, I asked Wendy, "Do you remember where it was?"

"I think it's on Memorial Drive," Wendy said. "We need to turn left up ahead."

While commercial development near the highways leading to and from Houston seemed outsized and imposing, after turning onto Memorial Drive and going a mile or so, the surroundings became more relaxed. We found tree-lined streets and neighborhoods much like those at home, although the architecture used more stucco and roof tiles and the plants were tropical.

"There it is," Wendy said after a couple of miles.

"Is it?" I wondered out loud, slowing down. The sign read, "Terry Hershey Park."

"That's it," Neil agreed.

There were pull-offs on both sides of the street, it being a long narrow park that runs north to south, sandwiched between alternating blocks of homes and small office buildings along the Buffalo Bayou. We pulled off to the right and got out to walk on a paved path running alongside the bayou. On its opposite bank, the vegetation was lush and tumbling down to the slow muddy water. Birds flitted over the water catching insects. The path we were on went down a shallow incline and under the overpass we had just driven over. As soon as we got underneath, we noticed a faint smell of guano, and in the crevices between the expansion joints above, we could see huddled bats.

"Wow," Neil mused quietly, "It would be fun to see them come out at night."

I gave him a small nod and held a finger to my lips. The last thing we

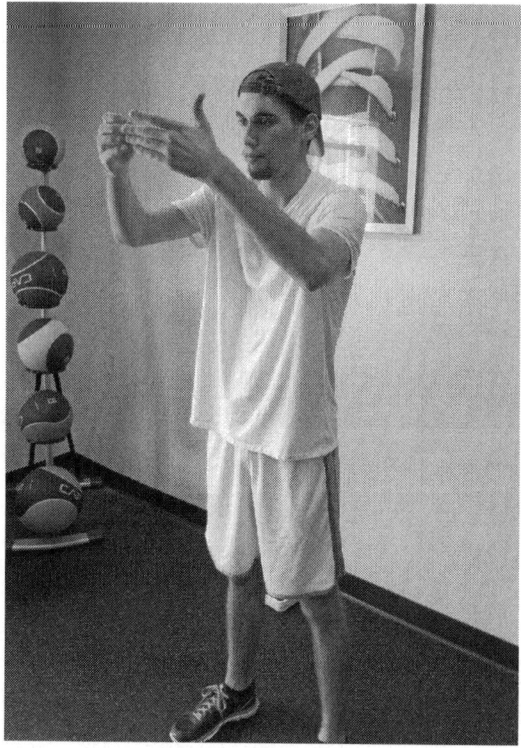

needed was startled bats taking flight all around us! We slowly ambled to the other side of the park and found a bench, so we plunked down to just sit and observe. The contrast between park and suburbs — cheek-by-jowl as they were — was almost surreal. Bicyclists whizzed by and small groups of pedestrians were just out for a stroll, yet we half-expected an alligator to climb up the bayou's embankment.

"It's a bit different from home," I observed.

"A bit," Wendy nodded. "The sun sure feels good. I like it."

"Me too," agreed Neil.

After half an hour of soaking up the sun, breathing in the tropical humidity, listening to the insects and birds, and just watching the world go by, we went back to the car. Our last stop for the day was the H-E-B to get groceries for dinner, then we returned to our suite.

While Wendy prepared dinner, Neil and I hit the gym. He followed the same routine as before – the elliptical bike, some gentle lifting, and some balance exercises. I was honestly amazed and impressed with his coordination and strength. The single biggest giveaway of his illness was the eye patch.

As with previous days, over dinner, we made plans for the following day. There was another park — a large one just north of Route 10 — called Bear Creek Pioneer Park.

"It's bounded by Addick's Dam Road," Wendy said as she looked at the map.

"Another catch basin for stormwater run off?" I wondered.

"I would guess," Wendy nodded. "It features a small zoo, an aviary, several playing fields, and walking paths through the woods."

"Sounds like a good place to check out," Neil agreed.

After finishing dinner and cleaning up the kitchen, we played a board game, something we've enjoyed doing since Evie and Neil were little. We brought one Neil's favorites, *Ticket to Ride*, and he gleefully set up the board. Over the next forty-five minutes, he smiled and joked as he kicked our butts, always seeming to be two or three steps ahead in his strategy.

"Do you ever stop playing chess?" I asked.

"Nope," he smirked. "I like finding the unique strategies of different games."

We played one more game, then wrapped it up for the night. Wendy and I put things away, and Neil went to his room to do some eye exercises. Twenty minutes later, he checked his email and the MGH portal.

"I got the results from MGH," he announced. "The spinal MRI back on March 31."

"What?" Wendy asked.

"The repeat spinal MRI," Neil reminded her. "It was negative."

As we had assumed. Good "bad news" or bad "good news." Take your pick. It underscored Neil's diagnosis. He spent some time on the phone, texting and chatting with friends, while Wendy and I checked emails and watched a bit of news, then we all turned in for the night.

APRIL 17, 2016

Sunday dawned brightly; another good weather day was on tap. We were lucky! We slept late, and after breakfast and the normal routine, Neil shared his important news with Sheryll:

> **To: Sheryll**
> **From: "Eugene (Neil) Fachon"**
> **Subject: Spinal MRI**
> **Date: April 17, 2016**
>
> Hello Sheryll,
>
> This is Neil Fachon; below I pasted the results from my recent spinal MRI. It seems to have turned up clear, so I hope shouldn't need to redo this. Please let me know if you need a more official copy of this transcript, as this is cut and pasted from my MGH patient portal.
>
> Cheers,
> Neil
>
> *Results:*
>
> > Exam Number: 19174559 Report Status: Final
> > Type: MRISpEvMetWWO
> > Date/Time: 03/31/2016 16:36
> > Exam Code: MRICRDWWO
> > Ordering Provider: Ly, Kien-Ninh I
> >
> > HISTORY:
> > Spinal Anomaly: retention - Neoplasm: initial staging or surveillance on treatment: Malignant Brain Tumor NOS - Likely has diffuse intrinsic pontine glioma. Reporting difficulties with urination and defecation. Please do screening spine MRI

REPORT Reviewed by Dr. Jennifer Chang with Dr. Otto Rapalino (Attending Radiologist)

TECHNIQUE: MRI of the entire spine with and without contrast, with FIESTA and Sagittal post-contrast sequences obtained.

COMPARISON: MRI of the spine performed 3/16/2016. MRI of the brain performed on 3/3/2016

FINDINGS:
Focused examination for the purposes of screening for metastatic disease in conjunction with MRI of the spine performed on 3/16/2016 demonstrates no evidence of drop metastasis.

There is a focal linear T2 hyperintensity at the C6-7 level, likely reflect a focal prominence of the central canal. Otherwise, there is no definite evidence of T2 abnormality within the cord.

There is normal anatomic alignment of the spine. Vertebral body heights are preserved. Intervertebral disc spaces are maintained. The conus terminates at the level of L1. The cauda equina and conus medullaris appear unremarkable.

There is redemonstration of mass-like lesion involving the pons and upper medulla oblongata, better characterized on recent MRI of the brain performed on 3/3/2016.

The visualized paraspinal structures are unremarkable.

IMPRESSION:
No evidence of drop metastases.

PROVIDERS: SIGNATURES:
Chang, Jennifer MD
Rapalino, Otto MD Rapalino, Otto MD

With this report, a small "point of order" reared its head. MGH referenced the spinal MRI taken on March 16. That was Neil's first spinal MRI, the one they told him was no good, hence the need for a retake — which took them two weeks to reschedule! Now they were citing the first MRI in the March 31 report?! We had no time to look back, but this peculiarity was annoying.

Neil heard back promptly from Sheryll: *"I will have to verify this with Dr. B and our Regulatory Officer who oversees the study. We cannot deviate from the protocol."*

With that, we set out for Bear Creek Pioneer Park. It wasn't far "as the crow flies," but just like going to the clinic, we had to drive east on Route 10 far enough to take an underpass U-turn and come back west to the park entrance. As soon as we entered the park, we saw acres and acres of cultivated space, including soccer fields, baseball diamonds and a tennis court complex. A bit further on, we saw a small zoo/aviary and a variety of park buildings.

We drove around a few minutes — passing a soccer field with two girls' teams warming up — as we searched for one of those walking paths through the woods. We found an area where a few cars were parked near a trailhead, so we parked and got out to walk. Once again, the trees and foliage were much like Florida, with several swampy areas that looked perfect for alligators. After twenty minutes of slow meandering, Neil had enough.

"Let's watch some soccer," he requested.

I knew that caught his eye, too, so we drove back to the field where the teams were now playing. In my mind's eye, I saw Neil running swiftly, his loose jersey flapping like a flag at his back, a ball at his feet.

"I'd love to see you playing again," Wendy smiled at Neil in the rearview mirror.

"I'll do my best," he nodded.

After half an hour or so, Wendy suggested we go see the zoo, so we drove back towards the entrance and parked near the buildings. The displays were arrayed along a sidewalk, and we strolled in the company of families with infants in strollers and toddlers in hand, some seeing these animals for the first time in their lives. "Wook Mommy, a tuhtul."

Those were the days! Blessed innocence.

"I'm getting a little tired," Neil announced.

"It's time for lunch too," Wendy added, so we headed back to the hotel.

After lunch, Neil took a nap while Wendy sent an update to Dr. Elinzano's office, still hoping they might sign on to help with Neil's treatment.

To: Stephanie, (Dr. Elinzano's assistant)
From: Wendy
Subject: Eugene Fachon: Houston ANP Study for DIPG Patients
Date: 4/17/16

Hi Stephanie!

Greetings from Houston. Here's a quick update to keep you all in the loop.
Today is Eugene's (Neil's) fifth day taking 3mg of dexamethasone. Over the next couple of days, he will undergo baseline tests – brain MRI, PET scan, etc.

Neil is the first to volunteer and sign on to this Phase 2 clinical trial on the study of ANP therapy on DIPG, which was announced this past week. If Neil qualifies for the trial, Anti-neoplaston (ANP) treatment will begin at the end of the week.

More details at http://www.burzynskiresearch.com/research-development.html

Blessings!
Wendy Fachon

Wendy never heard back from Stephanie, but a reply from Sheryll was waiting for Neil when he woke up from his nap:

To: Eugene Fachon, Dean Fachon
From: Sheryll
Subject: RE: Spinal MRI
Date: April 17, 2016

Hello Neil,

Unfortunately, the scans must be within 14 days of starting treatment. Because your last spinal MRI was on 3/31, we will need another. I have called Houston Medical Imaging. Since there are three scans to do, they will be done on Tuesday and Wednesday.

We would like to see you tomorrow and I will give you the rest of the information.
Please come to the clinic at 1pm

Sheryll

Neil would have to take yet another spinal MRI! I was annoyed, but Neil took it in stride — just one more step on a journey he was determined to take. The rest of the day passed quietly. We were enveloped in feelings of comfortable routine and eager anticipation. Tomorrow, the final countdown would be at hand. We spent the evening at our various computers, sending updates and sharing hopes, then we turned in.

SEVERE WEATHER
APRIL 18, 2016

As we slept, the clouds above Houston piled into a Jovian mountain range that let loose a prolonged thunderstorm in the middle of the night. Rain fell as if tipped from a great overhead lake. Fractal streaks of electricity lit the dome of the sky in relentless succession, accompanied by deep ripping sounds like giant redwood trees being torn in half, punctuated by drumbeats of thunder that shook the building's foundation. Once we were awake, there was no going back to sleep, only watching in astonishment and wondering how high the water behind the levee was getting.

The thunder and lightning eased slightly as dawn broke, but the rain kept falling in buckets. We turned on the TV and were greeted with, "We interrupt our normal broadcast with this urgent alert! Nine inches of rain has fallen overnight in the Houston area. Downtown Houston is closed due to flooding." The picture cut to images of car roofs like lily pads where major intersections were flooded, and people being evacuated from rooftops using whatever could float; one man had lashed a dozen milk bottles together. Airport runways were closed, and critical parts of the highway were submerged. Heavy rain was forecast to continue.

"Oh my God," Wendy said for the lot of us.

The Mayor of Houston came on next to explain that flash flooding had caused seven bayous to exceed the capacity of their channels, thus overflowing their banks. Downtown Houston was completely flooded, and businesses were all closed. Residents in areas not flooded were urged to stay home and barricade vulnerable areas with sandbags, then the broadcast switched briefly to show volunteers filling sandbags. Anyone whose home was flooded or in immediate danger of flooding was urged to evacuate. Emergency agencies were responding to calls as quickly as possible.

"Holy mackerel," Neil looked out through the waterfalls running down our windows. We were barely able to discern the levee surrounding George Bush Park. "I wonder how high it's getting," he said, tipping his head toward the levee.

We all had the same thought. We were next to a body of water which, if the levee failed or spilled over, the hotel's first floor would be flooded, at least. Even the drainage ditch on our side of the levee had transformed into a small angry river, but it had not overflowed into the street. For the moment, we were dry, unlike so much of the rest of the city.

"I guess we're not going anywhere today," Neil shook his head ruefully. He was ready for action!

"I would say not," Wendy agreed. "I'm sorry. But at least we're safe here. All we can do is hunker down. I'll get breakfast going and heat up some water for your coffee," she added.

"Just hold the pot out the window," Neil suggested.

"Ha ha," Wendy chuckled.

"Yes, get the coffee going," I nodded. "While we still have power, I'm gonna walk down to the lobby to see if anyone has more news."

The night manager was still on duty, but some of the day help had managed to get through the flooding, and the kitchen was up and running, if scaled back a bit.

"This is wild," I mentioned to the women setting up breakfast.

"Oh, this happens," she said. "But we deal with it. This is a bad one, though."

When I returned to our suite, an email from Sheryll had arrived.

To: Neil, Dean
From: "Sheryll S. Acelar"
Subject: flood
Date: April 18, 2016

Hi,

I will be out of the office today. My area is completely flooded. Please do not try to get to the clinic. Due to weather, there is a flood warning and the clinic may close for the day since half of the workers called in. It is flooded everywhere, so I it's best to see you Tuesday.

I'll email you the address for the scans so you have it.

Best,
Sheryll

I replied: *"Understood. We are in a good spot so far, but flooding all around. We are standing by and will plan on tomorrow."*

Sheryll answered: *"Great! Be safe! We can see you tomorrow morning."*

We remained cloistered in our rooms as the rain kept on pouring. We played games, did some reading, watched the latest reports on TV, and napped. The weather continued through much of the day, dropping nearly twenty inches before tapering off. In the storm's wake, a town familiar with flood emergencies went into recovery mode.

> ***Excerpt from Dr. Burzynski's report, April-18-2016***
>
> The patient is being prepared for administration of antineoplastons according to protocol BT-55. He already read, understood and signed the informed consent documents and complied with all provisions of the protocol BT-55 necessary for admission to the clinical study. He is scheduled to have an MRI of head with and without contrast, PET/CT scan of head and placement of subclavian vein catheter. Soon after evaluation of his MRI and PET/CT scan by his neuro-oncologist and providing that he will fulfill all entrance requirements, he will be started on antineoplastons A-10 and AS2-1 according to protocol.

"FOUR"
APRIL 19, 2016

When dawn broke, the skies were partly cloudy, and the forecast was fair. Neil checked in early with Sheryll, and she confirmed that Houston Medial Imaging (HMI) had survived unscathed by the flooding. *"All systems are go."* She also reminded Neil to forgo breakfast because his PET scan was scheduled for 11:30 a.m., and he wasn't supposed to eat anything for at least four hours beforehand. Almost immediately following the PET scan, he would get a baseline MRI of his brain, without contrast first, then with contrast. It would be a marathon day.

"Could you be at the clinic by 10:00 a.m. to pick up the referral paperwork?" she asked.

"You got it," he promised.

We had to detour around one flooded underpass to reach the clinic. Wendy called ahead when we were close, and Sheryll waited for us at the door. "How are you feeling, Neil?" she greeted him with a smile.

"Raring to go," he assured her. "I hope the weather cooperates."

"There's a slight chance of isolated storms north of the city," she shrugged. "But it should be okay here," then she handed Wendy a manila folder: "Here's the referral paperwork for the scans." Looking back at Neil, she added, "It's going to be a long day. I'm sorry Neil."

"No worries," he smiled. "I'll handle it."

"That's the spirit," Sheryll nodded. "If everything goes as we hope today, tomorrow will be busy too! You're scheduled to get the catheter implant in the morning, but they're still getting sorted out from the weather, so we don't have the exact time. A nurse named Rosie will call you when they know. If it's possible afterwards, the spinal MRI will be that afternoon."

"Yikes," I grimaced.

"I know," Sheryll cringed a little too. "That MRI will be without contrast, and then again with. Neil's cervical, thoracic, and lumbar spine. It will take some time."

"When will we know if Neil has met the requirements for the clinical trial?" Wendy asked.

"Dr. Burzynski will notify me immediately if there are any concerns," Sheryll said. "And of course, I'll call you right away."

"Let's do it," Neil gave Sheryll two thumbs up.

"Good luck, Neil," she waved goodbye, and we got back in the car and headed straight for Houston Medical Imaging (HMI), located much closer to downtown Houston.

The GPS wanted us to take many roadways and underpasses that were flooded, so we had to ad-lib a little, but we still made it with time to spare. There was a brief moment of anxiety when the clouds above thickened and a single clap of thunder rolled in the distance, but it steered clear to the north, as Sheryll had mentioned. Neil checked in, and they took his paperwork and insurance information, then we all sat together on a very plush sofa in the waiting area. To our surprise and delight, the waiting area featured a few display cases full of crystals and geodes.

"Someone here must be an ardent geologist," Wendy said, and we inspected the collection to help pass the time. Neil was called about half an hour later.

"Try to have a good nap in the torpedo tube," I kidded him.

He gave us two thumbs up and went with the nurse.

With a few hours on our hands, Wendy and I decided to go for a walk. On the ride to HMI, we had spotted a restaurant named Snap Kitchen. It looked like a candidate for some good organic Neil-food, so we wanted to check it out. We told the receptionist what we were planning, and she promised to call immediately if we were needed.

We strolled west on Richmond Street a few blocks to the intersection with Kiby Street, the road we drove in on. Amazingly, there had been no serious flooding in the area, and Snap Kitchen was open. As soon as we entered, we knew we'd hit pay dirt. Their menu was largely comprised of fresh locally grown organic veggies and pasture-raised meats. They also had a wall-length cooler filled with freshly prepared salads, wraps, meals and — hallelujah — a variety of cold-pressed veggie juices. They were bottled, but they were also labeled to indicate when they had been pressed — that morning. We bought salads and juices for lunch and sat down to eat.

"We definitely have to bring Neil here," Wendy nodded eagerly. "This is perfect!"

"I have to agree," I said between bites. Indeed, we would end up going back so often we got a discount card — a "buy ten, get one free" sort of thing.

After lunch, we headed back towards HMI. Along the way we noticed a pub that looked interesting, with a menu that boasted amazing gulf shrimp. Something to check out another time. We let the receptionist know we had returned, then we sat down. It was 3:00 p.m. by the time Neil stumbled back into the waiting area. He was tired, running on fumes, and feeling awful. We departed as quickly as possible and went straight to Snap Kitchen to get him a veggie juice and a power bar, then we headed for the hotel. We stopped once at the H-E-B, long enough for Wendy to run in and get some gulf shrimp since Neil had enjoyed them so much in Galveston.

Wendy sautéed the shrimp in coconut oil and topped them with lemon juice and garlic. Neil polished off a dozen in short order, accompanied by a dish of sautéed kale, sweet potatoes and onions, and a helping of leftover lemon chicken and rice. After eating all that, he was still hungry and ate a dish of buttered green beans. He topped the meal off with a bowl of whole milk yogurt mixed with sliced oranges and bananas.

"Whoa," Neil sighed, sitting back from the table. "That was great, Mom! Thanks."

"I'm glad you enjoyed it," Wendy smiled. "You earned it!"

"That was a long day," I nodded sympathetically.

Neil shrugged. "I was wiped out before, but my energy level has gone from a one to a ten. Let's go for a walk!"

"We can clean up later," Wendy said. "Sure, now's a good time!"

It was just after 7:00 p.m. when Neil put on his Boonie hat, and we headed out into the evening air. There was no traffic on Grisby Road, and the water in the drainage ditch had fallen to a heavy stream's volume. We strolled east until we were almost even with the edge of Bush Park. We paused for five minutes to enjoy the sunset colors, then we returned. We walked roughly half a mile each way, and Neil kept an eager pace, his stride strong, if a bit foot-draggy at times.

"Another big day tomorrow," I said as Neil marched up the stairs to the hotel's second floor. "You up for it?"

"Way up," he smiled. "Let's get'r done."

To: "Sheryll S. Acelar"
From: Dean
Subject: Catheter and MRI
Date: April 19, 2016

> Sheryll,
>
> Neil is getting his second wind and very much wants to do the double-header tomorrow. Please confirm where and when we need to be. Also, any special prep instructions? Eating breakfast okay, or prohibited? Liquids? We await instructions for tomorrow.
>
> God Bless,
> Dean

Sheryll replied: "*Great! Rosie will call to let you know when and where to report tomorrow. Neil should not eat anything for at least 8 hours prior to the procedure. I hope we can get this all done as soon as possible. I also need to complete all paper work before we can start.*"

Rosie called around 9:30 p.m. that night. Neil's surgery to have a catheter inserted into a vein under his left collarbone would be done by Dr. Younan Nowzaradan. We needed to have Neil at the Foundation Surgical Hospital on Fannin Street in Houston by 9:00 a.m. the following morning to check in.

"THREE"
APRIL 20, 2016

Neil slept well and awoke feeling refreshed. "All systems are go," he smiled. Unfortunately, he would have to skip breakfast again. Thank goodness he ate well the night before, leaving him with plenty of energy for the moment. We left the hotel at 7:15 a.m. and entered the address for the Foundation Surgical Hospital on our GPS. As with our ride to HMI, a few detours were needed to get around flooded areas, but we arrived at the hospital by 8:30 a.m. Wendy and Neil went ahead to check in, while I parked the car.

Parking presented a curious pickle, but not for the reason one might expect. The lot wasn't crowded, but when I pulled into a space, I noticed the car's odometer had just rolled over to a number ending with "666." So, I'm superstitious: I've disliked this number since I was a kid — maybe too many horror movies. It might have been less disconcerting if seeing it were just a one-off, but ever since arriving in Houston, I'd noticed it popping up more frequently than seemed probable — often on license plates. Seeing it on the odometer — leaving it sitting there frozen in place — gave me a creepy feeling, like being stalked, especially on the heels of that monster storm. *Don't be an idiot*, I told myself as I sat there, but I couldn't leave it, so I backed out of the space and drove up and down the garage until the odometer hit "667". It took a few minutes and must have looked very strange to anyone monitoring security cameras, but I felt better.

By the time I joined Neil and Wendy, they were seated with a nurse in a small office, going over the admission paperwork and insurance. Once check-in was done, we took an elevator up to the surgical floor. Neil informed the receptionist he was there, and we took seats in the waiting area with a handful of other patients. Soon thereafter, he was called. We wished him luck and gave him long hugs. He smiled his best toothy grin, gave us two thumbs up, and went with the nurse.

Neil was prepped and ready for surgery by 10:00 a.m. Unfortunately, the surgeon wasn't there. Due to the storm, Dr. Nowzaradan was delayed until noon, and by then we were worried we wouldn't make it back to HMI in time for Neil's spinal MRI. Fortunately, the surgeon had performed this procedure many times, and once surgery began, Neil's catheter was placed in half an hour. His sedation wore off quickly, and we had a chance to visit him briefly in recovery (a picture of which found its way to the front page of the *Boston Globe*). Neil was all smiles and thumbs up, ready for the next "event," but he had to wait for an X-ray to confirm the catheter's proper placement. At 2:30 p.m., this was confirmed, and we were given instructions on how to care for the incision — keep it bandaged, have a nurse check the dressing and change it as needed, and don't tug on the tube — then Neil was discharged.

He felt none the worse for the wear, and it was impossible to tell anything had been done once he put on his shirt, but now he had a flexible twenty-inch tube protruding from the upper left side of his chest. The clear tube terminated in a small plastic tip covered by a threaded endcap. The tube also incorporated a pinch clip, which served as a safety against blood flowing out. No, there was no blood in the tube. It had been back-flushed with saline solution, and blood could not flow out, nor medication in, without the pinch clip being open and a special fixture threaded onto the plastic tip to open its tiny internal valve. The incision site was covered by a bandage.

"Are you hungry?" Wendy asked on our way to the car.

"Ohhh yes," Neil nodded. "I'm hunnn-gry!"

Having nothing to eat since 8:00 p.m. the night before, Neil was obviously famished once again. Time was tight, but there was no food restriction for his spinal MRI, so we stopped at Snap Kitchen for a quick salad before returning to Houston Medical Imaging for his 4:00 p.m. appointment. We squeaked in just on time.

The spinal MRI took over two hours, so it was another long and difficult day for Neil, but he was getting into his stride, so he made light of it. "I feel good," he nodded when we departed, disk in hand. "Tired, yes, but I'm finally getting into the fight."

To say we were proud of our boy would be an absurd understatement. He was showing us "how things get done!" We stopped at Newk's for a quick dinner on the way home, then Neil was in bed and asleep by 8:30 p.m.

After he was sound asleep, Wendy and I sat up in our room.

"Where do we stand with our budget?" I wondered.

"Our imaging expenses have come to roughly three thousand two hundred dollars," Wendy replied after consulting her notebook. "HMI gave us a discount because we paid out of pocket. Besides that, Neil's health insurance is covering the blood tests, and it should cover the surgery."

"That's not bad," I held back a yawn. "Assuming Neil meets all the entry requirements, the clinic will cover the costs of all medications, equipment, and visits."

"That's a blessing," Wendy sighed gratefully.

"Indeed," I did yawn. "I need to send a couple of notes, then it's time to turn in."

To: "Sheryll S. Acelar"
From: Dean
Subject: Marathon two days...
Date: April 20, 2016

Sheryll,

Neil did it. We waited over 3 hours for the procedure this AM, and another two hours for x-rays and discharge. Long long time at the hospital. We stopped briefly to get some food into him, then we went straight to HMI. He 'cooked' for two hours and was done at 6:30. We have a disk with the images. I can deliver it early tomorrow morning, but I expect Neil will still be asleep – he needs it. I'm sure I can have him back at the clinic by 11AM, if that works. Let me know. Is everything a 'go?' We are eager to get started with the real work...

God Bless,
Dean

I also sent a quick update to family and friends, recounting our marathon days and Neil's amazing positivity: "*Like his Drill-sergeant told him, 'Never give up!'*" As my email disappeared into the ether, a note from Sheryll arrived:

To: "Dean"
From: "Sheryll S. Acelar"
Subject: RE: Marathon two days...
Date: April 20, 2016

> Hi,
>
> Yes! Neil has quailified. We are proud of him too! Of course, he can come at 11am. I am preparing the paperwork tonight so we can keep things going.
>
> Good night.
> Sheryll

"Neil did it," I announced to Wendy. "He's in the clinical trial."

"I knew he would," she smiled gratefully.

"Should we tell him?"

"Nooo," she shook her head. "He needs his sleep more than anything. Time enough tomorrow."

"TWO"
APRIL 21, 2016

I went downstairs early to grab a hotel breakfast — egg patties, sausage patties, yogurt, and coffee. Neil was still asleep when I returned to the suite, but Wendy was moving about quietly in the kitchen. There was an email from Sheryll waiting for me:

> **To: Dean**
> **From: "Sheryll S. Acelar"**
> **Subject: RE: Marathon two days...**
> **Date: April 21, 2016**
>
> Hi,
>
> When you get here to drop off the CDs, can you let me know? I have to give you a blood-work request form for Quest. We need baseline bloodwork before Neil starts.
>
> Thank you,
> Sheryll

"I'm heading into the clinic with the disk," I told Wendy. "It sounds like Neil will start treatment today, but we'll need to go back to Quest first, to get baselines."

"I'll get him fed as soon as he's up and ready," she replied.

"See you shortly," I smiled. "This is it!"

Morning traffic was in full rush hour mode when I merged onto Route 10. This was the one time I wished for that "speed pass." I called Sheryll as soon as I pulled into the clinic's parking lot.

"I'll meet you at the entrance," she told me. "I'll be right down."

A few minutes later, I exchanged the CD of Neil's spinal MRI for the lab paperwork.

"So this is the big day?" I could not quite believe it. "He'll start treatment?"

"That's the plan," Sheryll smiled. "Take Neil to Quest to get baseline measurements of his electrolytes, enzymes, and blood cell counts. Try to have him back here around noontime."

"FAN-TASTIC!" I nodded. "See you again soon."

Neil was awake and getting dressed when I returned from the clinic. He emerged from his room in game day spirits — anxious and excited. This was the day he would start hitting back at the invader lodged in the base of his skull.

"Sheryll said you'll start treatment this afternoon," I reported.

"Mom told me," he grinned.

"All systems go?"

"Way go!" he pumped his fists.

Neil wolfed down breakfast and was ready by 10:30 a.m. Traffic had thinned, and we had no trouble getting to Quest, but the lot was jammed once again, and this time no slots opened up. I dropped Wendy and Neil at the door and cruised the lot, waiting for someone to vacate a space. Of course, there were other cars doing the same thing, so it all came down to timing — who was closest to whatever spot opened up. It was like parking in Cambridge, Massachusetts on a Friday or Saturday evening. While I was still driving around, Wendy called for a pickup. Neil's blood was drawn, and a urine sample was provided.

"All good," I asked as they slid into their seats.

"No problemo," Neil smiled.

We drove to the Burzynski Clinic, navigating the traffic like old hands, and parked next to the Bougainvillea, as bright as Neil's spirits. Things were going his way!

TWO AND HOLDING

We had no particular expectation as to how things would unfold, so when Sheryll met us and escorted us to the small conference room we used when Neil first signed the consent forms, we thought nothing of it. A few moments later, Dr. Burzynski joined us.

"So how are you feeling?" he shook Neil's hand.

"Raring to go," Neil smiled.

"I'm glad," Dr. Burzynski smiled back. "Unfortunately, we may have a problem."

We all tensed. Neil's shoulders squared.

"I received a letter from FDA yesterday afternoon," Dr. Burzynski continued.

"Hmm. What's it say?" Neil asked politely.

Wendy and I just leaned forward, squeezing the armrests of our seats.

Dr. Burzynski placed a document on the table. "The FDA has placed a Full Clinical Hold on the trial."

You could've heard a pin drop.

"God D-" I started, but Neil quickly put a hand on my wrist.

"What does that mean?" he asked quietly.

Dr. Burzynski started reading the letter aloud[13], but it was difficult to quickly take in. Seeing the perplexed looks on our faces, Dr. Burzynski offered, "Let me try to explain. They cite two reasons for hold, one due to manufacturing process deficiencies identified in March of last year. We

13 The entire letter is included in the appendix at the end of this book.

took steps to address their concerns and responded a year ago. We heard nothing further."

"And since then, they approved the clinical trial," Neil observed.

Dr. Burzynski nodded.

"And they bring it up again now," Neil shook his head as if doing a double take at a chess move his opponent just made and took back. "After a year?!"

"Curious timing," Wendy frowned.

"The second reason," Dr. Burzynski continued, "is due to a change they are making in definition of 'ingredients' we use to make antineoplastons." He returned to reading the letter:

> *As per your submission, phenylacetic acid (PN) and phenylacetylglutamine (PG) cannot be considered as starting materials but are drug substances. Provide the name and physical location of the manufacturing facility(ies) for these drug substances. Confirm that these are manufactured under GMP conditions.*

"We have used these ingredients [PN and PG] for a decade," Dr. Burzynski explained. "They undergo many steps of processing and purification. The FDA knows this, but suddenly it decides these ingredients are 'drug substances.'"

"Which means they must be manufactured like they'll be administered directly to patients," Neil interpreted, speaking in a flat voice, his tension sublimating into "analyzing the board."

"Precisely," said Dr. Burzynski nodded.

"It sounds arbitrary," I shook my head cynically.

Dr. Burzynski read further:

> *In order to address these deficiencies, you must submit the following information:*

> *Identification of an alternative manufacturing facility and all required information regarding that facility and its manufacturing processes required under 21 CFR 312.23. The submission should contain detailed information to demonstrate that the alternative facility can manufacture ANP from an acceptable and qualified drug substance(s), the drug products (AS10/AS21-1) are sterile, meet established acceptance criteria, and the products are comparable to those manufactured by S.R. Burzynski Manufacturing Facility.*

"No such manufacturing facility exists," Dr. Burzynski frowned deeply. "It would cost millions of dollars and take years to build."

"May I see the letter?" Neil asked, and Dr. Burzynski handed it to him. Neil read for a minute, then said, "So the FDA is demanding you correct an ingredient deficiency by taking steps to ensure '*the products are comparable to those manufactured by S.R. Burzynski Manufacturing Facility.*'"

Dr. Burzynski nodded.

"Yet they're citing 'manufacturing deficiencies' in that very facility," Neil thumped the table with a fist. "I'm sorry, this is bogus!"

"Disingenuous," I agreed.

"And deficiencies were addressed," Dr. Burzynski shrugged with his hands. "A year ago."

Since the clinical trial was FDA-reviewed, IRB-approved. and listed on the government's own clinical trial website, the content and timing of the letter were suspicious at best.

"This just stinks," Neil pursed his lips, starting to tremble a little.

"After all these years," I looked at Dr. Burzynski. "The FDA is still playing 'Tom and Jerry' with you."

Dr. Burzynski tipped his head to the side with a questioning look.

"Cat and mouse," I elaborated.

"But you're a clever mouse," Neil looked up hopefully.

Dr. Burzynski's eyes twinkled. "The letter says I may not enroll any new patients."

"But I'm already enrolled," Neil picked up the thread, his chess-head kicking up another notch. Looking back at the letter, he added, "It also says '*you may not resume administration of ANP in any adult or pediatric patients previously treated.*' But I haven't started the actual treatment, so you would not be 'resuming.'"

"That could work," Dr. Burzynski nodded. "You enrolled on thirteenth. You went through all exams and passed all requirements. Your catheter is in place..."

"All before this letter arrived," Neil slapped his hands on the table. "Let's do it! I didn't come this far to turn around and go home with my tail between my legs just to die!"

Neil was strategically positioned in a gray area. He was enrolled in the trial and ready to start, and he was in Texas, a state where "Right to Try" was the law.

"I agree completely with Neil," I said simply.

"So do I," Wendy nodded.

Dr. Burzynski nodded too. "Alright. I'll draft a document saying we've discussed all of this, and you want to proceed. We start treatment under the protocol today, and I will inform FDA, but I cannot predict what they will do. You may want to talk to your lawyer."

"Ugh," we exhaled in unison. "Let's not go there just yet. Let's hope it doesn't come to that."

Dr. Burzynski raised an eyebrow that hinted it most likely would.

"I could also write to the FDA," I suggested, "pleading Neil's case directly."

"They don't like dealing with patients," Dr. Burzynski shook his head. "But you can try." Then, he called Sheryll in, "Please take them to treatment room three."

Sheryll escorted us down the hall, while Dr. Burzynski returned to his private office. This turn of events, though unpleasant, was probably no surprise to him. He had been defending himself against similar interference from the FDA and the Texas Medical Board (TMB) for thirty years.

"ONE"

"Treatment room three" would be Neil's private abode at the clinic for the next three weeks. On our way to his room, we passed a large room populated by a handful of patients and nurses. Neil gave Sheryll an inquiring look.

"These patients are only getting AS2-1," Sheryll explained. "You're the only patient who will get AS2-1 and A-10 together. That's what we're testing in the clinical trial."

"Aha," Neil nodded.

"And here we are," Sheryll announced as she opened a door, "Treatment room three."

He stood at the entrance to a room that was roughly fifteen feet by fifteen feet and brightly lit. As we filed in, we noticed a window overlooking the indoor arboretum on the opposite wall. Along the left side wall was a counter and supply cabinets. Along the right wall was a couch and side table. On the inside wall to the left of the door was a recliner, and in the middle of the room was a simple white table, a working surface with no drawers or trim and with two folding chairs pulled up to it. All the surfaces were vinyl, plastic, or metal — easily cleaned. Very practical.

"Take a seat," Sheryll motioned Neil to the couch. "I'll go find Julian."

Neil and Wendy took the couch, and I sat on the recliner.

"So this is it, Buddy," I smiled at Neil, pushing the FDA's machinations completely aside.

"Yup," he nodded. "Hard to believe we made it this far."

"Yes it is," Wendy added. "It's exciting!"

"I'll say," Neil agreed, struggling back a contradictory yawn. "I'm happy to be here. I'm just tired."

"Put your head down," Wendy smiled and moved to a chair so he could stretch out.

He crumped over and fell asleep almost instantly. After all the heartache, uncertainty, and confrontation, Wendy and I just sat there, trying to block the FDA from our thoughts and recapture our feelings of hope.

Ten or fifteen minutes later, there was a knock on the door.

"Wake up Buddy," we told Neil.

He pulled himself upright as the door opened, and in walked a male nurse. He was roughly my age, a little shorter than average with a lean build and silver hair parted in the middle and swept back to just over his ears. He wore glasses, a small hoop earring in his left ear, and a silver scorpion pendant dangled from a long chain around his neck. He also wore a tie-dyed Grateful Dead T-shirt and "pogo sneakers" — crazy-looking walking shoes with spring loaded heels that gave him almost two inches of lift and a springy step. He fairly hopped into the room, his open and friendly face radiating so much humor and kindness that he could actually get away with asking, "So, Mr. Fachon, what brings you here?"

Neil picked up immediately, arching an eyebrow and yawning deadpan, "The weather. It's good for my arthritis."

The nurse laughed and bowed theatrically. "I'm Julian," he shook Neil's hand. "I'm sorry you've got to be here, but you've come to the right place. I'll do my best to take good care of you the whole time you're here."

"I'm sure you will," Neil smiled, immediately comforted by this new companion.

"And I'll train your parents on how to do everything I'm about to do," Julian added.

Things were about to get as real as it gets.

"First things first," Julian began. "We need to change the dressing on your surgical wound," and he went to the supply cabinet to get a package containing the sterilized bandages, gloves, cleansing wipes, and antibiotic ointment he would need.

"Could you guys step outside for a few minutes?" he asked us. "This needs to be as sterile as possible." Then, he asked Neil to put on a mask and take off his shirt.

We stepped outside the room and closed the door as Julian began to open and spread out a dressing change kit. This was our first hint of the many procedures we would encounter and have to learn how to master. Several minutes later, Julian invited us back into the room.

Wendy asked, "How does the incision wound look?"

"Fine," Julian nodded. "A little redness and swelling at the sutures, but that's normal. I cleaned the area and spread antibiotic ointment before dressing it back up. We'll need to change the dressing on a regular basis for a while — until the stitches come out and the healing is fully resolved. In the meantime, when he wants to take a shower, you'll need to seal the entire area, including the catheter, with a waterproof covering."

"How do we do that?" I wondered.

"When he's disconnected from the pump," Julian started, "you'll cap the catheter with a sterile green tip, coil the tube, and tape a sterile plastic covering over the tube and the dressing."

"Okay," I shrugged uncertainly.

"Don't worry," Julian reassured us. "I know this is all new and seems complicated, but it's easy," he promised. "I'll teach you everything."

Next, Julian took Neil's baseline vital signs and introduced him to his new constant companion, a dual channel "BodyGuard 121 Twins Infusion System."

"This pump will administer the ANPs through your catheter," Julian explained. "It gets programmed to deliver an exact dose at four-hour intervals. Once Dr. Burzynski decides on your dosage for the day, we use one of these pump sheets to determine the parameters for distributing the dose across six separate infusions," and he showed us a worksheet with the tables and formulas needed to perform the calculations for flow rate and duration. The worksheet incorporated a half-sized picture of the pump face in the lower right corner.

The pump itself was a solid brick of mechanical and electronic technology, roughly six inches by four inches and two inches thick. In the center of its face was a numerical keypad along with "start," "stop," "channel," "prime bolus," "on/off," and "power" buttons, and to each side was a hinged cover plate, which opened to expose the mechanical workings for massaging liquid medications through thin IV tubes at a very precise volume and rate. The whole thing was powered by an internal rechargeable battery. At night, when Neil slept, the pump would be plugged into an outlet and placed on the table beside his bed, delivering ANPs as it charged up for the next day.

"You'll typically get a few hours each morning when he can disconnect from the pump altogether," Julian continued. "Otherwise, the pump and the ANPs will get tucked in this pump case, and you'll carry them with you." Julian held up what looked like a small black camera case — roughly ten inches by six inches by six inches — with a clear plastic window on top, through which to see the pump's face. Inside the case was a set of hook-and-loop straps to hold the pump firmly in place. The case also had an adjustable clip-on shoulder strap.

"Are you taking notes?" I asked Wendy.

"Don't worry," Julian soothed again. "When I'm done training you, this will all be routine."

"Considering the clinical trial could last up to two years," I nodded, "I imagine you're right."

"We'll go over this as many times as it takes for you to be completely comfortable with the process," Julian promised emphatically.

Sheryll stepped into the room around 2:00 p.m. to deliver the intravenous bags of ANPs from a secure dispensary. These clear liquids were the product of a highly regulated month-long manufacturing and quality -assurance process. There were two IV bags – Atengenal (A-10) and Astugenal (AS2-1). The A-10 bag held roughly one and a half pints of liquid, the AS2-1 roughly half of a pint. Each bag was sealed inside its own sterile Mylar bag and labeled with a unique peel-off sticker indicating the date of manufacture and lot number.

Sheryll told Julian the dosages Dr. Burzynski wanted to start with, and Julian used this information to complete Neil's first pump sheet. We would need to fill out a sheet every day for the duration of Neil's treatment. Julian explained the details as he completed the sheet, but seeing our "you're going too fast" expressions, he paused. "It's a lot to take in all at once," he smiled. "I know. But we'll keep going over everything until you're so comfortable you can do it in your sleep."

When he was done with the sheet, Julian got up to excuse himself for a moment. "I need to go wash my hands with antibacterial soap before spiking the bags and clearing air bubbles," he explained. "Just to be extra careful there is no contamination at this stage of preparation."

When he returned, Julian sat at the treatment table and cleaned the surface and edges with alcohol wipes to ensure the entire working surface was freshly sterilized. Next, he arrayed the pump, IV tubes (which had covered "spikes" on one end and threaded connectors with sterile caps on the other), a Y-adapter in a sterile pouch, and all the attendant tips, surgical clamps, medical tape, and a pair of scissors on the table. These were laid out strategically, like puzzle pieces, each piece placed where it would fit with another.

For the final steps in the set-up procedure, Julian snipped open the protective Mylar bags and removed the IV bags of ANPs, positioning the A-10 to the left of the pump and the AS2-1 to the right. Each IV bag had a twist-off cap covering a nipple, which would be "spiked" at the time of use. Julian peeled the lot labels off each Mylar bag and adhered them to the pump sheet, right beneath the image of the pump, then he took the smaller of the two discarded Mylar bags and taped the open side to the lip of the table so it hung in front of him, the bag's mouth open and facing up. "This is to catch excess fluid as I clear air from the IV bags and lines," he explained.

We nodded in anticipation.

Next, Julian unwrapped the Y-adapter, connected the threaded ends of the IV tubes to the top-prongs of the "Y" and tucked the assembly into the Mylar bag hanging in front of him. He also taped the tubes down to the end of the table to ensure the assembly couldn't slip out of the bag while the lines were being cleared.

"We try to avoid spillage," he explained. "The ANPs are nontoxic. I've gotten them all over my hands many times, but you've noticed the smell."

"Yup," we nodded, Neil chuckling to himself, no doubt thinking, *the piss doctor*.

"It's not really bad," he reassured Julian.

Julian smiled appreciatively. "Now comes the fun part!"

In a very deft and practiced sequence, Julian twisted the nipple cap off the IV bag of AS2-1, removed the sterile tip from the spike on the IV tube and quickly inserted the spike into the nipple, breaking the bags inner seal and pressing the spike firmly into place. This had to be done quickly while allowing nothing to contact the spike, thus minimizing any chance of contamination. Once the bag was "spiked," Julian pulled on the spike to show that no amount of tugging could separate the union. The IV tube would snap first. Then, Julian laid the spiked A-10 bag on the table next to the pump and went through the same process with the AS2-1.

With both bags spiked, Julian opened the left side of the pump and ran the A-10's IV tube through the pump's left channel mechanism. There were small collars on the tube to get it properly aligned. Then, he used the pump's priming function to bleed out any air trapped inside the IV bag and tube, right down to the tiniest bubble. (This was an elaborate and painstaking procedure, which will be described in greater detail a bit later.) Once complete, the entire process was repeated for the AS2-1.

When both sides were purged of air, Julian tucked the ANP bags into the bottom of the pump case and "dressed" the IV tubes so they would not crimp, then he programmed the pump — referring to the pump sheet prepared earlier — and strapped the pump into the case so its face was visible through a plastic window in the lid. Next, Julian neatly threaded the IV tubes through a padded slot at the back of the case, then he zipped the case closed, leaving the ends of the tubes that would connect to Neil's catheter laying coiled on the table.

IGNITION

At roughly 3:30 p.m., Julian used an alcohol wipe to clean the bottom end of the Y-adapter, then he removed the sterile cap from the blue tip on Neil's catheter, used a sterile wipe to clean it, snugly threaded the end of the Y-adapter to it, and opened the catheter's safety clip.

"And that's it," Julian smiled. "You're ready to go."

"That's all," Wendy and I rolled our eyes.

Julian chuckled. "Would you like to do the honors?" he asked Neil, motioning to the pump face. "Just press the 'start' button."

Without a moment's hesitation, Neil pressed the button, sending his first dose of antineoplastons into his body and giving us two thumbs up, grinning ear to ear, eyes twinkling.

20

LIFT OFF

"Making complex thoughts simple to think about is a really great feeling!" NF

Neil's first dose of A-10 would take several minutes, to be followed almost immediately by AS2-1.

"Okay, we're going to keep you here for the first infusion cycle," Julian said. "I'm going to check on my other patients, but holler immediately if you feel any nausea or sickness. In the meantime, drink water anytime you feel thirsty, and oh," Julian went back to the storage cabinet. From the bottom shelf, he took a quart-sized plastic urinal marked in cubic centimeter increments. He handed the urinal to Neil. "From now on, use this to measure how much you pee. We need to keep track of your total fluid intake — water, juice, whatever you drink — and your total output."

"Even rental beers," Neil chuckled.

It was Julian's turn to raise an eyebrow. "I'll pretend I didn't hear that," he smiled, then he gave Neil a worksheet to record his liquid input/output. "Come get me when the infusion is done," he said before leaving the room. "And holler immediately if you need me sooner."

We remained at the clinic throughout Neil's first infusion, and Sheryll popped in a few times to check in. He remained stretched out on the couch and asleep for a good part of the time. When he wasn't snoozing, he sipped down a bottle of water, which we dutifully recorded on his record sheet, and he made one trip to the bathroom, recording that too.

When his first infusion cycle was complete, I went to find Julian. He was just down the hall in the large treatment room. "I'll be right there," he nodded.

"Nap time is over," Wendy coaxed Neil awake.

He slowly sat up, stretched cat-like and yawned, smacked his lips, and looked for his bottle of water, then he took a deep gulp.

"How do you feel?" I asked him.

He smiled quizzically, searching a moment for words. "It feels like a waterfall in the back of my head."

What a good feeling that must have been!

Upon returning to the room, Julian checked Neil's vital signs again and inspected the intake/output sheet. "Good," he nodded. "You must need to pee."

"Yep," Neil nodded, "but I can wait a little longer."

"Okay. We're almost done for the day," Julian told him. "So how do you feel?"

"We were just talking about that," Neil rubbed his hands together. "It feels like a waterfall in the back of my head."

Julian nodded, looking pleased. "That sounds encouraging."

"Have you heard that before?" Neil wondered.

"Not exactly, but I like how you put it," Julian answered, then he turned to us. "In the morning when he's done with this round of infusions, you can disconnect him from the pump to give him some free time. Just record the total amounts of ANPs delivered. The numbers will be displayed on the pump's readout. Write them below the lot number stickers on the pump sheet. You can turn off the pump, but leave it charging until you come back to the clinic."

"Okay," we nodded. "And how do we disconnect him?"

"Whenever the pump is on 'hold' between infusion cycles," Julian explained, "and at the end of a complete series of infusions, he can be disconnected," and he demonstrated. "This may look a bit scary, but it's easy! Get one of the prepackaged saline syringes; close the safety clip on the catheter; disconnect the catheter's blue tip from the Y-adapter and wipe the blue tip with a sterile pad; evacuate any air from the syringe — to do so, point the syringe upwards and plink it to coax bubbles to the top, then squeeze the plunger until a few drops of fluid come out — then screw the syringe onto the blue tip; undo the safety clip; invert the syringe so the plunger is up and flick it a few more times in case there are any last bubbles; push the plunger in, not all at once but in two or three spurts over five seconds until the syringe is almost empty. This will purge ANPs from the line. Once that's done, close the safety clip, unscrew the syringe, and screw a sterile cap onto the blue tip, and voila!"

"Oh yeh," I puffed. "That looks easy!"

"He makes it look easy," Wendy shook her head, just as daunted.

"None of this is rocket science," Julian smiled reassuringly. "It just takes practice and attention to detail."

"And a checklist," I nodded.

After this demonstration, Julian needed to take a blood sample through Neil's catheter — to check his electrolyte levels. This required drawing the saline solution back out of the IV line until some blood made it all the way to the syringe, then unscrewing that syringe and attaching another to draw a pure blood sample.

"Did you feel any of that?" I asked Neil.

"Not a thing," he shrugged.

Once Julian had the sample he needed, he walked me through purging the IV line, and I reconnected the pump. It would deliver five more dual infusions throughout the remainder of the day and into the wee hours of the following morning.

"Now," Julian continued, "be careful with the IV lines. Try not to let anything tug them."

The IV lines emerged from the bottom of Neil's untucked T-shirt. Julian looped a foot of slack in the lines and secured the loop to the hem of Neil's shirt with a pinch clip like the ones used to hang a "visitor" name tag.

"This is a safety loop," Julian explained. From the clip, the IV lines were still long enough for Neil to stand up while the pump case was on the ground. "If you try to walk off without picking up the case, or if you snag the lines on something, you'll feel the tug on your shirt. A gentle reminder to pick up the case."

"And if I don't," Neil cringed.

"You'll know it," Julian grimaced. "Just don't do that. I'm sure you'll get used to it quick."

"I'm sure I will," Neil agreed. "It's my lifeline."

Julian nodded with compassion. "Now just give me a moment to check your electrolyte levels," he said and left the room.

"We've got a lot to learn," Wendy said.

"I'll say," I agreed, a bit intimidated.

"I think you can handle it," Neil reassured us.

Julian returned a few minutes later. "You're good to go," he smiled. "Just keep drinking water, and if you run into any difficulty — anything at all, no matter what time — just give me a call."

"Let me just use the bathroom once more before we go," Neil said, picking up the pump case and slinging it over his shoulder, then grabbing the plastic urinal.

"Be my guest," Julian held open the door. "Meanwhile, I'll get Sheryll."

She and Julian returned at about the same time as Neil. "Three hundred twenty-five cc," he announced.

"Good," Julian nodded, jotting it down on the record sheet and handing it to Wendy. "Make sure you write it all down."

"Oh we will," she assured him.

Sheryll smiled, "So how are you feeling, Neil?"

"FAN-TASTIC," he gave two thumbs up. "And I'm hungry!"

"That's good," she beamed. "Very good!" Then, she turned to us. "We'll do bloodwork here tomorrow. Can you bring him at 9:30 a.m.?"

"No problem," we all nodded. "And we'll start drafting a letter to the FDA."

She nodded, a shadow of concern briefly crossing her face, then she smiled. "Call with any issues or questions — anything at all — day or night!"

"We got it," Neil nodded to her and Julian, then he slung the pump case over his shoulder with an easy grace, and they escorted us to the clinic's door.

"Do you have any other suggestions for eating out?" Wendy asked. "We love Newk's, but it's time for a little more variety."

"I like the Movable Feast," Sheryll recommended.

"Ruggle's Green," Julian added. "Both are fairly close."

"I'd try Movable Feast if you just want a really nice meal," Sheryll said. "Ruggle's Green can be a wait, and there's a lot more going on. It's more of a party."

"Yeh, maybe the Feast to keep it simple," agreed Julian. "But you'll love Ruggles Green when you go there!"

"Movable Feast sounds like the move," Neil looked at us.

"And so it shall be," Wendy agreed. We said our goodbyes for the day and trundled out to the elevator.

"How is it?" I asked Neil, nodding at the bag.

"Sorta like a backpack," he smiled. "No biggie."

"You're taking ANPs," I reminded him, "and you say 'no biggie.'"

"Meant to be," Neil smiled. "Feels meant to be."

"To the Movable Feast," Wendy smiled. "Life is a movable feast!"

"Who said that?" Neil asked.

"Hemingway," she smiled.

We walked into the bright afternoon sun, flanked by colorful bougainvilleas — silent fireworks in celebration of the moment — and piled into the car. I entered the address for the Movable Feast into the GPS, and it took us west on Route 10 to a turnaround, then east a few miles to exit onto the access road. We continued a short way and turned into a standard-looking shopping plaza anchored by a supermarket and a long building lined with several individual shops facing the parking lot.

Movable Feast was at the left end of this building. The restaurant had outdoor seating beneath an overhang adorned with hanging tropical plants. A wrought iron railing and several plantings cordoned this area off, so it could only be entered through a doorway from inside the restaurant. Half health food store and half restaurant, the Movable Feasts décor was classic Tex-Mex with accents of Hemingway-bohemian. The vibe was suggestive of just kicking back to enjoy the world going by. Standard menus were located on a side table near the entrance, and daily specials were written on a chalkboard behind a dessert display case, which also served as a walk-up counter for placing orders. Everything was made with fresh organic ingredients. What we had that first dinner I cannot recall, but before we had taken our second bites, we were all in agreement, Movable Feast would become a regular visit. Neil was famished and ate his fill, also drinking plenty of water, especially while the pump was running. After finishing, we went straight "home." Neil's "back teeth were floating."

After such a hectic schedule the last few days, bedtime came early. We arranged Neil's side table to accommodate the pump's charging station and a bottle of water for over-night sipping, and we put the plastic urinal on the floor alongside the table within easy reach. The priority in setting things up was to give Neil as much scope in his IV lines as possible. It would be a challenge to sleep tethered like that. He was a bit uncertain to start, but he was sure that he could adjust.

"We're very proud of you," we told him. "Sleep tight. And holler if you need anything."

"I'm proud of you two, too," he hugged us. "Thank you."

I sent a quick email to family and friends:

To: Family and friends
From: Dean
Subject: Next hurdle...
Date: Thu, 21 Apr 2016

Dearest Family and Friends,

Although he was formally enrolled over a week ago, Neil still had to undergo a battery of testing to satisfy the protocol for the trial. Now, after all the poking, needles, scans and surgery, Neil has passed all the requirements, but ironically there has been a last minute regulatory complication. I cannot go into detail as it's an issue Dr. Burzynski must address, and it will hopefully be settled in short order, but in the meantime Neil is getting infusions of antineoplastons and he's quite happy about it. We all have a good feeling about the prospect for success with Dr.Burzynski, and Neil aims to fight with everything he's got. For those of you who have played a game of chess with Neil – or watched him play – you know he packs some serious fight. And of course we will be at his side, as will you. We thank you from the bottom of our hearts for your love and support, and most of all for your prayers. So many people need help from above – all the more so when we find ourselves in real trouble – and prayers do make a difference. Hugs and kisses to you all! You are in our prayers too.

God Bless,
Dean

After that, Wendy and I tucked in for the night. We both checked on Neil at different times during the night, and all seemed quiet. Buoyed by hope, the night passed peacefully.

Excerpt from first of two Doctor Burzynski reports, April-21-2016

The patient successfully completed the requirement of the pretreatment MRI of the head with and without contrast, the PET/CT scan and underwent the placement of the subclavian vein catheter. I explained to the patient and his parents that yesterday afternoon on April 20, 2016, we received a letter from the FDA directed to the Burzynski Research Institute as the Sponsor of the Investigational

Drug Application. I read the letter to the patient and his parents and explained in lay terms that the investigational New Drug Application was placed on full clinical hold and I may not enroll new adult or pediatric patients in any protocol under the IND. I explained that according to the FDA, the reason behind the hold is [concern about] unreasonable and significant risk of illness and injury to a human subject [due to ingredients used to manufacture ANPs]. I also explained that the process of manufacturing of antineoplastons and the suppliers of chemicals used for manufacturing have remained the same over 10 years. The patient and his parents believed that they were already admitted to the clinical study since the patient was properly examined on April 13, 2016 and signed the informed-consent documents on April 13, 2016. They requested to commence with administration of antineoplastons. I informed the patient and his parents about possible risk of the treatment and also informed them that we are going to notify the FDA about this patient's treatment and we will ask them for clarification. It is possible that the FDA will request discontinuation of the treatment. The patient and his parents fully understood the content of the FDA letter and they requested to proceed with the treatment of antineoplastons and signed this progress note.

Excerpt from second Doctor Burzynski report, April-21-2016

Subject came in for Week 1 Day 1. PI was available to assess clinical disease status. Vital signs were taken and were stable. Subject reported grade 1 fatigue today, 04/21/2016, attributed to the hectic schedule of completing all the requirements for the screening visit. PI made the clinical decision on dose adjustments. First dose of antineoplastons were received at the clinic. No adverse reaction or allergic reaction reported. Electrolytes were drawn and showed no clinical significance. Subject did not have any other issues or further questions for PI. Subject was advised to call for any other issues or symptoms. All procedures were done according to protocol.

LEARNING BY DOING
APRIL 22, 2016

Wendy and I awoke feeling more rested than we had in days. The last dose of Neil's first infusion was done when I went quietly into his room to shut off the pump, disconnect the IV lines, and flush the catheter as Julian had instructed. Doing this for the first time, my hands shook a little, but I managed. Neil was awake, but his head was still mashed in his pillow.

"You look groggy. Need to sleep more?"

"D'ya mine if I do," he mumbled. "I dint konk out 'til afta 'leven. Tough get'n comfable wifou'tuggin' the tubes."

"I'll bet," I nodded, noting the empty water bottle and the urinal that was over half full. "Not to mention having to drink and pee throughout the night." This would all take getting used to. "Sure thing, you go back to sleep."

To: "Sheryll S. Acelar"
From: Dean
Subject: RE: Marathon two days...
Date: 4/22/2016 8:11 AM

Good morning Sheryll,

Neil is asking for little more sleep this AM. He did not get to sleep until after 11 last night, then he went through the night just fine, but after the last few days he is still exhausted. Could we come in at 10:30 instead of 9:30?

Thanks,
Dean

* * *

To: Dean
From: "Sheryll S. Acelar"
Subject: RE: Marathon two days...
Date: April 22, 2016

That's fine.

The extra hour helped, especially with the pump disconnected. Neil slept a bit more, then he did a few eye exercises to help wake up before emerging from his room. "I'd like to take a shower," he announced.

"You could use it," Wendy held her nose, goofing. "And a shave."

I coiled the catheter and covered it and the bandage with a six inch by six inch square of clear plastic, then I taped each side carefully to his chest. "You're good to go."

Neil enjoyed his first shower since getting the catheter. "That really felt good," he smiled, emerging in a cloud of steam from the bathroom. He had a fresh shave as well.

"FAN-TASTIC," Wendy beamed. "Now get dressed and have some breakfast. It's ready."

By 10:00 a.m., we were ready to go. Since the clinic would be doing the bloodwork, there would be no need to stop at Quest Lab. Traffic was still heavy — even if "rush hour" was technically over — so we arrived a few minutes late.

"Good morning Neil," Irena greeted him brightly and opened the door into the inner sanctum.

Sheryll met us and brought us back to our room. "Dr. B will be right in," she smiled.

We were familiar with Dr. Burzynski's nickname, of course, but we had not presumed to use it. Now, it seemed as if Sheryll was giving us permission. A moment later, Dr. B knocked on the door and came in.

"Good morning," he smiled to everyone, then he gave Neil a quick exam. "How was your night?"

"Not bad," Neil replied. "I did okay, but it's a little difficult to keep from rolling around while you're sleeping," he admitted.

"Yes," Dr. B nodded. "You will adapt. Did you drink plenty of water?"

"He sure did," Wendy handed over intake/output worksheet.

"Any nausea or dizziness?"

Neil shook his head no. "Just sleepy."

"That's fine," Dr. B smiled. "And we have results from your baseline MRI. It looks good. No significant change from Boston."

"Wow!" we all clapped.

"You must be doing something right," Neil smiled at Wendy.

"The diet must help," Wendy nodded. "Cutting out processed food and sugar, just for starters."

"That is helpful," Dr. Burzynski nodded. "Unfortunately, the tumor is quite large already, so we have no time to lose. I will increase your dose just a little today, to help you acclimate more, then we increase according to protocol."

"Got it," Neil nodded. "Sounds good."

With that, Dr. B wished us a good day and departed, and Sheryll returned. "Today, we'll have you do the prepping under Julian's supervision."

Right on cue, Julian walked in. Sheryll carefully handed over the bags of ANPs and told him Neil's dosage for the day.

"Here we go," Wendy and I exchanged nervous glances.

"Good morning, Campers," Julian smiled and gave us another little bow. He chatted with Neil about how the night went, then Julian turned to us. "Now it's time to wash your hands," he ordered Wendy and I, giving Neil a conspiratorial wink. "You get to relax."

"Fine with me," Neil smiled and leaned back in the couch. He and

Julian discussed rock bands — the Grateful Dead, mostly, and also The Who — while Wendy and I washed up carefully.

Upon our return, Julian instructed us to start with cleaning the treatment area using alcohol wipes. I went to the cabinet for some wipes, and we proceeded as Julian had done the day before.

"Now let's set up the equipment," he continued.

Like setting up a board to play chess, each piece had its place. We put Neil's pump in the middle of the table, then we gathered what we needed from the cabinet and arrayed it as Julian had yesterday. He made a few small adjustments, but for the most part, we had it correct. Everything was ready to "spike the bags."

"This part seems pretty difficult," we both hesitated.

Julian cleaned his hands with an alcohol wipe, then we let him sit at the table and demonstrate once again how to remove the spike covering, twist off the cover on the IV bag's nipple, and insert the spike, all in a swift set of graceful motions.

"That's gonna take practice," we nodded, admiring Julian's skill.

"You'll get this too, I promise," Julian nodded us back to our seats.

With the bags spiked, Wendy suggested I work on my own for the moment. "It will be awkward for two side-by-side."

"Yeh," I nodded. "You're probably right." I sat down and began by running the IV lines through the pump, aligning the collars as Julian had done.

"That looks good," Julian nodded. "It takes just the right amount of gentle tension on the tubes to get them aligned."

The next part of the entire procedure would be the most time consuming — clearing air from the IV bags and lines. It was a painstaking process of "ploinking" the soft IV bags with an index finger to get the bubbles out of every corner and crevice, coaxing them to float to the top of the bag, then using the pump's priming feature to pump that air out of the bag. Eliminating all the bubbles, including minuscule bubble specks, which had a stubborn way of sticking in the corners and along the seams of the bags, was an iterative process.

"No wonder you guys all wear glasses," I joked with Julian as I squinted into the corner of the A-10 bag. It took me three or four cycles before he was satisfied.

Once air was cleared from the bag, the IV line had to be cleared as well. This entailed holding a segment of line vertically (starting nearest to the bag) and flicking the line with a finger so any bubbles inside the tube would break loose and rise, then taking the next length of IV line and continuing, segment by segment, until all the bubbles were collected at the end of the IV line, in or near the Y-adapter. For the last step in this process, I laid the IV line on the table and ran the pump while using the flat of the scissor handles to rap on the IV line and the Y-adapter, pumping all the air out. I had to keep the pump running until the line was filled with clear liquid. In the process, several cc of ANPs were pushed out as well, hence the need for the catch bag taped to the edge of the table.

Throughout this time, Julian kept a watchful eye on me while kibitzing with Neil. They were becoming good buddies.

Once the first line was clear, the entire process had to be repeated for the bag of AS2-1 and its IV line. At this point, Wendy took over, and she was going into the second hour of ploinking and flicking when Julian interjected, "You guys are doing great."

"You think?" Wendy paused.

"Absolutely," Julian nodded. "You'll have this in no time. Once you get the hang of it. You won't have to obsess quite so much with the bubbles. Get what you can see, but if you miss something, this little trap on the Y-attachment is there to catch it," and he pointed at a small bell-shaped fixture on the Y-adapter.

"Ah-ha," Wendy blinked. "Good to know."

Once our preparations were complete, Julian gave everything a final inspection, then he walked us through the pump sheet, showing us the calculation for dividing total dosage, the flow rates, and the delay between intervals. With that, it was time to program the pump, tuck the IV bags into the pump case, dress the IV lines to emerge through the chafe slot,

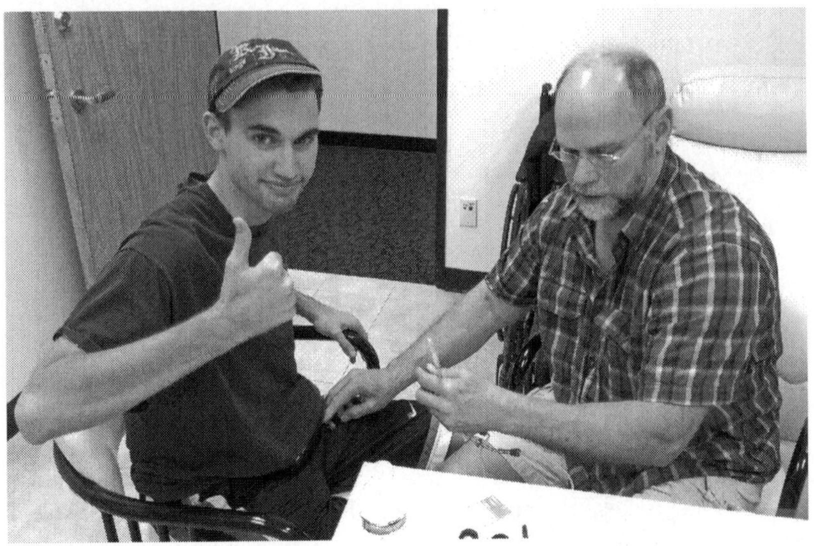

and strap the pump into place so its face was readable through the plastic window in the lid of the case.

"We're all set," Julian smiled. "Great job! Who wants to do the honors?"

I looked at Wendy, but she nodded at me.

"Okay Neil," I said, "let's saddle up."

He grinned and plunked down in the chair next to me.

"Have an alcohol wipe open and ready," Julian coached. "Wipe the end of the Y-adapter, remove the sterile cap from the catheter's blue tip, wipe the receiving end of the blue tip, and thread it onto the Y-adapter. Twist it on snugly, but not too hard."

The ballet of fingers was almost like spiking a bag, but my hands were quickly adapting. The very last task was to undo the catheter's safety clip.

"Are you ready?" I asked Neil. He gave me two thumbs way up, Wendy took a picture, then I connected the pump and pressed the start button.

A FUTURE FEELS POSSIBLE

We were fairly buzzing with hope when we departed the clinic. A small celebration was called for, so we went to Newk's for lunch, then we checked out the iFLY Indoor Skydiving facility we'd seen across the parking lot. It was almost like entering a movie theater, but we could hear the muffled sound of air being driven by a massive fan. There was a staircase leading up two flights to a landing, which was glassed off from the 'flight room.' In the center of the room was a Plexiglas chamber. It was cylindrical, aligned vertically, and about twenty feet in diameter. The chamber had a small entrance, and inside was an open mesh trampoline for a floor. A huge high-speed fan was blowing up from beneath.

Visitors were welcome to watch, so we went into the flight room while a first-time skydiver suited up and an instructor reviewed basic procedures.

"More lessons," I said to Neil.

"I'm down," he nodded eagerly.

A moment later the instructor backed up to the chamber's entrance and stood at the threshold holding the student's hands. They nodded to each other, then the instructor stepped back into the airstream and lifted off into a layout position almost instantly. Next, the student leaned into the airstream and lifted off with a screech of delight. The instructor brought her to the center of the chamber and helped her get used to the airstream. After a few minutes, he guided her back out of the chamber so he would have room for a demonstration. Using his hands and body like flaps, he did flips and spins, and he moved side to side and forward and back.

Neil chuckled. "That's totally cool!"

"I always wanted to try skydiving," I told him as we left the building. "Before Mom and I got married, I had some friends who invited me."

"Why didn't you?" Neil asked.

"I just never quite had the nerve."

"Too bad," Neil shrugged. "This looks like a safe way to get a taste."

"For you," I agreed, "once you're done with this treatment."

"That's a plan," Neil smiled.

After leaving iFLY, we stopped at the H-E-B for fresh fruit, then we returned to the hotel and took it easy for the rest of the day — napping, hanging out by the pool, reading and writing emails, and watching a house-flipping show on TV. Wendy completed the day with a delicious home-cooked meal.

"What say we watch a movie," I suggested after dinner.

"Sounds good," all agreed.

Wendy did cleanup; Neil used his new HDMI cable to connect his computer to the TV in our room; and I pulled an armchair in from the living room for him to have some place to sit. Once Neil sorted out the connections, we all settled in to watch *Revanant.*

At the end of what proved to be a gruesome saga of early frontier days in the US, Neil commented, "There's no way he survived all of that. Jumping off a cliff and falling into a tree?!"

"Not to mention getting mauled by a grizzly bear," I added.

"Well, that's Hollywood for you," Wendy shrugged. "But he survived. That's the point."

"Touché," Neil hugged her and yawned. All the while, the pump was doing its thing, and Neil had been all but oblivious, save for sipping from a bottle of water. What a great day! But it was after 9:00 p.m., and he was ready for bed.

Going through the evening routine for a second time helped us start finding our rhythm. Neil had less of a struggle falling asleep, although he would have to wake up intermittently to use his urinal and drink water. At one point, I heard a clunk from his room.

"You okay?" I asked softly.

"A-yuh," Neil replied. "Knocked the water bottle off the table."

"Just don't knock over the urinal," I chuckled, as did he.

Both times Wendy and I got up to use the bathroom that night, Neil seemed to be sound asleep.

Excerpt Doctor Burzynski Report, April 22, 2016

Subject came in for Week 1, Day 2. PI was available to assess clinical disease status. Vital signs were taken and were stable. Subject reported grade 1 fatigue on 04/21/2016 which

> resolved this morning by 10:30AM, 04/22/2016. This was attributed to the hectic schedule of completing all the requirements for the screening visit. Dose of antineoplastons from yesterday were recorded and received 5 doses due to early stop for blood test. PI made the clinical decision on dose adjustments. Astugenal will be increased at a slower pace than recommended in the protocol for the safety of the subject. Atengenal will be increased by PI according to protocol. AE for grade 1 fatigue recorded in CRF. Electrolytes were drawn which showed no clinical significance. It was decided by the PI to do electrolytes daily in the next three days for the safety of the subject. Subject did not have any other issues or further questions for the PI. Subject was advised to call for any other issues or symptoms. All procedures were done according to protocol.

DOSING UP
APRIL 23, 2016

The alarm was set for 7:00 p.m. The pump would be done with Neil's last dose, so I went to his room to turn it off, disconnect the lines, and flush the catheter. This activity was enough to wake Neil.

"Good morning Buddy," I smiled. "How'd you do?"

"Better," he yawned.

"You're free to move about the cabin," I joked. "All disconnected and flushed." I noticed his urinal was almost full, and he'd gone through two water bottles. "You must have been up a few times."

He nodded.

"Any trouble falling back to sleep?"

"Not really," he shook his head. "Konked back out pretty quick."

"Fantastic."

That earned me a smile as I picked up the urinal and recorded the volume on the worksheet. I took the urinal to the bathroom to empty and rinse, closing Neil's door to give him some privacy. He emerged a few minutes later.

"It's nice to have some extra mobility for a while," he said, stretching out his arms.

"Enjoy it," I nodded.

The morning routine was just that. After the normal "ablutions," Neil downed his juice and supplements, had some herbal tea, and ate breakfast by 9:00 a.m., then we were off to the clinic.

Neil's visit would begin with a blood test and another dressing change. After drawing the blood through the catheter, Julian excused himself to take the sample for analysis. "I'll be back," he intoned.

When he returned, Julian asked me to put on a mask and stay to watch the dressing change. He sat on a chair in front of Neil and talked me through everything as he did it: He asked Neil to put on a mask; Julian donned his own mask and gloves; he opened the dressing change kit and spread the contents on the sterile surface of the open kit; he donned a second set of gloves; he removed Neil's old bandage; then he cleaned the wound, applied antibiotic ointment, and re-bandaged the wound. Everything had a prescribed method and order to minimize any chance of infection. The wound was a bit red and swollen — not unusual — but Neil was developing a slight rash under the bandage adhesive.

"It's a bit of an allergic reaction," Julian explained. "If it gets worse, we have an ointment for it." Another wrinkle to iron. Lastly, Julian changed the blue tip on Neil's catheter.

"The blue tip is a one-way valve to prevent blood flowing out when the pump is disconnected," Julian explained. "Have I mentioned that already?" he crimped his face quizzically. "Anyway, it should get changed periodically. Just make sure the safety clip is closed when you do!"

I cringed at the thought of leaving it open. "I guess so!"

Neil's bloodwork came back quickly. His sodium and potassium numbers were "in the zone." Dr. B stopped in to evaluate Neil's progress, and based on his good spirits and renewed energy, Dr. B decided to proceed with upping the dose according to the protocol — 208 ml of A10 and

56ml for AS2-1. Sheryll stopped by shortly thereafter with the new bags of ANPs.

"That seems like a pretty big increase," I raised my eyebrows questioningly.

"That's the protocol," she replied. "Let's see how he does."

Because this was a substantial dose increase above what Neil received the first two days, we would have to prepare two sets of bags, the second to be swapped in after Neil's third infusion, which Julian calculated would be at 8:16 p.m. in the evening. Wendy and I both worked on preparing. Doing two sets of bags back-to-back helped establish "best practices." We were getting the knack. Of course, doing two sets also meant it would take twice as long, but Julian had a second pump we could use to clear air from the lines, so Neil was back up and running while we finished getting the second set of bags and IV-tubes ready.

"With the increase in dose," Julian told Neil, "you'll need to be more conscious of drinking water and staying close to bathroom facilities."

"Duly noted," Neil nodded.

The weather was hot and muggy, and there wasn't much interest in being outside, so we headed back to the hotel to take things slow and give Neil a chance to adjust to the dose increase. He did fine throughout the day, drinking and peeing more often for sure. When 8:16 p.m. came around, I stopped the pump, closed the safety clip on the catheter, unscrewed and detached the Y-adapter from the used set of bags, attached the new Y-adapter from the second set of bags, opened the safety clip, and hit "start." Simple enough, but the pump lights just blinked red and green intermittently.

"That doesn't look right," I frowned.

"Let's call Julian," Wendy and Neil said together.

The phone rang at most twice and Julian picked up. After I described the situation, he told me to switch channels on the pump and "start" the second channel as well. Boom. That was it. I thanked him, and he reminded us to call any time. "Have a great night."

Throughout the day, we had tracked Neil's increased fluid input and output. This would be a significant adjustment for him to "sleep with," but he was up for the task. After sending an update to family and friends, we turned in early:

To: Family and Friends
From: Dean
Subject: Day three of treatment
Date: 23 Apr 2016

Dearest Family and Friends,

These last few days have been very eventful. We meet with Dr. Burzynski every day, and we have met many of the staff who work at the clinic, as well as some patients. Our nurse, Julian, has a heart of gold and a sense of humor to match. This becomes evident the moment you meet him and see his pogo-shoes with rainbow laces and the Grateful Dead t-shirts he likes to wear. In addition to taking care of Neil, he is teaching Wendy and I how to prepare the medication bags, the pump, and all the connecting equipment so we can maintain treatment once we return home. It is quite an involved and time-consuming process requiring certification.

Neil is on his third day of treatment with antineoplastons – each day the dose is increased. He is getting infusions from the aforementioned pump which connects to his vascular access catheter and delivers the antineoplastons in six doses spread throughout 24 hours. He is taking it well, but until he reaches a stable dose it will take getting used to. So how is he doing? It is way too early to say anything for sure, but he is noticing some improvements in his vision, and his energy level seems to be improving after bottoming out the morning after the first day of treatment. We are documenting his symptoms as best we can to chart changes. That's about all for now. We are turning in early – still catching up on lost sleep but making some progress. We need to be at the clinic tomorrow at 9:30AM, and that will pretty much be our schedule for the next few weeks. Sending hugs and kisses to you all!

God Bless,
Dean

Excerpt Doctor Burzynski Report, April-23-2016

Subject came in for Week 1, Day 3. PI was available to assess clinical disease status. Vital signs were taken and were stable. Subject did not report any new symptoms. Fatigue reported yesterday, resolved on 04/22/2016 with no recurrence since then. Subject stated that double vision and walking slightly improved from the baseline. Doses from yesterday were recorded and received 5 doses due to blood test required today. PI made clinical decision on dose adjustments. Astugenal and Atengenal will be increased to the recommended dose based on the protocol. Electrolytes were drawn which showed no clinical significance. Subject did not have any other issues or further questions for the PI. Subject was advised to call for any other issues or symptoms. All procedures were done according to protocol.

21

WARNING LIGHT

"Failure is an important part of growth." NF

SUNDAY, APRIL 24, 2016

The night passed quietly, but a little after 8:00 a.m., we heard stirring from Neil's room, then a weak voice, "Mom, Dad, can you come in here?"

We never got up so fast. "What's up, Honey?" Wendy asked.

"Not feeling too good," Neil told her. "Like I'm going to throw up."

"I'll turn off the pump," I said, which had almost completed his last dose.

After disconnecting the pump and flushing the line, Neil tried to sit up and was immediately gripped by heaving. Wendy held his shoulders, and I grabbed the wastebasket next to his bed. Most of the previous night's dinner splattered into it. A moment later, he laid back down exhausted.

"I couldn't drink enough water," he sighed. "I need to just chill."

"Okay," we agreed. "Try to sip a little when you feel up to it."

I called Sheryll to let her know what had happened. "Neil is having a tough morning. I had to stop the pump just before the last infusion was done. He threw up a minute later."

"I'm sorry," she commiserated. "This can happen as patients adjust. I'll let Dr. B know. Please come in as soon as Neil feels up to it. We need to check him and do bloodwork."

"He's still laying now, but will do," I agreed.

After resting several minutes, Neil tried to sit up again, and just as quickly, he threw up again, ending with dry heaves and leaving him shaken.

"Oh boy," he muttered, as if his DIPG had just made a move he hadn't expected, laying bare a new vulnerability. "My head hurts."

"You'll be fine," Wendy coached him.

"Sheryll said this is not too unusual as patients adjust," I added. "Keep resting, and when you feel ready, we'll head to the clinic so they can give you a checkup and do bloodwork."

"Rest as long as you need to," Wendy reiterated and made sure he had plenty of fresh water by his side. "Sip slowly, just a little at a time."

He nodded weakly. "I wish I'd stopped the pump sooner. I just couldn't keep up."

"Too big an increase too fast," I consoled him. "This is a balancing act — like the slackline. It'll take time to figure it out."

Neil gave a small nod, and Wendy sat with him while I sent a follow-up email to Sheryll.

To: "Sheryll S. Acelar"
From: Dean
Subject: Rough morning...
Date: April 24, 2016

Hi Sheryll,

As discussed on the phone, Neil awoke feeling nauseous and threw up a considerable amount of last night's dinner. He threw up again after we tried to sit him back up. Now he is dressed and sitting up. Once he feels up to it, we will head to the clinic. His comment this AM was that he felt like he should have stopped the pump sooner – that he was getting too much salt and just could not drink enough water to keep up with it. This is partially exacerbated by the fact he has had trouble swallowing for several weeks. While it may be his dinner did not agree with him, I think it likely his dosage was increased too much too quickly. I'm not sure he will want

> to re-connect to the pump right away – not until he's feeling himself again...
>
> Otherwise, attached is the draft of the letter I mentioned to you. We will see you at the clinic as soon as possible.
>
> God Bless,
> Dean

The "letter" referred to was a response we were drafting to the FDA. As a veteran of many FDA-tussles, Dr. Burzynski's comments would be invaluable, and we wanted to do whatever we could to reinforce his response to the FDA's clinical "hold." We wanted the FDA to know Neil was fully appraised of their concerns; he was fully "informed" and had given his "consent;" and he very much wanted to continue the trial. The letter would go through multiple iterations on its way to becoming an appeal written to a variety of bureaucratic and political figures. First and foremost, however, Neil had to recover from this morning's setback.

SUCKING IT UP

After half an hour, Neil managed to sit up and hold down a few sips of water.

"I think I'm okay," he told Wendy. "But I'm not sure I can go back on the pump today."

Wendy nodded and gave him some privacy to get dressed. Shortly thereafter, he emerged from his room looking pale and dispirited. Nonetheless, he was ready to leave for the clinic at roughly 10:00 a.m. I called Sheryll to let her know we were on our way, and she and Julian greeted us at the door to shepherd Neil back to his treatment room. As soon as he stepped into the room, he felt sick and threw up again, only a little water, fortunately, in another handy wastebasket.

"Just lay down on the couch," Julian soothed him. "Rest easy while I get your vital signs and draw some blood to check your electrolytes."

"You'll be okay Neil," Sheryll touched his shoulder gently, easing him back on the couch. "This isn't unusual when patients are first adjusting."

Neil lay back and dozed off. Ten minutes later, Julian returned to announce Neil's sodium levels were fine, but his potassium levels were off, and he was dehydrated. Dr. Burzynski prescribed some IV dexamethasone to reduce swelling, and some D5W hydration, which Julian administered intravenously. Since we arrived late to the clinic, Julian had already prepped a new set of bags, which lay ready and waiting. Neil rested another half an hour or so, then Dr. Burzynski came in to see him.

"How are you feeling now?" he asked as Neil sat up slowly.

"A little better," he tried to smile. "Tough to process enough water when you're sleeping," he shook his head gently. "I'd like to hold off for today if that's okay," he added, looking at the prepped bags.

"That's fine," Dr. Burzynski agreed without hesitation. "We can resume tomorrow. Take today to recover your strength. You'll be fine."

So, that was the plan for the rest of the day. We were back at the hotel by mid-afternoon. Neil managed to eat a little boiled rice, two slices of plain turkey, and a small bowl of lettuce. He also sipped some water. Even though he held it all down, he seemed to be staring into the abyss when he curled up to nap in his bed. This setback had rattled him.

"It'll be okay," Wendy soothed him again.

PREPARING TO JOUST

Throughout the remainder of the day and into the evening, I exchanged several emails with Sheryll — alternating between how Neil was doing and composing the FDA letter. Sheryll relayed my draft to Dr. B, and he replied through her. This was the start of an increasingly direct conversation between Dr. B and us. We were on the same page: with a death sentence hanging over Neil's head, there had to be some way to convince the FDA to let him follow through with the treatment he'd chosen — to accord him his "right to try."

To: "Sheryll S. Acelar"
From: "Dr. Stanislaw R. Burzynski"
Subject: Re: Rough morning...
Date: 4/24/2016

Please tell Mr. Fachon's father that the letter is very good, but the ending is too weak. I'm afraid his son may quickly deteriorate if the FDA forces us to stop. This should be spelled out in the letter. The vomiting he experienced could indicate swelling of the tumor as a reaction to ANPs. The tumor tissue could be starting to die. Dead tissue causes inflammation and swelling, which should decrease soon.

I think the letter should go to VP Joe Biden ASAP. He is now at the annual cancer congress (AACR). I will try to get the contact information.

SRB

* * *

To: "Sheryll S. Acelar"
From: "Dr. Stanislaw R. Burzynski"
Subject: Re: Rough morning...
Date: 4/24/2016

Please mention also to Mr. Fachon that the letter should be addressed to VP because he is in charge on the National Cancer Program and he is also a father who lost one of his sons to brain cancer. I have a friend who will get contact information to reach VP effectively. He also suggested that Mr. Fachon make it an open letter and send to the major newspapers.

SRB

VP Biden? Oh brother! "All of a suddenly," this letter was taking on discouraging proportions.

To: "Sheryll S. Acelar"
From: Dean
Subject: Re: Rough morning...
Date: Sun, 24 Apr 2016

Hi Sheryll,

Does Dr. Burzynski want to include the letter with his response to the FDA? That was my original intent. If the ending seems restrained or weak, I wanted to conclude with a grace note, a fig leaf for the person most immediately responsible for making this decision. Nonetheless, I have sharpened the conclusion:

> "While we can appreciate the FDA's concerns about safety, in a situation where death is imminent, please do not let an excess of caution jeopardize what we believe to be Neil's best hope, not just for prolonging his life, but for renewing his "Lease." Absent sustained treatment, there is every reason to believe Neil will succumb to this cancer within weeks, as per the original prognosis.
>
> Thank you for your prompt attention. Time is of the essence. My son's life is truly at stake."

If we get slammed, we can take the FDA to task in the next round, but some diplomacy now might be expedient. I would prefer addressing the letter to the FDA and "CCing" or "BCCing" the VP, if Dr. Burzynski is amenable. I'll need contact info for the FDA and the best contact info for the VP, then I will finalize, save as a .pdf and send to you. I can also write a separate letter for the VP. As for making any letter an open letter, I have no qualms, but my gut still tells me to attempt defusing the situation at its source before escalating.

I certainly recognize that my son's life is on the line; that has been at the front of our minds since March 4th! We are all very grateful to Dr. Burzynski, to you, to Julian and the rest of the clinic for what you are doing, and I'm very sorry we all have this new problem to cope with. It's needed like the proverbial hole in the head, but if we pull together we will surmount it, God willing.

God Bless,
Dean

* * *

To: "Sheryll S. Acelar"
From: "Dr. Stanislaw R. Burzynski"
Subject: Re: Fwd: Rough morning...
Date: 4/24/2016

The FDA does not like to deal with patients. I think it will be best if Mr. Fachon sends the letter to VP Biden asking for immediate intervention. This way the legal action can hopefully be avoided and the issue resolved quickly and quietly.

SRB

* * *

To: "Sheryll S. Acelar"
From: Dean
Subject: Re: Fwd: Rough morning...

Date: Sun, 24 Apr 2016

This afternoon Neil is still pretty wiped out. He's feeling somewhat defeated and frightened, and his headache is a little worse. Yes, he has been taking some food and water and potassium supplements, but is there anything else you'd recommend for his headache?

Between us, I can't help but wonder, after the good day he had, if we had just maintained dosage whether this would have happened. I recall mentioning to Julian that I thought the dose was a pretty big increase...

I know how important this clinical trial is and how distracting this FDA intrusion has become. I want the trial to succeed for the clinic's sake almost as much as I do for my son's. Tomorrow will be a crucial day. I pray we can make it a good one.

Please let me know the most expedient way to send a letter or email to the VP, and I will CC Dr. Burzynski.

Thank you so much for all you are doing!
God Bless,
Dean

* * *

Via Sheryll
To: "Sheryll S. Acelar"
From: "Dr. Stanislaw R. Burzynski"
Subject: Re: Rough morning...
Date: 4/24/2016

Please also assure Mr. Fachon that patients typically experience such symptoms when the tumor is responding.

We have to protect him from swelling of the tumor. The symptoms should pass.

SRB

* * *

To: Dean
From: "Sheryll S. Acelar"
Subject: RE: Fwd: Rough morning...
Date: April 24, 2016

Hi,

Dr. B is trying to get the contact info as we speak. Also, he would like to discuss with Neil about increasing the dose of dexamethasone, if he agrees.

Sheryll

* * *

To: Dean
From: "Sheryll S. Acelar"
Subject: RE: Fwd: Rough morning...
Date: April 24, 2016

Hi,

For the headache he can take 2 advil tabs.

I'm sorry he feels defeated. Hopefully that does not discourage him from moving forward. We can adjust the dose tomorrow. For now let him rest.

Also, remember that Dr. B would like you to CC him on the final FDA letter.

Best,
Sheryll

PERSPECTIVE

By evening, Neil's appetite and spirits had recovered enough to eat a small dinner. Wendy cooked up some rice, chicken, and green beans.

"You're doing better," she smiled hopefully after Neil polished off his meal.

"You're not as green," I smiled. "JK."

"Much better," he nodded. "I think I just need to ramp up a bit slower."

He had come to terms with this setback and wasn't about to throw in the towel.

"Yup. That was a pretty big increase after just getting started," I agreed. "Sheryll says Dr. B will make some adjustments tomorrow. She also said he would like to increase your dose of dexamethasone, if you're willing," I shrugged. "For a little while, to help you adjust to increasing the ANPs."

"I guess so," Neil frowned. "For a little while."

"I don't like the dexamethasone either," Wendy cringed. "The side effects get nasty if it's taken too long."

"If it helps you acclimate to the dose of ANPs Dr. B hopes you to reach, it's worth it," I reasoned. "Then you can taper off again."

"Sounds like a plan," Neil acquiesced.

After finishing his meal, Neil got up from the table. "I'd like to catch up with some friends," he said, retiring to his room and his laptop.

Wendy took care of cleanup, and I sent another note to Sheryll.

To: "Sheryll S. Acelar"
From: Dean
Subject: RE: Fwd: Rough morning...
Date: 4/24/2016

I will certainly send a copy Dr. Burzynski. I doubt very much I can send anything to Joe Biden that he'll actually see in a timely fashion, if at all... Neil is doing a bit better now, with some dinner in him. I think any sense of defeat is temporary, so long as there is no repeat anytime soon. See you tomorrow.

God Bless,
Dean

Before turning in for the night, we called Evie to confirm her visit to Houston for Neil's upcoming birthday. Yes, she planned to come stay for a week, leaving the day after Neil's birthday. Thank goodness. Neil needed to see her. He wouldn't say it, but he was doubtless getting a little bit bored with our company.

Excerpt, Doctor Burzynski reports, April-24-2016

Subject came in for Week 1, Day 4. PI was available to assess clinical disease status. Vital signs were taken and were stable. At 8:30 AM the subject experienced 2 episodes of vomiting with a 30 minute interval. The antineoplastons was stopped at 8:25 AM and vomiting occurred after. Subject presented to the clinic at 10:30AM and at 10:40AM subject had one more episode of vomiting. Grade 2 vomiting recorded. Subject also complained of a grade 1 frontal headache after the vomiting. Subject was given dexamethasone 3mg intravenously for possible increase intra-cranial pressure as recommended by the PI. Electorates were drawn and showed normal sodium and grade 1 hypokalemia of 3.4 mmol/L. For the safety of the subject, PI ordered for D5W IV hydration which was administered at the clinic. Due to the vomiting episodes, potassium chloride 10meq p.o. b.i.d. was prescribed for the hypokalemia. Doses from yesterday were recorded and received all six doses. PI made the clinical decision on the Antineoplaston dose adjustments. Atengenal and Astugenal will be reduced today,

> however, the subject requested to be off the antineoplastons for today and rest. The ANP bags were already spiked and since the subject opted to be off, the ANPs will be disposed of accordingly. PI approved request. Subject was advised to call for any other issues or symptoms. All procedures were done according to protocol and for the safety of the subject.

RE-BOOT
APRIL 25, 2016

Neil slept well, waking up Monday morning in much improved spirits and ready for breakfast. With his meal he took three milligrams of dexamethasone as per usual, and he took a potassium supplement to maintain his electrolyte balance. After breakfast he was ready for a shower and the rest of his morning routine. Once complete, we hopped in the car and headed back to the clinic, handling Houston traffic like old pros.

It was once again time to change the dressing on Neil's surgical incision. This time, I did so while Julian observed, making corrections as needed. "You did fine," he pronounced when we unmasked. Neil gave me a high five.

"Honestly," I said, trying to peel off the gloves, "this second set of gloves is a bitch."

Neil and Julian both chuckled.

With the dressing change complete, Dr. B came in. "How are you doing today?" he smiled brightly. "Much better, I hope."

"Very much so," Neil agreed. "But that was a bit frightening," he admitted.

"Yes," Dr. B nodded. "It can be, but it's not unusual. Nonetheless, we will reduce dosage to get you back up and running, and I would increase dexamethasone to eight milligrams per day"

This seemed prudent given the episode Neil had just endured. "I'm not real keen on dexamethasone," he frowned. "Hopefully it's temporary."

"We'll hope so," Dr B agreed, and with that, he shook Neil's hand and departed. A moment later, Julian came in.

"It should be quick today," Neil observed. "We can use the bags you prepped yesterday."

"Oh no," Julian frowned. "Those were discarded. Once spiked, ANPs need to get used that day."

So, it had been an expensive decision to give Neil a day off — two sets of bags down the proverbial drain. And Wendy and I were back to prepping. Julian watched as we coached each other through the process almost flawlessly, and Neil was up and running by 11:00 a.m., giving us two thumbs up.

"I'm hungry," he added. "Can we go to the Movable Feast?"

That we did, and he ate well. By mid-afternoon, he said his eyes were tracking better and his energy was good. He wanted to go for a walk. As far as we were concerned, the ANPs were kicking in, and Neil's positivity was back!

When we returned from our walk, the FDA situation went on the front burner. Dr. Burzynski was convinced we should approach VP Biden to intervene — that we might find a sympathetic ear because his son, Beau, had succumbed to a brain tumor. VP Biden had since been appointed to head the "Cancer Moonshot" program, an effort intended to improve cancer prevention and early detection, to accelerate cancer research, and to make more therapies available to more patients. It seemed logical to at least try making contact, so the FDA letter began to transform into a personal letter to VP Biden. After I made some changes, I gave Neil a copy to review. Half an hour later, I knocked on his door.

"Have you reviewed the letter?"

"Yup, it's fine," he shrugged. "I just wish we didn't have to deal with this crap. It's a waste of time and energy, as if we have either to spare."

"I know... Let's hope we get lucky."

"It's chess Dad. Not much luck in a game between experts."

"You think they're experts, the FDA?"

"Maybe not," Neil frowned, "but they have the power."

"The board is tipped," I agreed.

"Just a bit," Neil scoffed sarcastically.

The next half an hour saw a small volley of additional emails from Sheryll. Dr. B wanted to send a copy of the letter to an unnamed confidant for review. If it passed muster, this person could possibly facilitate contact with VP Biden. Dr. B also decided he would like to include the letter with his own response to the FDA's action. Of course we would be happy to oblige Dr. B's request, but Neil's care was foremost, and we were getting too sidetracked:

To: "Sheryll S. Acelar"
From: Dean
Subject: Steroid dose and timing...
Date: April 25, 2016

Sheryll,

We gave Neil 3 mg dexa this AM. Dr. B wants to up dosage to 8 per day. I wonder if just doubling the dose would be fine. I hate to adjust things so abruptly unless deemed absolutely necessary. The next question is when should we give it, with lunch or dinner?

I will send the final draft of the letter shortly.

God Bless,
Dean

Sheryll replied: *"Dr. B stated that we can try 3mg twice a day, and he can take it with dinner. If it's not enough we can follow with another increase."*

I answered: *"That sounds good...The letter is coming in the next few moments. We're just trying to put in a few finishing touches and make sure there are no typos!"*

"Okay," I announced. "Dr. B is fine with just upping the dexamethasone to six milligrams per day – three with breakfast and three with dinner. We'll hope that's enough. You can always add more if needed."

"Sounds okay," Neil agreed reluctantly. "Let's hope it's enough."

Wendy nodded.

"And I'm sending the draft unless there are any last comments or changes."

"Let her rip," Neil puffed.

"Okay," Wendy nodded.

I pressed "send," and we silently prayed for a successful "Hail Mary."

> **To: "Sheryll S. Acelar"**
> **From: Dean**
> **Subject: Letter appealing for assistance**
> **Date: April 25, 2016**
>
> Dear Sheryll and Dr. Burzynski,
>
> The final draft is attached. As it seems you have someone else who wishes to vet the letter, please let me know if I should make any further changes. Also, will it be forwarded via email? Thank you. I hope it helps.
>
> God Bless,
> Dean

With the day's work done, we made a quick trip to the H-E-B to stock up on fruit and get something for dinner, and the evening passed in good spirits. Neil was back up and running.

"How are you feeling?" Wendy asked him after dinner.

"The waterfall is back," he smiled.

> ***Excerpt Doctor Burzynski report, April-25-2016***
>
> Subject came in for Week 1, Day 5. PI was available to assess clinical disease status. Vital signs were taken and were stable. Subject reported that vomiting and headache

> resolved since 04/24/16. Subject was off antineoplastons since 4/24/16. PI made the clinical decision on dose adjustments and Atengenal and Astugenal will be restarted today at reduced dosages. Electrolytes were drawn which showed no clinical significance. Grade 1 hypokalemia resolved today. It was decided by the PI to do electrolytes daily until further notice...

FINAL VERSION
APRIL 26, 2016

I awoke early to check my email in case there were any more comments from Dr. B. Indeed there were:

> **To: "Sheryll S. Acelar"**
> **From: "Dr. Stanislaw R. Burzynski"**
> **Subject: Re: Letter appealing for assistance**
> **Date: 4/26/2016**
>
> Hi,
>
> The letter is very good but a few things should be corrected.
>
> 1. We are not "alternative"
>   - Pre-clinical research was funded by the grant coming from "War on Cancer" fund and performed at Baylor College of Medicine and M.D. Anderson Cancer Center. I was a Principal Investigator and faculty member at Baylor. The final results of pre-clinical work were presented in 1976 and coincided with 200 Anniversary of US. Currently I'm holding the title of Professor of Neuro-oncology of respected foreign university.

- Fourteen separate Phase 2 trials sanctioned by FDA in DIPG, GBM, Anaplastic Astrocytoma and a number of other brain tumors proved response rate required by protocols and tumor free survival over twenty years. The results are published in peer-revised journals and reported at the congresses of neuro-oncology.

2. For over 20 years the details of manufacturing of the medications were known to the FDA and the company used the same suppliers of raw chemicals for 10 years.

- Suddenly in March 2015, FDA decided that raw chemicals are "ingredients" of the medications. It was immediately explained to the FDA that this is not true and that the raw chemicals are submitted to a number of steps of chemical process which delivers final ingredients.
- In the letter received on 3/21/16 FDA placed complete hold on enrollment of new patients to clinical trials until a new manufacturer of raw chemicals will be found and these chemicals produced by the methods required for medications.
- To comply with FDAs requests would require construction of a new factory, will take many years and will multiply the cost of medications. The approval of medications which cured many brain tumor patients in Phase 2 trials will be delayed for many years and many patients will die needlessly.

This is long explanation. I would recommend to revise the letter and use the most important fragments of the above. VP should know more about our treatment from you, because he will be immediately "swamped" by "1001 lies" of our adversaries.

I would cc the letter to Dr. at FDA who placed the hold. I will give the name and address when I come to the office. The letter to Biden should be sent today, but the copy will be attached tomorrow to the letter to FDA.

Best,
SRB

Wow! Those were some "marching orders." I spent the next hour doing my best to capture the essence of Dr. B's comments without making the letter too much longer.

To: "Sheryll S. Acelar"
From: Dean
Subject: Re: Fwd: Letter appealing for assistance
Date: April 26, 2016

Sheryll,

Attached is the final letter based on this AM's suggestions from Dr. B.. It's still long, but at least its formatted to fit on one page, cc's included. I am on my way back to the clinic with the file and PC in case any further changes or typos need correcting. I would normally sit on something like this for a day and then edit to tighten further, but we are in a time-crunch. I will need to make use of your printer, and I'll need paper, envelopes and express shipping labels. See you shortly. In the meantime, please print and give to anyone who needs to do a quick final proof read. If anyone thinks there are things we could cut, that's fine too.

Thank you and God Bless,
Dean

After sending the email and attachment, I went to the clinic. Carolyn Powers, Dr. Burzynski's personal secretary, met me at the elevator and escorted me to the executive office wing of the clinic. This included her office — with one wall like a library, filled with publications and journals — Dr. Burzynski's office and a large conference room. Carolyn had cleared a side table in her office, so I pulled up a chair, and she gave me all the materials and assistance I needed. Fortunately, there were no more changes, so it was just a matter of printing copies and assembling the mailings. This is the letter as sent:

April 26, 2016

Vice President Biden, Chairman Cancer Moonshot Task Force
The White House
1600 Pennsylvania Avenue NW
Washington, DC 20500

Dear Vice President Biden:

I am very sorry for the recent loss of your son, Beau. I'm writing in hopes you might lend your voice to help my son, Eugene "Neil" Fachon, avoid a similarly premature fate. On March 4th 2016, Neil was diagnosed with Diffuse Intrinsic Pontine Glioma (DIPG), a rare, intractable and aggressive form of brain cancer. Neil, age 19, is a highly motivated sophomore in the College of Engineering at Northeastern University. Being in Boston, Neil was seen by Neuro-Oncologists at Massachusetts General Hospital and the DANA Farber Cancer Institute. Both gave him 3 months to live. Using a "standard" course of radiation, they could extend his life another 3 months.

Experimental treatments were also discussed, none of which have yielded significantly different results from standard therapy.

Faced with a short-term death sentence or a slightly prolonged death sentence, it seemed clear we needed to look further for help. Fortunately, there are a great many books and videos about cancer, and the Burzynski Clinic features prominently among many – especially where brain cancer is concerned. We contacted the clinic and learned they were about to begin an FDA-approved clinical-trial specifically for DIPG patients who had not undergone "standard" care. After doing extensive research – including speaking with an Argentinian girl who was successfully treated for DIPG at the Burzynski Clinic – Neil decided to enroll in the clinic's new trial.

Neil signed the enrollment agreement on April 13th 2016, but he still had to undergo a battery of tests to comply with FDA regulations. Finally, after all the poking, needles, scans and surgery to place an arterial catheter, Neil passed the requirements in time to begin treatment on April 21st 2016. On the same day, Dr. Burzynski told us about a letter he received from the FDA the prior afternoon (April 20th) placing a hold on enrolling new patients in this trial. Dr. Burzynski explained the FDA's concerns stem from its re-classification as "ingredients" of some of the raw materials the Burzynski Research Institute uses to synthesize antineoplastons. Dr. Burzynski also explained these raw materials undergo several complex chemical processes to create the actual ingredients for antineoplastons. Unprocessed, these raw materials would be useless. Dr. Burzynski also told us the FDA has been fully apprised of his manufacturing procedures for 20 years, and he has been using the same suppliers for the last 10 or more years with no adverse effects. Given these facts and Dr. Buzynski's well documented history of success with intractable brain cancers (in many FDA-approved trials, no less) we enthusiastically elected to proceed with the clinic's DIPG trial.

Neil is now on his fifth day of treatment at the Burzynski Clinic. He seems to be doing well, but until he reaches a stable dose it will take some getting used to. While it is way too early to say anything for sure, Neil has noticed some early signs of improvement in his vision, energy level and overall alertness. We are documenting his symptoms as best we can to chart changes, but for the time being we are encouraged, as these early signs suggest he is getting some relief from the worst of his symptoms. While we can appreciate the FDA's concerns about safety, this reclassification of raw materials as "ingredients" could not come at a worse time. At best it seems an excess of caution that will effectively terminate a clinical trial for a proven therapy, thus also terminating what we believe to be Neil's best hope, not just for prolonging his life, but for renewing his "Lease." Absent sustained treatment – which will not be possible should this FDA re-classification remain – there is every reason to believe Neil will succumb to this cancer within weeks, as per the original prognosis.

Could you please put in a word at the FDA to help amend this situation which not only threatens the life of my son, but of others who are caught in this needless and seemingly arbitrary circumstance?

Thank you for your consideration, and God Bless,
Emil "Dean" Fachon

CC:
Dr. Stanislaw Burzynski, MD, PhD, Founder and Director of the Burzynski Research Institute
Dr. Patricia Keegan, Director Division of Oncology Products 2, FDA Center for Drug Evaluation and Research
Ms. Deanne Varney, Lead Regulatory Project Manager, FDA Center for Drug Eval and Research

ONWARD AND UPWARD

Having done all I could, I went back to the hotel. The monkey was off our backs for the moment, and spirits were good. Wendy and Neil had tackled the morning routine without a hitch, and all lights were "green." As soon as I had some breakfast and the dishes were cleaned, we headed back to the clinic. Irena greeted us with her warm smile and held open the door to the inner sanctum.

"He's just so handsome," she reminded us, veritably pinching Neil's cheek with her smile.

Neil chuckled into his hand.

We went straight to the treatment room. As soon as Neil settled on the couch, Sheryll entered with Julian on her heels to do a quick blood draw — to check Neil's electrolytes.

"Hello Neil," Sheryll said brightly. "How are you doing?"

"FAN-TASTIC," he beamed.

"That's the spirit," she smiled. "I think Dr. B plans to maintain the same dose for another day to help you adjust."

"Sounds good to me," Neil gave her thumbs up.

Julian quickly extracted a blood sample and promised, "I'll be right back!"

"I'll be right back too," Sheryll said, "with today's ANPs." She opened the door to find Dr. B just reaching for the doorknob.

"Good morning," he smiled, eyes twinkling. "How are you today?"

"I'm well," Neil shook his hand. "Yesterday was a good day. How are you?"

"Very good," Dr. B nodded thanks and proceeded to give Neil an exam while Wendy and I washed our hands and started getting the prep table cleaned and all the equipment laid out.

"You guys are looking like pros," Julian commented upon his return, with Sheryll right behind holding the day's ANPs.

"We'll maintain same dose," Dr. B confirmed to Sheryll. "Tomorrow, we advance." Then, he took a look at our work with a nod of approval.

"I'll be ready," Neil smiled his thanks as Dr. B left.

While Wendy and I were working out the bubbles, Sheryll invited Neil to the common-treatment area to meet some of the other patients — patients receiving AS2-1 only.

"I'd love to," Neil jumped at the chance.

COMMUNITY

There were three or four wheelchair- or stroller-bound patients in the common room, along with an assortment of parents, siblings, spouses, and dear friends. Most were in various stages of training. One of the patients was a young African American girl, Chloé. She was roughly seven years old and had been through multiple surgeries, radiation, and chemotherapy. Each time, the tumor returned. Her parents, not wanting to give up, discovered the Burzynski Clinic and decided they had to give it a chance. Chloé's little brother was with her — full of energy and smiles — and while their parents were learning the prepping routine, Neil sat down to quietly talk and play with the children.

When Wendy and I finished prepping, she went to find Neil ensconced in a game of chess with Chloé's little brother. Wendy touched Neil's shoulder, "I hate to interrupt, but we're ready for you."

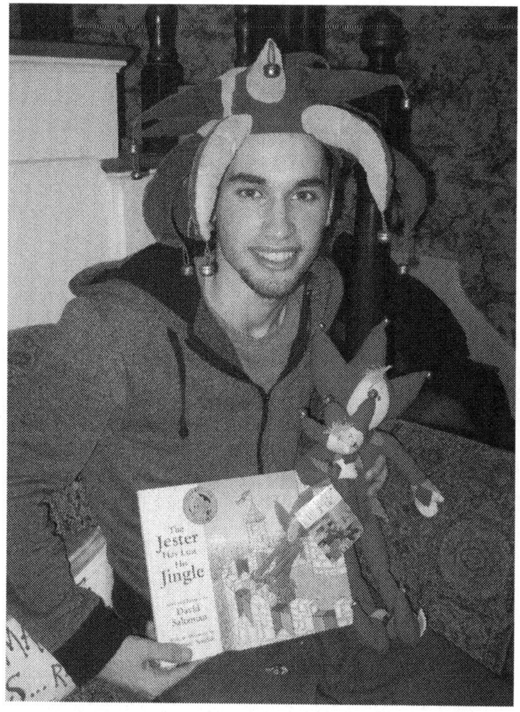

"It's a good thing," Neil smiled. "He's got me in a bit of a pickle," then he winked at the boy. "Let's play again tomorrow."

"You bet!"

On their way back to the treatment room, Neil commented, "I wish we'd brought a copy of *The Jester Lost His Jingle*. I'd like to read it to the kids." Thinking of the laughter he'd helped bring to dozens of children who were struggling with life-threatening illnesses made him smile. Sharing the *Jester* was one of his happiest high school achievements.

"I'm sure The Jester & Pharley Phund would be delighted to send a copy," Wendy replied.

"Let's call them," he agreed.

Neil sat down next to me, and I hooked him up. "You ready?"

He gave me two thumbs up, and I pushed "start" with confidence. Julian did not have to lift a finger or say a single word the entire time. "You guys are certifiable," he punned.

Neil chuckled, "I'll say."

"HEY NOW," I grumbled and chuckled at the same time.

"J-K," Neil's eyes twinkled.

"But seriously," Julian added, "you're doing very well with your training. You guys are good."

We were in the groove!

The day drew to a close with another wonderful home-cooked meal and discussions about "the letter" — mostly about the sad absurdity of having to write it.

"Uh," Neil finally waved an exasperated hand to dismiss the topic. "Let's go for a walk."

"Good idea," we agreed.

As soon as the kitchen was tidied up, we were down the stairs and out the door, Neil with his pump case slung over his shoulder with practiced ease. The "backyard" of the hotel was becoming quite familiar, and Neil's stride was strong as we followed our usual route heading east on the sidewalk.

"I can't wait to see Evie," he commented as we strolled.

"Getting a bit stir crazy, are we," I patted his shoulder.

"Just a few days," Wendy nodded. "It will be fun!"

"Like the 'good old days' on the boat," I added, "playing games and taking adventures."

"Good times," Neil purred.

After our walk, Neil settled into his room to do eye exercises and spend online time with his friends. Wendy sat down with a book, and I sent an important update to family and friends.

To: Family and friends
From: Dean
Subject: You can't make this stuff up...
Date: Tue, 26 Apr 2016

Dearest Family and Friends,

We are on day 5 of Neil's treatment. We hit a bump on Sunday – a very tough day due to issues with adjusting to the medication – but Neil is doing much better these last two days. FYI: We got the results of Neil's MRI a week ago, and there wasn't any noticeable change in the tumor! That is good news! In another few weeks we will see how the tumor is reacting to the Antineoplastons. Signs are hopeful, even given the rough day Sunday.

You may recall I mentioned an issue that had cropped up – something Dr. Burzynski was addressing. Things have taken a difficult turn, and we are trying to do all we can to help. Read the attached letter to VP Biden and you will know as much as we do. If you can think of any way to help expedite this message to it's intended recipient, let us know. We will take all the help we can get.

That's it for the moment. You might think we have quite enough on our plate, and you would be correct. But we are doing okay, due in large part to the prayers so many of you are sending to heaven on our behalf...

Much love and God Bless,
Dean

Excerpt Doctor Burzynski report, April-26-2016

Subject overall feels well with no new symptoms to report. Doses from yesterday were recorded and all six doses were received. PI made clinical decision on maintaining the same dose of Atengenal and Astugenal today. Electrolytes were drawn which showed no clinical significance. Subject did not have any other issues or further questions for the PI.

TEAM NEIL
APRIL 27, 2016

Forwarding "the letter" to family and friends sparked an uproar, some replies arriving within minutes:

To: Dean
From: Charles
Subject: Re: You can't make this stuff up...
Date: Tue, 26 Apr 2016

Dean and Wendy,
Oh my goodness! I have shared this with my brother-in-law, Ron. He is an attorney and likely knows someone or someone who knows someone...
Charles

* * *

To: Dean
From: Stephen N.
Subject: Re: You can't make this stuff up...
Date: Tue, 26 Apr 2016

Would it make sense to copy your congressman in Washington?
Love,
Steve

More suggestions and offers of assistance poured in the following morning:

To: Dean
From: Bill
Subject: Re: You can't make this stuff up...
Date: Wed, 27 Apr 2016

How do you feel about allowing this to be shared on social-media and/or email to mobilize power from people's support everywhere. It would spread very quickly. I'm sure if you have been researching the alternative remedies, you have seen this scenario happen over & over to stop the programs that are so often the lifeline. Thank you federal gov. and big business. Maybe a world of support can help in this day and age.

Love & hugs, Tammy & Bill

* * *

To: Dean
From: Carl
Subject: Re: You can't make this stuff up...
Date: Wed, 27 Apr 2016

Dean,

This is so frustrating. I can only imagine your feelings. Why shut down a program without an alternative?? Suggest you post on social media to help get the word out. We can all share. May just lead to other avenues of appeal as well. I'm sure you have been in direct contact as well with the FDA.

Very best,
Carl

* * *

To: Dean
From: Tim
Subject: Re: You can't make this stuff up...
Date: Wed, 27 Apr 2016

Hi Dean,

This is a horrible turn of events. The frustration levels you have been forced to deal with are off the charts. I hope this can be overturned quickly!

I've asked around my office and another advisor has a client who works on the Food side of the FDA... I have forwarded your letter to this advisor and he will see about sending it to his contact.

Sherri has her team scanning their contacts and brainstorming. They might be able to forward this letter or have further suggestions.

Neil is strong and 'Team Neil' will do what it can to help!

Tim

"Tim says 'Team Neil' is on the job," I told Neil that morning while disconnecting him from the pump, the previous day's infusions complete. "How are you feeling?"

"I'm good," he nodded, then he grinned. "'Team Neil.' I like it. Way to go, Tim!"

There was a sense of relief in Neil's eyes, knowing good folks were pulling for him.

"We'll cross our fingers and say our prayers," I nodded. "We'll see what happens."

"Indeed we will," he agreed. And it was back to routine. "I need a shower."

I sealed up the incision area, and he jumped in for a nice long hot shower while I quickly touched base with Bill, Tammy, and Carl.

To: Bill, Tammy, Carl
From: Dean

Subject: Re: You can't make this stuff up...
Date: Wed, 27 Apr 2016

Social media is a good possibility, but let's wait before taking that path while we give private channels a chance. More soon.

Love you, and God Bless!
Dean

After Neil's shower, we enjoyed scrambled eggs and fresh fruit for breakfast. Table conversation centered around "social media," and we agreed we might need to prepare for a full-court press, but we fervently hoped we would not. It just seemed absurd to think the FDA wouldn't see Neil's perspective and let him soldier on: They had nothing to lose, and he had everything to gain. We would just keep thinking positive.

Soon, it was time to head back to the clinic. Julian met us promptly to take a blood sample. "I'm just going to take this to the lab," he said as soon as he had the sample. "I'll be right back. And we need to check Neil's incision, too."

I wasn't real comfortable with the dressing change process, so upon his return, I asked Julian to take charge. We all put on masks, and Wendy and I stepped back to observe.

"It's still a bit itchy," Neil noted.

"I have something for that," Julian said as he gently lifted the bandage. "Yup, contact dermatitis, and the wound is a little scabby and red." He cleaned the wound carefully and applied a dab of antibiotic ointment, then he cleaned where the bandage adhered to Neil's skin and applied some sort of topical treatment. "We'll need to change this more often," Julian nodded, gently pressing the new bandage into place.

"I'm glad you're good at doing it," I said, removing my mask. "I really get flummoxed with the extra set of gloves."

Julian laughed.

Sheryll delivered the day's ANPS, and Wendy and I got busy with what we were getting good at — prepping for infusion.

"You're ready to be 'certified,'" Julian gently applauded. "You could get jobs at the clinic!"

"Well, we wouldn't want to cramp your style," I joked. "But it would be great to get certified!" Certification would mean we could administer Neil's treatment unsupervised — as in when we were home.

We had winnowed the prep time down to just over an hour, and that would pretty much be the norm going forward. Almost like clockwork, Sheryll came in as we finished, with Dr. B right behind.

"Good morning," he beamed at Neil. "How are you feeling?"

"I'm fantastic," Neil smiled.

Dr. B smiled his twinkling smile in return. "Good. Good. Your bloodwork is fine, so if you feel ready, I'd like to increase your dose."

Neil nodded. "It was just too much too fast before, but I think I'm ready."

"Okay," Dr. B understood. "But we need to keep climbing at a steady rate. You need to drink plenty of water."

Neil shook Dr. B's hand, "Let's do it!"

With that, Dr. B nodded to me in silent acknowledgment of the letter and took his leave.

We programmed the pump and connected the IV lines, and Neil hit "start."

"You're doing great, Neil," Sheryll said. "And your parents. We need to keep monitoring you for another week or ten days, but as long as your incision is healing and you're able to take the dose increases, you should be able to go home."

"FAN-TASTIC," Neil hoisted his grin like a flag, "not that we aren't having fun here," he demurred.

"That would be good timing," Wendy said. "In a few days, Neil's sister comes for a week. It would be great to return home with her."

"You'll need a doctor at home," Sheryll reminded us. "A 'sub-investigator' to perform regular physical and neurological assessments, order tests, and report back to the clinic."

"We have some ideas," Wendy replied, "but we haven't really asked anyone yet."

"You should do that," Sheryll said. "We can't let you leave until you have someone keeping tabs on you locally. That's a trial requirement."

"Of course we'd like someone local to help anyway," I added to nods of agreement from Wendy and Neil.

"Of course," Sheryll agreed. "I'll send you a link to the form your sub-investigator will need to complete for the FDA."

"So, I guess we're done for the day," Neil concluded.

"Yup," Sheryll smiled. "Have a great afternoon, Neil."

"You too," he replied.

"We're going to start by trying lunch at the café downstairs," Wendy added.

"Great idea," Sheryll agreed. "Wanda's Polish specials are fabulous!"

"Sounds like yum," Neil rubbed his belly. "Until tomorrow."

VONDERFUL VANDA

The clinic's café was opposite the lobby on the ground floor, directly down the hall from the elevator doors, on the left. It was a clean simple space with four or five tables and picture windows overlooking the arboretum. Opposite the windows was a counter with a cash register and a display case. Behind the counter was a door to a small kitchen. As soon as we entered, a woman emerged from the kitchen to greet us with an Aunt-like smile.

"Welcome," she said, "I'm Wanda," pronouncing her "W's" more like "V" — an accent with which we were now quite familiar. Many of the people at the clinic were Polish, making our visit like a brief foray into the heart of Europe.

"It's a pleasure to meet you, 'Vanda,'" Neil smiled.

"And you young man," she smiled back. "I still have some stuffed Polish cabbage rolls — today's special. Or I can make you a sandwich."

"I think we'll have three cabbage rolls, please," I smiled to nods of agreement from Neil and Wendy.

“I’m sorry,” she frowned. “I have only two servings left.”

“Then we’ll take those,” I said, “and I’ll take a sandwich — ham, cheese, lettuce, and tomato on rye bread?”

“Please take a seat,” Wanda gestured to the tables. “What type of cheese?”

“Cheddar.”

“Mustard?”

“Yes please!”

“It will just take a moment,” and she went into the kitchen.

We grabbed bottled waters from the cooler in the corner and took a table next to the arboretum windows. A few minutes later, Wanda brought two plates with two cabbage rolls each and potato pancakes.

“That smells good,” Neil inhaled as she put plates in front of him and Wendy.

“I’ll be right back with yours,” she nodded to me and breezed back to the kitchen.

“Go ahead and dig in,” I said.

Neil was famished and didn’t need telling twice. “Wow this is good,” he managed between his first and second bites.

“Here,” Wendy said to me, “try mine.”

It indeed was delicious, and I wished we had gotten there half an hour sooner. A few minutes later, Wanda delivered my sandwich along with two potato pancakes. “I had some extra of those,” she smiled.

“Polish comfort food,” Neil smacked his lips, “served up homestyle with a helping of love!”

Wanda smiled her thanks, and from then on, we made a point of knowing when her café would be open. Some of the dishes were not really ideal for Neil’s diet, but her cooking was worth the occasional exception.

When we returned to the hotel, more emails were waiting:

To: Dean
From: Tim
Subject: Re: You can’t make this stuff up...
Date: Wed, 27 Apr 2016

> Sherri has found another potential resource. She sent your letter to the VP of Government Relations at Brown University who will be forwarding it to the RI Congressional Delegation. We'll see what that can do.
>
> We are praying for you.
> Tim

I replied: *"Sounds great Tim! Neil is tickled by the thought of 'Team Neil.' Please thank Sherri for us. Our fingers are crossed."*

And there was a notification from FedEx:

> **To: Fachon**
> **From: trackingupdates@fedex.com**
> **Subject: FedEx Shipment 776199542540 Delivered**
> **Date: Wed, 27 Apr 2016**
>
> Your package has been delivered
>
> Tracking # 776199542540
>
> Ship date:
> Tue, 4/26/2016
>
> Delivery date:
> Wed, 4/27/2016 10:38 am
> VP Joe Biden

"Hey, the letter was delivered," I hollered. "Whether or not the vice president ever sees it, who knows? But it's there."

"Here's hoping," Neil chimed in.

There wasn't much more to say, and the rest of the day was spent lounging by the pool, doing some light exercise in the gym, and reading/writing emails before dinner.

To: Dean
From: "Sheryll S. Acelar"
Subject: please see link for the form needed for a doctor in your state to sign
Date: April 27, 2016

www.fda.gov/downloads/AboutFDA/ReportsManuals-Forms/Forms/UCM074728.pdf

We also received a call from Dr. Burzynski's wife and colleague, "Dr. Barbara," requesting a copy of the final letter to VP Biden. She, too, had some contacts who might be sympathetic. Over the course of our stay in Houston, Dr. Barbara would become much like a Great Aunt to Neil, in keeping with the familial feel of the clinic.

To: Dr. Barbara
From: Dean
Subject: Letter to VP
Date: April 27, 2016

Dear Dr. Barbara,
Attached is the final version of the letter that went out yesterday. Our network of friends is working on it too. Vice President Biden may get more than one copy... Just hope he gets at least one, and soon...Thank you for your thoughtful words and support, and God Bless!
The Fachons

She promptly replied: *"Thank you very much!"*
And I replied to Sheryll:

To: "Sheryll S. Acelar"
From: Dean

Subject: Re: please see link for the form needed for a doctor in your state to sign
Date: Wed, 27 Apr 2016

Thank you for the link. We have one particular candidate in mind – but he's someone we have not met with personally – so we'll put out additional feelers. One way or another, we should hopefully be covered....

Do you happen to know Neil's potassium level in today's blood work? Just want to be sure that number is good or whether we need to give him an extra supplement before bed. I hope we can proceed uninterrupted with incremental dose increases to reach optimum levels over the next several days.

God Bless,
Dean

She replied: *"Potassium levels were normal. I do not recall the exact number, but assuredly, it was good... We are hoping so too! Just keep on doing what you are doing for Neil. We will see you tomorrow."*

After dinner, we played another board game, and Neil crushed us with good-natured zeal. Before retiring for the night, however, he wanted to talk. "Not to spoil the mood," he said, "but what do we do if the FDA shuts me down?"

The question had been lurking like a thief in the back of our minds. We had suppressed our worries as we devised our plea for commonsense sympathy, but the possibility could not be avoided.

"We'll leave the country if we have to," I told him. "You're getting this treatment."

"Maybe we could go to one of those clinics in Mexico," Neil wondered.

"Possibly," I agreed. ""Or Switzerland. I'm sure Raffaele would help."

"We shouldn't have to," Wendy said bitterly. "This is supposed to be a free country."

"Indeed," Neil shook his head in dismay.

Of course, even if we left the country to escape the FDA's clutches, there was no guarantee Dr. B would be able to continue manufacturing ANPs, let alone ship them to us. We left this unspoken, however, not wanting to extinguish all hope. We got Neil settled in for the night, connected the pump to the charger, and made sure he had plenty of water. He spent another hour or so with his friends on social media, while my attention turned to the day's final emails.

To: Dean
From: "Sheryll S. Acelar"
Subject: RE: please see link for the form needed for a doctor in your state to sign
Date: April 27, 2016

Hi

Just want to let you know, Dr. B will be leaving at 10:30am tomorrow, so if you can come before then, that will be great.

Sheryll

I replied: *"We disconnect and flush at 9:05, so we will try to be there a shade after 9:30. Working on some options for doctors to monitor Neil once we return home. Too early to discuss, but we hope to have some options that will please Dr. B."*

The "possibility" I referred to was Dr. Kieran. He would be the best person by far to oversee Neil's progress, and he seemed to leave the door ajar just enough to ask. We crossed our fingers. Wendy would try again to reach Dr. Heinrich Elinzano's administrative assistant back at Rhode Island Hospital. If these two fell through, we would ask Neil's GP, Dr. John Slattery.

To: Dr. Mark Kieran
From: Dean
Subject: Eugene Fachon's status
Date: Wed, 27 Apr 2016

Dear Dr. Kieran,

I hope this note finds you well. Since last visiting with you we have journeyed to Houston Texas. Eugene (Neil) is doing well – much better than his original prognosis suggested. His last MRI, taken about a week ago and just prior to commencing treatment at the Burzynski Clinic, showed his tumor unchanged. Stable. We were very encouraged by this result. This suggests the dietary, supplement, colon therapy and meditation regimens Neil is using have been beneficial.

So that is the baseline Dr. Burzynski began with. Neil is now on his 6th day of treatment with antineoplastons. While some might call this 'chemo-therapy,' that term is a misnomer for something so benign. We are being trained to administer Neil's treatment (so we can continue once we come home) and I can tell you first hand that antineoplastons are about as caustic as salt water. Yes, they have a distinct smell like urine which becomes imperceptible in short order, and as they dry they become sticky. That's about it. I have had antineoplastons on my hands without any burning, itching or noticeable discomfort of any kind, save for the aforementioned stickiness.

What results are we seeing? That's difficult to say. Neil has had some very good days, some average days, and one very bad day. Not in that order. Today has been a very good day. Although it varies day to day, some of his symptoms seem to be showing improvement. His energy levels, alertness, and ability to focus his eyes on objects more than a few feet away have all trended better. Of course, Neil commenced taking steroids five days prior to beginning treatment, and he will continue taking steroids until he reaches a stable daily dose of antineoplastons – at which time he will be weaned off the steroids – so it is difficult to parse what the steroids might be doing vs the antineoplastons, but by the time he's weaned off the steroids we should just about be ready for another set of pictures and we will get a better idea.

I wanted to share this with you and Dr. Plant (please forward, as I do not have her email with me) because you expressed a sincere interest in Neil's health, as well as a possible willingness to monitor Neil's progress even so he is not undergoing treatment at D/F. When we return home, would that be possible? As Neil is currently in a clinical trial, his treatment-related expenses are being covered by the clinic, and whoever oversees his progress will be compensated by the clinic as well. I know it may be a stretch for you to accommodate a situation like this, but I also imagine you will be very curious to see how this all plays out first-hand. Please give it some thought. We have other options, so do not feel obligated, but of all the doctors we spoke with, we were very comfortable with you and confident of your expertise, so I wanted to ask.

Yours and God Bless,
Dean Fachon

With this note to Dr. Kieran complete, we turned out the lights on April 27, 2016, not knowing that Dr. B's response to the FDA was winging its way as we slept:

Sent via Fed Ex
April 27, 2016

Patricia Keegan, M.D., Director
Food and Drug Administration
Center for Drug Evaluation and Research
Division of Oncology Products 2
5901-B Ammendale Road
Beltsville, MD 20795-1266

RE: IND # 43,742
Serial #: 2188 (L88)

Subject: Information Pertinent to the Full Clinical Hold Letter of 04/20/2016

Dear Dr. Keegan,

Please refer to the Burzynski Research Institute (BRI) Investigational New Drug Application (IND) submitted under section 505(i) of the Federal Food, Drug and Cosmetic Act for "Antineoplastons A10/AS2-1 Injections."

On April 13, 2016, prior to initiation of the agency's Full Clinical Hold, Mr. Eugene E. Fachon, a 19-year old male with a diffuse, intrinsic brain-stem glioma was enrolled in BRI-BT-55. He is currently receiving therapy according to that FDA-reviewed and IRB-approved protocol.

Mr. Fachon, who is from East Greenwich, Rhode Island, began developing symptoms in January 2016. On March 2, 2016, he was seen by Dr. Walter Panis with complaints of ataxia, dysarthria, headaches, and difficulties initiating urination and defecation. MRI at that time showed a non-enhancing 3.6 x 5.7 x 5/1 cm tumor arising in the pons, surrounding the basilar artery, and exhibiting as significant exophytic component. Mr. Fachon was then referred to neuro-oncologist Dr. Isabel Arrillaga-Romany and neurosurgeon Dr. Daniel Cahill at the Massachusetts General Hospital. A biopsy was not performed. Mr. Fachon was prescribed dexamethesone 3 mg p.o. daily. Standard therapy and protocol therapy for a diffuse, intrinsic, pontine glioma were discussed. Mr. Fachon elected to come to Houston for enrollment in BRI-BT-55, and upon receiving your letter of 04/20/2016, I read it in full to the patient and his parents. They then insisted that the administration of Atengenal and Astugenal be continued if at all possible. This interaction was duly noted in the patient's medical record.

Along with this letter, we are submitting the two-week documentation required by the Protocol (Section 11.1.1). Mr. Fachon is considering completing his treatment in Houston and has not yet selected a local doctor to act as sub-investigator. His training, and the training of his parents, in the home-administration of Atengenal and Astugenal is 70% complete. As soon as it is finished, documentation that Mr. Fachon and his parents have successfully completed this training will be forwarded to the agency.

With Mr. Fachon's full understanding and agreement, I request that the Full Clinical Hold be changed to a Partial Clinical Hold so that Mr. Fachon can complete Protocol therapy.

Sincerely,
Stanislaw R. Burzynski, M.D., PhD.
President
Burzynski Research Institute, Inc.

Enclosures:
FDA Form 1571
FDA Form 1572
Up-to-date CRF
An electronic copy of all images of the screening MRI and the neuro-radiologist report.

Formative communications had taken flight, with more to follow, triggering events we could never have dreamed of, certainly not on top of a situation already fraught with mortal hazard. For the time being, however, our sojourn in Houston continued with a guarded sense of hope.

Excerpt Doctor Burzynski report, April-27-2016

Subject came in for Week 1, Day 7. PI was available to assess clinical disease status. Vital signs were taken and stable. Subject feels well with no new symptoms to report. Doses from yesterday were recorded and subject received all six doses. PI made clinical decision on increasing the dose of Atengenal and maintaining same dose of Astugenal today. Electrolytes were drawn which showed no clinical significance...

22

CHOOSE ACTION

"There is a sense of knowing and confidence in action that wasn't there before, no fear of being judged, just confident in who and what you are." NF

THURSDAY, APRIL 28

We arrived early at the clinic, as promised, and Dr B joined us almost immediately.

"I've sent my reply to FDA," he nodded. "Now we hope for the best. Sadly, that doesn't always work, but we try, yes?"

"Our fingers are crossed," we all nodded.

Dr. B smiled his twinkling smile and gave Neil a quick exam. "How are you feeling?"

"Doing fantastic," Neil smiled. "A little nausea, but it passed quickly. Nothing like before."

"Good," Dr. B smiled. "That's good! I'd like to continue increasing dose if you feel ready."

Neil nodded, "I am, just not too much all at once."

Dr. B nodded in turn, then he said, "I'll be away for a few days. Dr. Gregory will look after you in my absence."

Dr. Gregory (Dr. B's son) had his own clinic on the floor above the Burzynski Clinic. Dr. Gregory's clinic practices integrative medical care, and we had met with him previously to discuss some holistic health questions. Dr. Gregory was very involved with his father's clinic, so we had every confidence Neil would be in good hands.

"That'll be fine," Neil assured him

"I will talk to Dr. Gregory and Sheryll every day while I'm gone," Dr. B promised, then we all shook hands with familial warmth, and he departed.

We commenced our daily ritual, and it was not until when we were getting ready to leave that we learned where Dr. B was going. Everyone was quietly buzzing about Austin and the conclusion of the Texas Medical Board's latest proceedings against Dr. B. His optimistic demeanor, ever congenial and solicitous, had given no hint of the pressure he was under: the Texas Medical Board on one hand, and the FDA on the other. The tag team was at it again, with Neil caught in the middle.

After learning about this, Neil observed, "From what I've seen, Dr. B will handle the situation very well. I think he's a Grandmaster at this particular game."

I nodded, "But he has a lot of threats on his board."

"So do we," Wendy grimaced.

From a medical standpoint, things seemed to be going as well as we could have hoped, but our position was precarious, and we knew it. With that sobering thought, we left the treatment side of the clinic and headed out through the waiting area.

A "PLAY DATE"

As we reached for the door, we were intercepted by the clinic's Public Relations Director, Brenda. She had previously mentioned wanting to introduce Neil to her daughter, and sure enough, a young woman was with her. "Anna likes to visit the clinic when she has time off from school," Brenda explained, pleased to introduce her daughter to Neil and to us.

Like Neil, Anna was a college sophomore, and it was apparent her empathy for the clinic's patients was much like her mom's. Anna and Neil split off to chat briefly, and when we were saying goodbye, he announced he would like to invite Anna over for lunch.

"That sounds great," Wendy smiled, pleased Neil would have a contemporary to spend some time with — an unexpected "twist" of the welcome kind.

"How about Saturday?" we suggested.

"Sounds good," Anna agreed, and she and Neil exchanged numbers so they could make plans.

From the clinic, we went straight to the Movable Feast. In addition to lunch, Wendy needed to replenish a few of Neil's supplements, so we spent half an hour perusing the health food side of the business. Wendy found most everything she wanted, and Neil spent quite a bit of time examining a display of Himalayan salt lamps.

"Do you want one?" I asked.

"Maybe," he said, "but I'm thinking on it."

After another fabulous lunch, our next stop would be groceries. Wendy had discovered a Whole Foods Market in Houston, and although the location was well off our beaten path, we enjoyed exploring and decided to see if they had a few things she hadn't been able to find at the H-E-B. This detour took another hour, and while driving back to the hotel, Neil complained of mild nausea again.

"Are you getting enough water?" Wendy and I asked at once.

"Doin' my best," he nodded, holding up a half-empty bottle of water. He also drank plenty of water at the restaurant, sufficient to need "the facilities" before we departed, and then again at the grocery store.

"Do you need to disconnect?" Wendy asked.

"I don't think so," he shook his head. "It's not too bad. I'm just sensitive, I guess."

"Understandable," I said. "The FDA situation doesn't help."

"No," Neil agreed, "but we've done all we can, so let's forget about that for now."

I nodded and decided to give Sheryll a quick call. "Neil's nausea is back," I told her. "Not too bad, but we may need to think about reprogramming the pump to a lesser dose."

"Call immediately if he gets any worse," she said. "I'll let Dr. Gregory know, and we'll discuss options."

"Okay."

Neil was about the same when we got back to the hotel. "I'm still a little queasy, but no need to disconnect."

"Maybe it would help to lie down for a while," Wendy suggested.

"Yup," he nodded and retired to his room while Wendy put groceries away and I checked email.

To: Dean Fachon
From: "Kieran, Mark W.,M.D.,Ph.D."
Subject: RE: Eugene Fachon's status
Date: Thu, 28 Apr 2016
CC: "Plant, Ashley"

Dean,

I am glad to hear that Eugene is doing well and glad the trip to Houston was uneventful. We are of course happy to follow along but as per our prior conversation, we cannot be involved in any of Burzynski's treatment. We can get normal blood work and scans if that would help.

Mark

"Well," I told Wendy, "Dr. Kieran can 'follow along.' Even order bloodwork and scans, but there's no way he can be Neil's sub-investigator."

"I didn't think he could," Wendy admitted. "But it's always worth asking."

By evening, Neil's nausea abated, and there was no need to adjust his dosage. The specter of FDA meddling still haunted our thoughts, but Neil held it at bay by making plans for his lunch date with Anna.

"We just wanna get takeout from Snap Kitchen," he requested. "Anna says there's one fairly close by. We can pick her up at the clinic and grab some food on the way home."

"Sounds like a plan," I said.

Neil nodded. “She and I can eat and hang out by the pool.”

Yes, indeed, Dean and Wendy would definitely be elsewhere.

> ***Excerpt Doctor Burzynski report, April-28-2016***
>
> Subject came in for Week 2, Day 8. PI was available to assess clinical disease status. Vital signs were taken and were stable. Subject overall feels well with no new symptoms to report... PI made the clinical decision on increasing the dose of Atengenal and maintaining the same dose of Astugenal today...PI appointed a sub-investigator, Gregory Burzynski, M.D. during time PI would be away next week. Form 1572 was updated to include Sub-investigator and signed by Principal Investigator. SI will oversee the subject's clinical condition and adjust dose of anti-neoplastons, prescribe medications and make clinical recommendations.

POINT OF ORDER FRIDAY, APRIL 29

The day began with more emails. Our neighbors, Tim and Sherri, were working their network to the max. This included a contact at Brown University who was in regular communication with Rhode Island Senator Jack Reed's office. Sherri forwarded a sequence of emails:

> **To: Dean**
> **From: Sherri**
> **Subject: Fwd: Letter on Clinical Trial for cancer drug**
> **Date: April 29, 2016**
> **CC: Tim**
>
> *Begin forwarded message:*

To: Christopher A.
From: Albert D.
Subject: Letter on Clinical Trial for cancer drug
Date: Thursday, April 28, 2016

Chris:

I received the attached letter from a Brown employee whose son has an advanced form of brain cancer and is enrolled in a clinical trial which the FDA suddenly halted.

Could you convey this letter to the proper authorities at the FDA, and maybe VP Biden's office, to whom it is addressed?

Thanks, Al

To: Albert D.
From: Christopher A.
Subject: Re: Letter on Clinical Trial for cancer drug
Date: Thu, Apr 28, 2016
CC: Jill Brimmer (Reed)

Al-

Is it possible to get a waiver from Dean (attached filled out, signed and scanned/ faxed back to me), contact info for the doctor, the name of the drug, and the drug manufacturer ASAP?

Jill from our DC office, cc'd, has been in contact with the FDA and has a call tomorrow morning to discuss the matter further.

Thanks,
Chris

Release Form attached

* * *

To: Sherri
From: Dean
Subject: Re: Fwd: Letter on Clinical Trial for cancer drug
Date: April 29, 2016
CC: Tim

Hi Sherri,

Looking at these emails, there is an error regarding who Neil is. He is not a son of a Brown employee. Also, all the information requested is in the letter. Lastly, there was no attached document to print and sign, but since the letter is apparently being discussed already, is a "waiver" required at all? We can send the same letter to Jill, just addressed to Sen. Reed, if that would be most expedient. Thank you and talk again soon.

God Bless,
Dean

* * *

To: Dean
From: Tim
Subject: Re: Fwd: Letter on Clinical Trial for cancer drug
Date: April 29, 2016

Hi Dean,

In response to your e-mail back to Sherri, disregard the dialog that occurred on Brown's side. No, Neil is not the child of a Brown employee...but at this point that was the discussion that occurred to get this to Jack Reed, and regardless, Neil is the topic of discussion.

My thought is that Sen. Reeds office is requesting a form to allow him to speak on Neil's behalf, so we might as well oblige to their request and send the signed release back. Ultimately it is your/Neil's decision to make if you are comfortable doing so...

Let me know if you have received the Release Form.

Good luck,
Tim

* * *

To: Tim
From: Dean
Subject: Re: Fwd: Letter on Clinical Trial for cancer drug
Date: Fri, 29 Apr 2016
CC: Sherri

Got it. So long as there is no chance of anyone thinking we're attempting to deceive anyone.

Regarding the current situation, the appeal letter is intended to avoid formal action. We want to avoid that for obvious reasons. As such, it may be inappropriate to engage Senator Reed in this fashion at this time. Dr. Burzynski is scheduled to teleconference with the FDA next week. We'll know more after that. Let's keep this on hold for now.

Thank you, and God Bless,
Dean

> PS. The original email exchange mentions that someone may have already spoken with someone at the FDA about this matter. If so, what was the context? I am concerned any intervention, though well-intentioned, could trigger a negative reaction. Please advise that person to tread lightly – in the spirit of the letter, no more.

At roughly 8:00 a.m., I went into Neil's room to disconnect the pump and flush the catheter. After his brush with nausea the day before, Neil had thankfully been able to drink plenty of water throughout the night, and he awoke feeling fine. Wendy made breakfast while Neil took care of his business, and I returned to email central.

> **To: "Kieran, Mark W.,M.D.,Ph.D."**
> **From: Dean Fachon**
> **Subject: RE: Eugene Fachon's status**
> **Date: Fri, 29 Apr 2016**
>
> Thank you Mark, and understood. I think we can get our bases covered locally, but if not and we need to schedule a test, I will let you know. If you would like, I will periodically send updates. All the best.
> God Bless,
> Dean

PROCEEDING WITH CAUTION

The clinic routine went without a hitch, but before programming the pump, Dr. Gregory asked Neil if he wanted to maintain the same dosage. He thought for a brief moment and decided that that would be prudent, so we programmed the pump accordingly. With everything else being relatively quiet — no news from Dr. B, and the café was closed — we headed to the H-E-B to get groceries.

About midway through Neil's first dose, his nausea returned. It was mild, but we called Sheryll to let her know, suggesting once again that we might need to reprogram the pump at a reduced dose. She asked us to keep her posted, and we went back to the hotel. Neil felt good enough to have a small lunch, but his nausea was back by the end of the second dose cycle, maybe even a bit worse. It did not improve as quickly as he hoped, so rather than push his luck, he wanted to stop for the rest of the day to regain his equilibrium.

"You sure you don't want to just reprogram?" I asked.

He shook his head no. "I'm sure I'll be fine to start back up tomorrow," he added, "but maybe a slightly lower dose. I just don't want to risk it today."

After the blowout he had suffered, we understood, but this hinted at an issue with which he would continue to struggle. We stopped the pump, flushed the line, and capped the end with a sterile green tip.

"You're free to move about the cabin," I joked. "I'll send Sheryll a quick note."

To: Sheryll
From: Dean
Subject: RE: Holding off...
Date: April 29, 2016

Hi Sheryll,

Unfortunately, about an hour after the second dose finished, Neil decided he had to stop. The nausea had returned, a bit more so, and he just did not want to risk another severe bout of vomiting. The pump is off and he is disconnected and flushed. We hope and expect the nausea to pass over the next few hours. Unless circumstances demand otherwise, we will come in tomorrow as planned and figure on lessening his dose on channel 1 to

> between 120 and 140, with your and Dr. B's approval, of course.
>
> God Bless,
> Dean

She replied: *"Okay. I hope he feels better soon. We'll discuss dose tomorrow."*

As we hoped, Neil's nausea abated after disconnecting him from the pump. By late afternoon, he even felt good enough to consider an outing. We had seen a drive-in entrance to Bush Park on a previous outing.

"Let's take a ride to that entrance to Bush Park we spotted," I suggested. "See if there's still any floodwater inside."

"That would be interesting," Neil agreed.

We entered the park and drove up the embankment. The road went right up and over the levee, but we parked before reaching the top, in a lot off to one side, and got out to walk the rest of the way up.

"Whoa!" Neil stood up straight. It had been a week since the deluge, but the road going down the inside embankment went straight into the water — like a boat ramp. Trees and plants stuck out of the surface on either side of the submerged road as it meandered into the distance and disappeared around a bend. "That's at least four or five feet deep!"

"At least," I agreed. "If the whole park is this deep, that's a lot of water!"

Nearby, an outflow — a controlled release culvert of sorts — spewed a steady stream from the park into a channel running alongside the base of the exterior embankment — like the drainage ditch near the hotel, but much bigger.

"That must lead to the bayou," I thought out loud.

"I wonder how long it will take to drain," Wendy shook her head.

"I wonder how high it got during the storm," Neil cut to the chase.

"Ooo," I used a Neil-hoot. "I hate to imagine how close it came to the top."

After five minutes of staring at this bizarre caricature of the Everglades

— and perhaps a metaphor for Neil's life at the moment — we returned to the hotel.

"How you doing?" Wendy asked him.

"Better by the minute," he smiled.

By dinnertime, he was hungry and ready to eat a good meal. That was a relief! And after dinner, we took another short walk.

"Anna visits tomorrow," I gave Neil a good-natured wink.

He gave me mild look of annoyance.

"So you think you'll be ready to get back up and running tomorrow," Wendy asked.

"Absolutely," he agreed. "Just a little bit slower."

"It's a balancing act," I observed once again.

"It's a learning curve," Wendy corrected. "We're proud of you!"

"And I'm proud of you," he smiled back.

Thus, our day ended quietly.

> ***Excerpt Sub-investigator's report, April-29-2016***
>
> Subject came in for Week 2, Day 9. The sub-investigator was available to assess clinical disease status. Subject overall feels well, however, he experienced grade 1 nausea on 4/28/16. No nausea reported today, 4/29/16. Doses recorded from yesterday were recorded and subject received all six doses. PI made clinical decision to maintain on same dose of Atengenal and Astugenal today.

PREPPING FOR REMOTE OPERATIONS APRIL 30

Neil slept well. Not having to wake up to drink and pee throughout the night was a big help, especially given his trouble with swallowing and initiating any form of elimination; his tumor was increasingly stressing those parts of his brain in control of such functions. This was the case even before he was diagnosed, and it would be an ongoing handicap.

For the moment, however, Neil was feeling good — ready to continue on the path he was on, and he was looking forward to his lunch date with Anna. He was especially eager to see Evie, who would arrive the following day. For the moment, however, we still had our morning at the clinic to contend with.

"Let's do a dressing change," Julian announced upon entering the treatment room. I deferred to his expertise once again, and he laughed. "Fortunately, this isn't something we'll have to do too much longer," and we "suited up." Julian gave Neil's incision a thorough inspection. The redness and swelling had gone down, and his rash was improving. "These stitches can come out pretty soon," Julian muffled through his mask.

"How soon?" Neil muffled back.

"Sometime in the next week to ten days," Julian said as finished his ministrations and re-bandaged the area.

Neil took off his mask and took a deep breath. "That's much better," he smiled.

"Isn't it though," Julian agreed.

"You'll get to meet my sister in two days," Neil added. "She arrives tomorrow."

"I look forward to meeting her," Julian nodded. "You'll take her to Ruggle's Green?"

"Yep," Neil agreed. "We've been saving that for her."

"You'll love it," Julian assured him.

With the dressing change complete, Wendy and I set up the table.

"I spoke with Dr. B about your nausea," Sheryll announced when she delivered the day's ANPs. "He agrees with lowering the dose of A10."

Even though he was under the gun in Austin, Dr. B kept in touch with Sheryll and Dr. Gregory.

"I'm glad," Neil nodded, as Wendy and I set about prepping for his next infusion. By this time, we were completely at ease with the process.

"I think we can do this on our own," I announced once the pump was programmed and running.

"Like I said before," Julian smiled. "You guys could get a job at the clinic. And speaking of doing this on your own," he added, "that's what you'll be doing tomorrow and Monday."

"How's that?" I wondered.

"The clinic would be closed as usual on Sunday," Julian explained, "and also on Monday in observance of Polish Constitution Day."

Dr. B and the staff at the clinic were very proud of their heritage!

"We're ready," Wendy nodded. "We've had a good teacher. You enjoy the time off."

"Flatter me all you want," Julian laughed. "But I'll still be on call if you need anything. Now hold on a moment while I put together the supplies you'll need to take with you."

A few minutes later, Julian delivered a box filled with all the prep supplies we would need, and Sheryll delivered four bags of ANPs — two Atengenal and two Astugenal — enough for the two days of infusions.

"What about dosage?" I asked.

"We'll hold at today's levels," Sheryll replied. "If all is well on Tuesday, we'll increase again."

Neil gave her two thumps way up.

"I'll be on call if you need me," Julian repeated. "Don't hesitate to call."

"You know we will," Neil smiled, eyebrows arched maniacally.

Julian just chuckled.

Wendy and I each took a box, and the three of us departed the inner sanctum in high spirits, confident we were up to the task. Neil was glad to be back up and running, and the pump bag slung over his shoulder was becoming a habit. He smiled broadly upon seeing Anna in her Mom's outer office, to the left of the "adult" area of the waiting room, and he ambled right over.

"Ready to go," he held out a hand to shake hers.

"Absolutely," she beamed.

"I'll pick you up at five o'clock," Anna's mom told her.

With lunchtime approaching, we headed straight for Snap Kitchen. The kids took our orders and went in to get food while we sat in the car.

"This will be a good day for Neil," I smiled, and Wendy agreed.

Back at the hotel, Neil and Anna brought their meals to a table next to the pool. What they talked about in the shade of an umbrella is anyone's guess. Wendy and I stayed up in our suite, out of their way. Wendy did some housekeeping and reading, and I stowed the medical supplies in our closet, then it was time to check emails — another note from Tim and Sherri was waiting.

To: Dean
From: Tim
Subject: Re: Letter on Clinical Trial for cancer drug
Date: Sat, 30 Apr 2016
CC: Sherri

Hi Dean,

Your well written letter is the only basis of any conversation. There is no deception intended at all.

Jill's email address is attached to this thread. We have only been introduced to her through the effort of passing on Neil's letter. Perhaps you would prefer to contact her directly before submitting the release?

Good luck Dean.
Tim

It seemed I had inadvertently touched a nerve in my last reply, so I quickly replied to clear up any misunderstanding.

To: Tim
From: Dean
Subject: Re: Letter on Clinical Trial for cancer drug

Date: April 30, 2016
CC: Sherri

Hi Tim,

Poor word choice. I'm sorry about that. We do not think anyone intended any deception! I just want to be sure no one thinks we were trying to leverage a Brown connection that does not exist. Obviously there was some initial miscommunication that propagated that erroneous connection. As for contacting Senator Reed, I would only send him that letter for now. Evidently he got a copy, so the connection is made. If it comes to more formal action, we will proceed. For now, it feels premature.

I apologize for any misunderstanding! Thank you very very much for your ongoing help!!!

Love to you all, and God Bless,
Dean

With the misunderstanding with "Team Neil" hopefully smoothed over, my attention turned to Evie's upcoming visit:

To: Dean, Wendy
From: Evie Fachon
Subject: Fwd: Travelocity travel confirmation - May 1
Date: Sat, 30 Apr 2016

Arriving at 1:55PM : ^)

"Your reservation is booked and confirmed: Houston, May 1, 2016 - May 9, 2016."

Having Evie in Houston would be such a breath of fresh air! We planned to show her around town — at least the parts that we knew —

and take her to our favorite places to eat, and we were saving Ruggle's Green for something to experience for the first time together. Of course, Neil was just eager to have his oldest best friend at his side. Evie's visit would be a vacation, like the "old days" when the four of us took off on our sailboat and holed up overnight in places like Mackerel Cove and Dutch Harbor. We would play games for hours as the stars winked into life, and on clear nights, the kids would sleep out in the cockpit under that heavenly canopy.

Back at the poolside, 5:00 p.m. came all too soon, and with it, Anna's Mom arrived to pick her up. She and Neil parted with a hug and the promise to see each other again, and he was a bit melancholy when she left.

"Don't forget, Evie flies in tomorrow afternoon," Wendy reminded him.

"I'll be glad to see her," his face brightened.

"Like old times," I smiled.

The remainder of the day was mostly consumed with talking about Evie's visit. Not once did Neil complain of nausea. Reducing the dose of Atengenal did the trick. Neil knew he still needed to up-dose, and he was committed to trying, but he was relieved he could do so a little more slowly.

"Tomorrow is our first real solo flight," I said as we sat around the dinner table, digesting another fine meal.

"You guys got this," Neil said with an "are you kidding me" smirk.

"We do," Wendy agreed. "But we need to be extra careful we don't spill. It wouldn't do for the room to smell like someone couldn't hold it."

"No," Neil scrunched his nose. "That wouldn't be optimal."

"Maybe we should get a small rug to put under the table, and a tablecloth for the table itself," I suggested. "To 'cover' the bases."

"That couldn't hurt," Wendy nodded.

After dinner, while Wendy cleaned up, I took a quick trip to Walmart. I purchased a plastic picnic table cloth to tape over the table and a small area rug to spread underneath. In the event of a spill, there would be no lingering odor.

Excerpt Sub-investigator's report, April-30-2016

Subject came in for Week 2, Day 10. The sub-investigator was available to assess clinical disease status. Subject overall feels well, however, he experienced grade 1 nausea on 4/29/16 and parents stated that subject self-disconnected the antineoplastons yesterday receiving only two doses of each. No nausea reported today, 4/30/2016. SI made the clinical decision to reduce the dose of Atengenal and maintain on same Astugenal dose...

23

EVIE!

"I SO GLAD TO SEE YOU!![14]*"*

SUNDAY, MAY 1, 2016

Not having to go to the clinic meant we could sleep in an extra half hour, but once breakfast was done, we got busy with prepping. We started by spreading the area rug under the table and taping the tablecloth securely in place over the working surface. We then proceeded as we normally would at the clinic. Everything went smoothly until it was time to program the pump. We could not get it to reset from the previous day, so we had to call Julian. As promised, he picked up immediately and had us sorted out in less than a minute. Just when we thought everything was all set, however, we kept getting a warning light about a "downside occlusion" — air in the line. We had to re-lead one of the lines to get it cleared, but once over these speed bumps, Neil was up and running, and the decks were cleared for Evie's arrival! She would land that afternoon, and she planned to stay through Neil's birthday on the eighth

Neil's twentieth birthday: According to his original prognosis, as of May 8, he would have roughly one month left to live. If he had taken the recommended course of radiation, maybe another four months. Being in his company these last two months, however, and seeing how well he was doing, it seemed likely he would significantly outlive his best-case progno-

14 A phrase coined by me as a toddler, with regards to my own big sister, Suzanne. It was exactly how Neil felt.

sis. Following his chosen path of treatment was having an impact. Would it be enough to save his life? Maybe, but we knew it was a long shot, so every day with him, especially a birthday, was a treasure. And there would be no better present than his sister!

As the time to leave for the airport drew near, I offered to go alone to get Evie. "You don't need to schlep around in the car for two or three hours."

"Okay," Neil nodded. "I'd like to go, but it might be tough finding "facilities" if I need them."

"That too," I nodded.

"We'll have her for a full week," Wendy reminded him. "You'll get plenty of together-time."

"Okay then," I said. "I'm on my way." I gave Neil and Wendy a hug and departed.

It was warm and muggy as I hopped into our Toyota Corolla and headed east on Route 10, then north up Route 69 to the George Bush Intercontinental Airport. There was plenty of traffic the whole way, and power lines traced a landscape of commercial development. The cloverleaf turn-offs, highway splits, and merges were just as confusing as the night we arrived. How we managed to navigate to the hotel without any missteps was a small miracle.

The airport's pickup areas were partitioned by airlines, so I cued up for American and took a drive through to get the lay of the land. Police officers kept waving the traffic along with little or no wait-time allowed. Get your passenger and scoot! On my second pass through, I saw Evie coming out a door. As luck would have it, a space opened up at just the same moment, and I pulled over just long enough to load her backpack into the trunk and give her a quick hug before the police started shooing us out.

"It's great to see you," I beamed. "We've been looking forward to this!"

"Me too," Evie smiled. "How's it going?"

"Pretty well, really," I nodded. "We're anxious about the FDA situation."

"Of course," Evie huffed. "I don't understand why they'd try to do that to one person — someone who is terminally ill."

"Join the club, Sweetheart," I said. "Neither do we."

Having Evie in the car was an instant cure for homesickness, and as we drove back, I got caught up on school news, we discussed Neil's progress, and we exchanged comments on the Texas-huge roadways and scenery.

"It's so good to see you," I smiled. "Did I tell you that?"

Evie chuckled. "You too."

At ten minutes out, I called ahead, and the welcome committee was waiting outside. Evie jumped out of the car and flung her arms around Neil. He shut his eyes, and his smile reached his ears.

"It's good to see you," he hugged her tight.

After several seconds, they released each other, and Evie held Neil at arm's length. "You look great," she told him. "How are they treating you?" she playfully nodded at us.

"You know," he arched a sage eyebrow. "They take good care of me, but thank God we now have a fourth player to do some real gaming!"

We all laughed.

"Can I get a hug too?" Wendy pouted.

Evie wrapped her Mom in her arms. "I've missed you," they said almost in unison.

With greetings complete, Evie turned back to Neil and nodded to his pump case. "So you have a constant companion?"

"I do," Neil nodded. "Can you believe it? I'm still here," and he lifted his shirt to show her the lines.

"Of course you are," she scolded. "You're not going anywhere."

"Not anytime soon," Neil smiled.

"Elise is sending a special present for your birthday," Evie changed the subject.

"What's that?"

"It's when you celebrate the day you were born," Evie dead panned.

Neil chuckled.

"Oh, you mean the present," Evie smiled and shook her head no. "I can't tell you. Even if I knew. But she says we'll recognize it when we see it."

I pulled Evie's backpack from the car. "Okay, shall we head up?"

We trekked up the stairs, Neil taking them with a purposeful stride, then down the hall to the far end.

Wendy opened the door with a flourish. "Here's our digs."

"Wow," Evie approved as she stepped over the threshold. "It looks pretty nice!"

"It suits our needs pretty well," Wendy agreed.

"This will be your bed," I said, putting her backpack next to the fold out sofa.

Evie made her camp in the living room, laying her things in the corner or on the side table and placing some clothes in the lower drawer of the TV stand. After she settled in, we were a cozy family once again, very much like sharing the confines of our little sailboat. She and Neil spent some time holed up in his bedroom catching up, while Wendy and I checked our emails, and I sent an update to Sheryll.

Before long, it was time to think about dinner. "How about a trip to get some fresh groceries for dinner?" Wendy asked Evie. "You won't believe the grocery store we go to, the H-E-B. I got lost the first time we went!"

"Sure!" Evie agreed eagerly.

Neil rolled his eyes — "here we go again" — and we took a short expedition, sort of like taking the dinghy ashore to go shopping.

Evie was duly impressed as she and Wendy picked out some fresh organic veggies and chicken, along with a treat for dessert. Upon returning to the hotel, the girls "rolled up their sleeves" to prepare a wonderful dinner, and the kids discussed Evie's classes as we ate. After dinner, Neil begged for a game of *Ticket to Ride*, which he won with a chuckle.

"Some things don't change," Evie chuckled with him.

Soon thereafter, it was time to turn in. We settled into our normal routine, and Evie opened the fold-out couch to find a surprisingly comfortable mattress.

Excerpt Sub-investigator's report, May 1, 2016

Week 2, Day 11. The sub-investigator was available to assess clinical disease status. Subject overall feels well with

> no new symptoms to report. Doses from yesterday were recorded. SI made the clinical decision to maintain on the same antineoplaston doses...

POLISH INDEPENDENCE DAY

May 2, 2017: The night passed uneventfully. Neil kept up with his infusions, drank plenty of water, filled his bedside urinal, and still managed to get some good sleep. Knowing Evie was there must have been a relief. As for her, being adaptable by nature and always ready to "camp out," she seemed to sleep well in her temporary abode. After getting up and disconnecting Neil from the pump, we followed the normal routine. With breakfast tucked into their bellies, the kids enjoyed a couple of hours of him not being tethered.

While the clinic celebrated Polish Independence Day — Dr. B had served in the Polish Army — we set up to prep. Evie, ever the scientist, intently followed the procedure, asking questions and observing our techniques all along. By the time the pump was programmed and Neil was hooked up and running, she was fairly amazed.

"Wow, that's one heck of a procedure," she shook her head. "You guys could practically be nurses."

"It is," Wendy agreed. "But we're getting so used to doing it that it's almost routine."

"We actually had some hiccups yesterday," I admitted.

"What happened?" Evie asked.

"We had trouble resetting the pump," I told her.

"But a call to Julian and some creative persistence got it all sorted out," Wendy said.

"And then we got a warning about a 'downside occlusion,'" I added.

"Air bubbles in the line," Wendy explained.

"We figured that one out on our own," I said. "We had to open the pump and clear the segment of IV line running through it. Once that was done, Neil was back up and running."

Evie nodded in approval. "Good for you!"

"Good for me," Neil grinned.

"So how does it feel?" Evie asked, "when the pump is running?"

"It feels like a waterfall in the back of my head," Neil closed his eyes, feeling. "It feels like something is happening."

"That sounds encouraging."

"But if I up-dose too fast," Neil added, "I get nauseous."

"It's a balancing act," I observed once again.

"A learning curve," Wendy added.

"Take your pick," I said. "Either way, Dr. B wants Neil to work up to a significantly higher dose, but if the leap is too big, that's a problem."

"I think Dr. B gets it," Neil offered.

"Right you are, Buddy," Wendy smiled. "So that's the strategy."

"Actually Mom," Neil grinned, "it's more of a tactic."

"Smart ass," I laughed.

"I get the idea," Evie smiled at her brother's dry humor.

After getting Neil up and running, we cleaned the prep area and carefully put everything away in our bedroom the closet.

"How about a walk," Neil suggested.

"Would you like to check out the levee in back?" Wendy asked Evie. "We've only been up there once."

"Sure," she nodded, and Neil eagerly agreed.

In short order, we were out the door, through the parking lot, and stepping over the low guardrail across the street. Water from the storm still flowed in the drainage ditch, but there was a stone sticking up in the middle, so we stepped across carefully and meandered up the twenty foot embankment strewn with wildflowers. The water level inside the park was still high — not as high as it had been, but the trunks of the trees were still half-submerged.

Evie's mouth dropped open. "That's a lot of water."

"You should have seen the roads the day after the storm," Neil nodded. "Highways were flooded and some of the underpasses were under ten feet of water!"

"We don't know how high it got here," Wendy gestured toward the park.

"That's probably a good thing," I cringed again at the thought.

"It's amazing you could get everything done when you did," Evie marveled.

"Indeed," Neil nodded. "Those were long days in the tube, not to mention the surgery."

"But you took it like a soldier," I gave him a thumbs up.

We took in the view a bit longer, then we descended the bank, crossed the stream, and walked along the sidewalk toward the east end of the levee.

"This is where we usually walk," Neil told Evie, striding with confidence. "It's a business district, but it's quiet at night and on the weekends."

Evie nodded. "Seems like a good place to exercise."

"And we have a small gym in the hotel," Neil added.

On our way back, Wendy asked, "What would you like to do for lunch?"

"The Feast," Neil didn't hesitate.

"The Movable Feast it is," we agreed.

We placed our orders at the counter. Evie wanted the "Veggie Bowl," Wendy the "Happy Veggie Patty Plate," Neil ordered the "Chili Pie," and I asked for one of the day's specials, a "Bison Burger" served with quinoa salad. Having been to the Feast enough for the servers to know us, we exchanged pleasantries, then we filled some large glasses with cool filtered water and found a table to wait.

"That's fun," Evie gestured to the straight-backed chair hanging high up on the wall nearby, then she admired the photos of Hemingway and the colorful art. Seeing the variety of hanging plants in the outside dining area, she added, "We'll have to eat outside sometime too."

"If you like that, wait 'til you see the arboretum at the clinic," Neil smiled.

We had plenty to admire and talk about as we waited, but soon our name was called, and Evie and I went up to the counter to collect our trays full of food and some silverware. We returned to our table and dug in.

"Wow," Evie exclaimed after a couple of bites, "I could eat here every day!"

"Couldn't you," I nodded.

"We just about do," Wendy laughed, and Neil nodded, his mouth full.

Because we were celebrating Evie's arrival, we indulged in dessert. They had some fresh lemon bars that were just about perfect — not too sweet, not too tart, and dusted with confectionery sugar.

After finishing our food and bussing our plates and silverware, we perused the health food-store. Evie needed some shampoo — her bottle was too big to bring on the plane — and Neil returned to the Himalayan salt lamps.

"The sunset glow is very soothing," he smiled.

"Pick one out this time," I told him, and he did.

"Feeling good?" Evie asked her brother when we climbed back in the car.

"Very," Neil nodded. "I am so glad to see you!"

"Me too," Evie beamed.

So, our day progressed blissfully into late afternoon, when talk turned to cooking a nice dinner at "home" and maybe a game. We also had *Heart of the Sea* to watch, and since Neil had trounced us at *Ticket to Ride* the night before, we opted for the video.

While Neil connected his PC, I pulled in an overstuffed chair from the living room for him to sit in, then Wendy, myself, and Evie propped our backs up with pillows on the bed. Neil hit the "play" button and sat in the chair close to Evie. Like *Revanant, Heart of the Sea* is a tale of loss, unlikely survival, and rebirth, this time based on true events, which inspired Herman Melville's *Moby Dick.* Deep in a corner of my heart, I hoped these stories would be metaphors for Neil's trajectory against his implacable foe(s). We all did.

24

"HOUSTON, WE HAVE A PROBLEM"

"Tell us about a tough time or problem in your life that you had to overcome.[15]" NF

MAY 3, 2016

We awoke to another bright morning of promise. After disconnecting the lines, Neil wanted a shower, so we got his catheter and bandages neatly sealed under plastic.

"That's elaborate," Evie observed as I taped down the plastic covering.

"Just need to keep it sterile and dry until it's fully healed," Neil told her.

"How's it doing?"

"The stitches should be coming out soon," he nodded, and with that, Neil was "off to the races."

While Evie and Wendy prepared to make breakfast, I set the table and then quickly checked emails. Finding nothing urgent, I sat down to watch a bit of news. Ten minutes later, Neil emerged from the bathroom in his usual cloud of steam with a towel wrapped around his waist.

"Did you leave any hot water for the rest of the hotel?" Evie ribbed him.

He chuckled and sat down so I could remove the plastic covering, then

15 A question Neil had posed to himself in training for eagerly anticipated co-op interviews.

he retired to his room to get dressed. In the interim, Wendy scrambled eggs with sautéed onions and peppers, and Evie cut up some fresh fruit. Everything arrived at the table about the same time Neil re-emerged from his room, looking like his old self without his constant companion.

"You look good," Evie told him.

"I feel FAN-TASTIC," he flashed his best impish grin, and we got through our normal routine in high spirits.

We left the hotel at roughly 9:30 a.m., stopped to get blood drawn at Quest lab, then went to the clinic, taking time in the waiting area for Evie to see some of the pictures of Dr. Burzynski with his various patients over the years, then we introduced her to Irena.

"Evie," she smiled, "It's wonderful to meet you. You have such a brave and handsome brother, and you're lovely too!"

"It's very nice to meet you," Evie smiled.

"I'm sorry he has to be here," Irena continued, opening the door to the inner sanctum, "but it's a good place to be," and she motioned us in.

Neil pointed out some of the doorways along the hallway to the left, but we turned right and went straight to his private room.

"Is this all for you?" Evie asked as she looked around the room.

"Special treatment," Neil raised his eyebrows and lifted his chin in a bit of "tut tut" theatrics. With a straight face, he continued. "It's because I'm on the clinical trial. I'm the only one getting A10." Then, he settled down on his couch. "Nothing for me to do now but relax."

Wendy and I went to the cabinet to get everything we needed to set up the prep table, and a moment later, Julian walked in. "Ahh," his face lit up seeing Evie, "you're Neil's sister."

"Evie," Neil stood up and held his hand out, "this is Julian. Julian, this is my sister Evie."

"A pleasure," Julian bowed with a smile. "I see some resemblance, but you're much better looking."

"Well thank you," Evie smiled. "I would hope so!"

"Hey now!" Neil jabbed back playfully.

"So how did the weekend go,? Julian turned to us.

"We did fine," I said, "except for the pump reset. Thank you for sorting that out."

"Not a problem," Julian nodded. "That's why I'm on call!"

"And we had some trouble getting one of the lines purged," Wendy added. "We ended up having to open the pump and plink the segment of line running through it. We couldn't see any bubbles, but that cleared the 'occlusion warning,' and we were good to go."

"You did exactly what I would have suggested," Julian nodded in approval. "Just like pros."

With the prep table ready, there was only so much we could do until Sheryll delivered the day's bags of antineoplastons. She was later than usual.

"She's probably caught up with something in the main treatment room," Julian offered. "I'll find her."

We waited another ten minutes, then Sheryll and Julian returned together.

"Hi Neil," she said, "could you come with me?"

"Sure," Neil replied. "What's up?"

"I'm not sure," Sheryll shook her head. Julian shrugged uncertainly.

Sheryll led us down the long hall and past the main treatment room where Julian turned in. "I'll be here when you need me."

Sheryll passed the nurse station and the short hallway leading to a pair of rooms — one in which Neil received his first examination at the clinic and another hardly bigger than a closet with the scale used to weigh patients. She continued past the little conference room where Neil signed the paperwork for the clinical trial. Except for the happy faces smiling at us from the photos the whole way, it seemed like a long sullen walk, but at last, we arrived at Dr. B's private office area. Sheryll stood at the entrance to his conference room and motioned us in.

"I'll talk to you later, Neil," she promised, a pensive look on her face, then she departed.

I waved to Carolyn Powers who was sitting at her desk as we filed into the conference room. It was divided by a long lozenge-shaped table with eight or so chairs on each side and a chair on each end. The room's sidewalls were covered with low shelves full of periodicals, and the upper walls held several framed presentation posters of clinical cases, many showing before-and-after images of brain tumors. The far wall was glass overlooking the parking lot. In the middle of the table was a speaker phone. A few people we had not met were already seated, and one of them motioned us to take seats.

"This is for you to listen," he told us. "Please don't say anything."

FDA/BURZYNSKI CLINIC TELECONFERENCE MAY 3, 2016

FDA Attendees:

- **Patricia Keegan, M.D. Director: Division of Oncology Products 2, Office of Hematology and Oncology Products, Center for Drug Evaluation and Research**
- **Deborah Miller, Ph.D., R.N. – Office of Health and Constituent Affairs**
- **Richard Klein**
- **Anuja Patel, MPH**
- **Joohee Sul – Medical Reviewer**
- **Suzanne Sensabaugh – Team Leader**

Burzynski Clinic and Burzynski Research Institute Attendees:

- **Carolyn Powers**
- **Tomasz Janicki,**
- **Samuel Beenken**

Carolyn followed us in a few moments later, a frown on her face. The gentleman who had seated us then pressed the button on the speaker phone:

> **Keegan:** So, we wanted to have this call to respond to your request that we modify the clinical hold from a full clinical hold to a partial clinical hold to accommodate the treatment of the patient whose therapy was initiated the day after the hold letter was issued. And based on the serious nature of the manufacturing defect identified, we do not think it is appropriate to modify the clinical hold, and we are not going to make any modifications at this time. So, we wanted to clarify that you understand that no patients are to be treated under the IND.
>
> **Beenken:** I would like to just say something on a personal basis. Um, I've been reassured by the manufacturer that the end product is the same A10 that has been used in the clinical trials right along. They view it as a manufacturing problem, not a patient safety issue. That's just a personal statement on my behalf. The other personal statement is that the patient will die shortly, and as you know, there are no other therapies for diffuse intrinsic brainstem glioma, and as you are aware, chemotherapy has shown no effect against this tumor. Again, two personal statements to be on the record. I am speaking for myself, not for the Burzynski Research Institute, but I think that sentiment is generally held.
>
> **Janicki:** My name is Tom. I am speaking as the Burzynski Research Institute. The entire process for this particular patient has started and has been submitted for registration process starting from April 13, so it was one week before the entire [hold] process started. The patient has been screened; the patient has been sent for the placement of the catheter, and this is a deadly disease.

Patel: I'm sorry. This is Anuja Patel with the FDA. Can you please introduce yourself and your affiliation?

Janicki: My name is Tomasz, T-O-M-A-S-Z, Janicki, J-A-N-I-C-K-I, and I am employed with Burzynski Research Institute.

Patel: Ok, great.

Beenken: The only reason that the patient wasn't on ANP therapy by the time the Full Clinical Hold letter was obtained was that there was a delay in inserting the central catheter.

Keegen: I think it is concerning that while you were in receipt of the Clinical Hold letter that you ignored it and started therapy anyway, and then came to us so that is of a concern in regard to the control and the management of this investigational product. So, I would like to make that statement clear that when we issue a letter, and you acknowledge receipt of it, that we expect that upon receipt, that you will act in accordance with that. So, this reflects a disturbing disregard for the regulations, but I think [we want] to pursue some comments with regard to individual patients, who as I understand it, have not been treated with standard of care.

Sul: Clearly, there wasn't a lot of clinical history provided, but based on the patient's history, we have some concerns regarding the fact that the patient has not received radiation therapy, which is an available therapy with a known survival advantage for gliomas, including brainstem gliomas. The other concern is that this patient is a bit atypical from the classic DIPG because of his age, and also, it appears from his notes and the radiology reports, they describe the significant exophytic components of the tumor.

Again, without all of the clinical details, we do, however, know that patients with an exophytic component can do better and often are actually recommended for surgical resections, so I think that these are additional concerns that the patient may not be aware of, and in fact, his understanding of the informed consent in terms of what kind of therapy he would be forgoing.

Keegen: Did you have a specific modification to the informed consent to cover the unusual circumstances of this patient's presentation, or did he sign a standard informed consent?

Beenken: He signed the standard informed consent on April 13. As you know, there are five cohorts to this phase II study, and he signed the consent form appropriate for his cohort. Dr. Burzynski did go over the letter and read it to him in full detail, and the patient and his family were very insistent that the therapy carry on if at all possible, and that was duly noted in the medical records.

Keegen: To clarify, you understand that a patient's consent does not override a clinical hold on an investigational drug trial.

Beenken: Yes, we understand that, and again, I'm speaking personally here. I believe Dr. Burzynski felt that the enrollment was already established, and your letter referred to no new enrollments and also suggested that you understood that there were no new enrollments. The registration process is just the legal aspect of defining that enrollment. So, Dr. Burzynski, I'm not speaking for him, this is just my personal opinion, felt that the patient was already enrolled and gave the patient every opportunity to back out of the therapy understanding that a clinical hold had been placed because of patient safety issues.

Keegen: And it had been placed because of patient safety issues, which you can't consent away by reading our letter. So, I think we have clarified our position, that the IND is on full clinical hold, and no patient may be treated until the manufacturing issues have been addressed.

Beenken: Well, we understand that.

Janicki: Yes, we understand this.

Beenken: And that message will be forwarded immediately.

Patel: Ok. So, that pretty much concludes our call today, and if there are any further questions or concerns, you may email me. You have my contact information, and I appreciate you getting on the phone with us and providing us dial up information this morning. Thank you, and have a wonderful day.

Janicki: Thank you.

Beenken: Thank you.

SLEDGEHAMMER TO HEAD

Neil slowly crumbled as this performance unfolded — all the promise and joy ebbing away, leaving him ashen and shaking as if he were back at Mass General being handed a death sentence, only this time it came through a speakerphone, which made it feel callous at best.

"Oh Buddy," Evie took her brother's hand in her own, holding back tears, and we just sat there, our hearts full of hope only moments before, now clenched in anguish. Everyone remained quiet.

"Oh my God," Wendy broke the silence, choking back tears. "These people have no idea what they're doing!"

"Unbelievable," I pounded a fist on the table. "What the," I began, then halted. "They doubt his 'informed consent?'" I asked myself out loud, unable to believe the things I'd just heard. Then, louder, I said, "We could line up a dozen oncologists and teach them more about DIPG and its treatment..." I clenched my fists. "They don't have a clue!"

"I'm so sorry," Carolyn shook her head despondently. "Dr. Burzynski would be here, but the Texas Medical Board has him tied down in Austin."

"What a coincidence," Neil spoke softly, a smoldering glint in his eyes.

"We'll let Dr. B know what has happened right away," she promised.

"He probably knows," Neil frowned. "He couldn't have changed this." Neil also realized that Dr. B would have recommendations about what to do next. "We need to talk with him."

I nodded as Sheryll opened the door. Someone must have paged her.

"They've shut down the trial completely," Carolyn told her.

"I'm so sorry Neil," Sheryll said, looking down for a moment and fidgeting with her hands. "I guess you should leave the clinic now."

"We have some things in his room," I snapped a bit harshly, but of course, it wasn't her fault. "I'm sorry."

"It's okay," Sheryll smiled thinly. "Of course, let's get your things."

"What about dressing changes and pulling the stitches?" Neil asked.

"We will assist with everything you need while you're in Houston," she said. "We'll need to continue monitoring your bloodwork for awhile as well."

We collected our things from Neil's room-no-longer, and Sheryll and Julian escorted us to the waiting area, their eyes moist. Word had spread throughout the clinic, and Irena was crying. She blew her nose, "This isn't right!"

We exchanged somber hugs, then Wendy, Evie, Neil, and I trudged out on leaden feet, deflated and adrift, like a family made suddenly homeless. I could imagine nothing more devastating being done to my son — being done by our government. He was marooned in the grip of a medical bureaucracy. The FDA might claim they were protecting the patient, or that we were indulging false hopes, but they gave no credit for the homework we'd done — no compassion for the distance we'd traveled to arrive at the pinnacle of "informed consent." Why does the mantle of authority corrupt Man's conscience so often? How could these people deny hope to a young man with his neck in a noose? They weren't just stopping Neil's treatment, they were killing his Hope.

There were so many things wrong with the FDA's decision. (It was the bookend to the vaccines that most likely kicked off Neil's nightmare.) But contesting the decision would take time and attorneys to parse it all out, time Neil couldn't spare. It was as if the FDA — whatever good intentions may have attended its creation — had become a DIPG itself, strangling the balance of Constitutional principles, that would otherwise mandate a deep and abiding respect for the freedom of an individual to make an informed choice for himself.

"The timing of this hold on the trial is truly unbearable.
DIPG is a rapidly progressing disease, and at this point,
I really don't have any time to be messing around.
Beyond this, the trial at the Burzynski Clinic is one
I carefully chose, was accepted into, and had already begun
the treatment protocol. I understand that it is by no means
a guaranty, but I truly believe it is my best chance." NF

Check.

Neil's saga will continue in the second book
of the Jester Knight Chronicles:

Itcōpō.

(In the Court of Public Opinion.)

POST SCRIPT

In 2016, the FDA shut down a clinical trial for one young man because it quibbled with the purity of an ingredient being used to make an experimental treatment, suddenly requiring this ingredient be manufactured as if it were a drug unto itself. The FDA offered no evidence of harm having ever been caused by the Burzynski Research Institute's decades old method of handling this ingredient. Fast forward to the early 2020s, when the FDA tried to cajole every adult and child in the country to take an experimental treatment while information about its ingredients was kept secret. Disregarding "informed consent," the FDA maintained its effort despite the unprecedented injuries and deaths that accrued in the wake of administering these so-called vaccines — injuries and deaths surpassing all other vaccines ever invented, combined! As much as authorities wish to disavow any causal connections, these facts are documented on the CDC's Vaccine Adverse Reaction Reporting System (VAERS) and by statistics from around the world. I shudder to think about how many Neils have been seeded with a premature demise.

APPENDIX

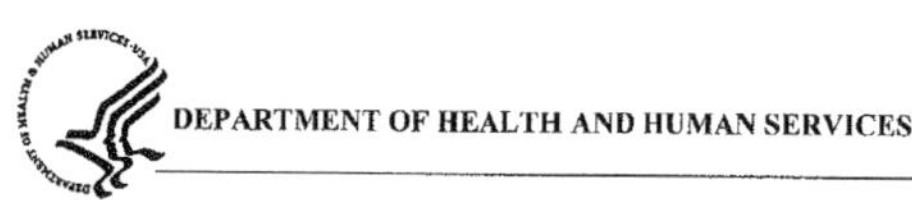

Food and Drug Administration
Silver Spring MD 20993

IND 43742

FULL CLINICAL HOLD

Burzynski Research Institute, Inc.
Attention: Stanislaw R. Burzynski, M.D., Ph.D.
President
9432 Katy Freeway
Houston, TX 77055

Dear Dr. Burzynski:

Please refer to your Investigational New Drug Application (IND) submitted under section 505(i) of the Federal Food, Drug, and Cosmetic Act for "Antineoplastons A10/AS2-1 Injections (ANP)".

We also refer to the inspection conducted at your S.R. Burzynski Manufacturing Facility located at 12707 Trinity Drive, Houston, TX 77477 from March 9, 2015 through March 19, 2015.

Your IND is on full clinical hold and you may not enroll new adult or pediatric patients in <u>any</u> protocol under this IND. In addition, you may not resume administration of ANP in any adult or pediatric patients previously treated. We note that there are no patients currently receiving ANP under this IND. The following are the specific deficiencies and the information needed to resolve the deficiencies.

21 CFR 312.42(b)(2)(i): Unreasonable and significant risk of illness or injury to human subjects.

1. Synthesis of the drug substances are not adequately described for A10 as well as AS2-1. As per your submission, phenylacetic acid (PN) and phenylacetylglutamine (PG) drug substances are provided by Spectrum Chemical, NJ and Kiangsu Group, Hong Kong respectively. Note that these cannot be considered as starting materials but are drug substances. Provide the name and physical location of the manufacturing facility(ies) for these drug substances. Confirm that these are manufactured under GMP conditions. Provide full characterization of the drug substances including optical purity data for PG.

2. The synthesis of isoPG is carried out by cyclization of PG followed by base catalyzed hydrolysis. Provide full characterization of isoPG and the ratio of PG vs isoPG. Provide batch to batch variation of this ratio. Provide data on process impurities during the synthesis of isoPG.

3. During the inspection of the S.R. Burzynski Manufacturing Facility on March 9, 2015 – March 19, 2015, deficiencies in your manufacturing process relating to the lack of sterility assurance, characterization of critical quality attributes, and inaccurate or unreliable data in records were identified. Our field investigator conveyed these

deficiencies to you on March 19, 2015. These inspectional findings are under review to determine the corrective actions necessary to address these issues.

In order to address these deficiencies, you must submit the following information:

a. Identification of an alternative manufacturing facility and all required information regarding that facility and its manufacturing processes required under 21 CFR 312.23. The submission should contain detailed information to demonstrate that the alternative facility can manufacture ANP from an acceptable and qualified drug substance(s), the drug products (AS10/AS21-1) are sterile, meet established acceptance criteria, and the products are comparable to those manufactured by S.R. Burzynski Manufacturing Facility.

Or

b. Information describing the corrective actions taken and demonstrating that these corrective actions have addressed all the deficiencies conveyed on the Form FDA-483.

Until you have submitted the required information and we notify you that you may resume clinical studies, you may not legally initiate or resume clinical studies under this IND.

Please identify your response to the clinical hold issues as a **"CLINICAL HOLD COMPLETE RESPONSE"**. An incomplete response will not start the review clock. Your complete response submission should reference, by date, any information previously submitted necessary to fully respond to these clinical hold issues. To facilitate a response to your submission, submit this information in triplicate to the IND. In addition, send a copy of the cover letter to Deanne Varney.

Following receipt of your complete response to these issues, we will notify you of our decision within 30 days.

If we have additional comments or information requests not related to this clinical hold, we will notify you. Your responses to any non-hold issues should be addressed in a separate amendment to the IND.

Please cite the IND number listed above at the top of the first page of any communications concerning this application. Each submission to this IND must be provided in triplicate, an original and two copies. Please include three originals of all illustrations which do not reproduce well. Send all submissions, electronic or paper, including those sent by overnight mail or courier, to the following address:

Food and Drug Administration
Center for Drug Evaluation and Research
Division of Oncology Products 2
5901-B Ammendale Road
Beltsville, MD 20705-1266

If you have any questions, call Deanne Varney, Lead Regulatory Project Manager, at (301) 796-0297.

Sincerely,

{See appended electronic signature page}

Patricia Keegan, M.D.
Director
Division of Oncology Products 2
Office of Hematology and Oncology Products
Center for Drug Evaluation and Research

This is a representation of an electronic record that was signed electronically and this page is the manifestation of the electronic signature.

/s/

PATRICIA KEEGAN
04/20/2016

Reference ID: 3919711

GLOSSARY

Anecdotal – based on personal observations in real-world situations, as opposed to scientifically established.

Antineoplaston (ANP) – the name given by Dr. Burzynski to the synthetic peptides he created. Antineoplastons is synonymous with anti-cancer.

Apoptosis – the process of genetically programmed cell death. In cancer cells, apoptosis inhibits uncontrolled cell division. This helps to suppress tumor development.

Astugenal A10 – one of two antineoplastons used in Neil's clinical trial.

Ashwaganda – an evergreen shrub that grows in Asia and Africa. It is commonly used for stress. Ashwagandha contains chemicals that might help calm the brain, reduce swelling, lower blood pressure, and alter the immune system.

Atengenal AS2-1 – one of two antineoplastons used in Neil's clinical trial.

Blood-brain barrier – a highly selective semipermeable border of endothelial cells that prevents some solutes in circulating blood from crossing into the extracellular fluid of the central nervous system.

Brainstem – located at the base of the brain, the brainstem is the stalk of the brain which connects it to the spinal cord. The brainstem sends messages throughout the body to regulate balance, breathing, heart rate and more. Sudden injuries and brain- or heart-conditions may affect how the brainstem works.

Biopsy – a surgical procedure (generally minor or done laproscopically) to remove a small piece of tissue or sample of cells from the body for testing in a laboratory to identify disease.

CBD – cannabidiol is one of more than 80 active compounds called cannabinoids found naturally in the cannabis sativa plant. CBD interacts with the endocannabinoid system, a network in the body that helps regulate many functions, including digestion, metabolism, mood, memory, sleep, motor control, pain perception, immune function, fertility, and pregnancy. Pain, anxiety, and depression are the top three conditions for which people report taking CBD. In addition, CBD effectively reduces seizures in two types of pediatric epilepsy.

Co-op – a co-op combines classroom-based education with practical work experience and provides academic credit for the experience. "Co-op"erative education helping young people to transition from school to a rewarding line of work.

Concussion – a concussion, also known as a mild traumatic brain injury (mTBI), is a head injury that temporarily affects brain functioning. Symptoms may include loss of consciousness (LOC); memory loss; headaches; difficulty with thinking, concentration, or balance; nausea; blurred vision; sleep disturbances, and mood changes.

Contact dermatitis – a localized allergic skin reaction affecting the outermost layer of skin, the epidermis, and the layer beneath, the dermis.

Chromosomes – threadlike structures made of protein and a single molecule of DNA that serve to carry the genomic information from cell to cell. In plants and animals (including humans), chromosomes reside in the nucleus of cells.

Curcumin – the primary bioactive substance in turmeric, curcumin has anti-inflammatory properties, and there is decent evidence that it can alleviate various conditions, from chronic pain to depression. Curcumin has poor bioavailability on its own, and thus it is often combined with Black Pepper or with lipids.

Dexamethasone – used to treat inflammatory conditions like cancer, arthritis, blood/hormone disorders, allergic reactions, skin diseases, eye problems, breathing problems, bowel disorders, and immune system disorders. Dexamethasone belongs to a class of drugs known as corticosteroids. It decreases your immune system's response to various diseases to reduce symptoms such as swelling and allergic-type reactions.

DANA Farber Cancer Institute – a premier cancer treatment and research institution, located in Boston, Massachusetts.

DIPG – diffuse intrinsic pontine glioma (DIPG) is a highly aggressive brain tumor which is difficult to treat. DIPG occurs in an area of the brainstem (the lowest, stem-like part of the brain) called the pons, which controls many of the body's most vital functions such as breathing, blood pressure, and heart rate. Because of its location in the brain and how rapidly it progresses, DIPG is a "high grade" malignant brain tumor.

DEC – Digital Equipment Corporation was a major American computer company and industry pioneer from the 1960s to the 1990s

Dandelion – leaves, roots, and flowers offer health benefits including promoting liver health and fighting inflammation.

D5W – Dextrose 5% in Water. Dextrose is a form of glucose (sugar). Dextrose 5% in water is injected into a vein through an IV to replace lost fluids and provide carbohydrates to the body. D5W is used to treat low blood sugar (hypoglycemia), insulin shock, or dehydration (fluid loss). Dextrose 5% in water is also given for nutritional support to patients who are unable to eat because of illness, injury, or other medical condition.

EKG/ECG – electrocardiogram

Endocrine System – the glands which secrete certain hormones into the bloodstream or tissues of the body.

Exocrine System – glands which secrete hormones onto the body's surfaces.

Endocannabinoid System (ECS) – a recently discovered biological system composed of endocannabinoids (endogenous lipid-based retrograde neurotransmitters) which bind to cannabinoid receptors (CBRs) and cannabinoid receptor proteins which are expressed throughout the vertebrate central nervous system (including the brain) and peripheral nervous system. The endocannabinoid system may be involved in regulating physiological and cognitive processes, including fertility, pregnancy, pre- and postnatal development, various activities of the immune system, appetite, pain-sensation, mood, and memory. The ECS plays an important role in multiple aspects of neural functions, including the control of movement and motor coordination, learning and memory, emotion and motivation, addictive-like behavior and pain modulation, among others.

Epigenetics – the study of how your behaviors and environment can cause changes which affect the way genes are expressed. Epigenetic changes are reversible and do not change your DNA sequence, but they can change how your body reads a DNA sequence.

FDA – the (United States) Food and Drug Administration is a federal agency of the Department of Health and Human Services. Among other things, the FDA is responsible for protecting the public health by ensuring the safety, efficacy and security of drugs and biological products.

GMP – Good Manufacturing Practices (GMPs) were developed by the FDA to ensure the integrity of industries creating food and drug products. The GMPs are listed in the Code of Federal Regulations (CFR) Title 21, Parts 210 & 211.

Glioma – a type of tumor which starts in the glial cells of the brain or the spine. Gliomas comprise about 30 percent of all brain and central nervous system tumors, and 80 percent of all malignant brain tumors.

HMI – Houston Medical Imaging, the location where all Neil's scans were taken while he was in Houston.

HPV – human papillomavirus

Histones – proteins that provide structural support for chromosomes. Each chromosome contains a long molecule of DNA which must fit into the cell nucleus. To do that, the DNA wraps around complexes of histone proteins, giving the chromosome a more compact shape. Histones also play a role in the regulation of gene expression.

Hormones – glandular secretions – are complex chemicals which help to coordinate different functions in organs throughout the body. Hormones are carried to distant organs – the skin, muscles and other tissues – by complex biological processes. A proper balance of hormones is required for the correct development of animals, plants and fungi.

IRB – Institutional Review Board. Under FDA regulations, an Institutional Review Board is a group that has been formally designated to review and monitor biomedical research involving human subjects. In accordance with FDA regulations, an IRB has the authority to approve, require modifications to secure approval, or disapprove research. This group review serves an important role in the protection of the rights and welfare of human research subjects.

Karnofsky Performance Scale Index – patient neurological classification according to functional impairment. The scale is used to compare effectiveness of different therapies and to assess the prognosis in individual patients. The lower the Karnofsky score, the worse the survival for most serious illnesses.

Lemon balm – *(Melissa officinalis)*, a member of the mint family, is considered a calming herb. It was used as far back as the Middle Ages to reduce stress and anxiety, promote sleep, improve appetite, and ease pain and discomfort from indigestion (including gas and bloating, as well as colic).

MGH – Massachusetts General Hospital (Mass General), a world-renowned medical facility located in Boston Massachusetts.

MD Andersen – the University of Texas MD Anderson Cancer Center is a comprehensive cancer center in Houston, Texas. It is the largest cancer center and one of the original three comprehensive cancer centers in the United States.

Methylation – DNA consists of four bases – cytosine, guanine, adenine, and thymine. Methylation is when a chemical unit called a methyl group (which contains one carbon and three hydrogen atoms) is added to cytosine. Healthy methylation supports proper gene expression. DNA methylation often inhibits the expression of certain genes. This can change how the body functions, potentially affecting health in many different ways.

MRNA – Messenger RNA (abbreviated mRNA) is a type of single-stranded RNA affecting protein synthesis. mRNA is made from a DNA template during the process of transcription. The role of mRNA is to carry protein information from the DNA in a cell's nucleus to the cell's cytoplasm (watery interior), where the protein-making machinery reads the mRNA sequence and translates each three-base codon into its corresponding amino acid in a growing protein chain.

MTHFR – Methylenetetrahydrofolate reductase (MTHFR) is a gene and an enzyme. The gene is named for the enzyme it produces, an enzyme that breaks down the amino acid homocysteine. If the MTHFR gene that codes for this enzyme is mutated, this may contribute to a variety of health-conditions ranging from depression to some cancers.

NIH – the Natioal Institutes of Health, commonly referred to as NIH, is the primary agency of the United States government responsible for biomedical and public health research.

Nettle – stinging nettle has been used for hundreds of years to treat painful muscles and joints, eczema, arthritis, gout, and anemia. It has also been used as a diuretic.

Occipital Lobe – the smallest and rear-most of the lobes in the brain, the occipital lobe is the brain's visual processing hub. It processes visual signals and works cooperatively with many other brain areas. The occipital lobe plays a crucial role in language and reading, storing memories, recognizing familiar places and faces, and much more.

Physiological Displopia – is a phenomenon where objects are doubled, either in front of or behind, whatever target you are focusing on – normal double vision. On the sub-conscious level, the brain actually uses the difference in the double vision in front of and behind the target object to help with determining depth perception.

PCP – primary care physician

PI – Primary Investigator (in a clinical trial. Dr. Burzynski was the PI in Neil's clinical trial.)

Pons – the largest part of the brainstem, located above the medulla and below the midbrain. The pons is a bundle of nerves that provides critical communication between the cerebrum and cerebellum.

Poke root – a powerful purifier and lymphatic. It can have a strong purgative effect; its power should be respected, and it must be dosed very carefully. It is most often used when there is lymph stagnation and congestion, often during viral illness.

Red Clover – is used to support lymphatic function, general immune support, healthy skin, and proper endocrine function. It contains genistein, daidzein, and biochannin-A among other isoflavones. Red Clover is often used in its unadulterated form as an extract or tea.

Stereotactic biopsy – guided by imaging technology, a sterotactic biopsy is a surgical procedure in which a sterotactic frame is attached to the patient's head to precisely control where a neurosurgeon inserts a biopsy needle into the patients brain to collect small or deep samples for later examination under a microscope.

SLTP – the Student Leadership Training Program which Neil attended and dearly loved during his high school years.

St. John's Wort – derived from a flowering plant known as *Hypericum perforatum,* St. John's wort is an herb people commonly use as a part of alternative medicine to treat depression, anxiety, and attention deficit hyperactivity disorder (ADHD).

Sub-Investigator – (SI or Sub-I) constitutes any member of a team of individuals, other than the Principal Investigator (PI), conducting investigational research.

Turmeric – may have anti-inflammatory, anticancer, antioxidant, and other benefits. Many high-quality studies show turmeric's active ingredient, curcumin, has significant benefits for the body and brain.

THC – tetrahydrocannabinol is the main psychoactive compound in cannabis which produces the sensation of feeling "high." THC can be injested via smoking, oils, edibles, tinctures and capsules. It is widely used for symptomatic relief from severe illness, and it has shown some potential as an anti-caner agent.

TMB – the Texas Medical Board is the state's version of the FDA:

> "Our mission is to protect and enhance the public's health, safety and welfare by establishing and maintaining standards of excellence used in regulating the practice of medicine and ensuring quality health care for the citizens of Texas through licensure, discipline and education."

Vestibular – the "vestibular system" includes the parts of the inner ear and brain which process the sensory information involved with controlling balance and eye movements. If disease or injury damages these processing areas, disorders of dizziness, balance and vision can occur.

Vaccine – Prior to August 26, 2021:

> A product that stimulates a person's immune system to produce immunity to a specific disease, protecting the person from that disease.

> As of September 1, 2021:
>
> A preparation that is used to stimulate the body's immune response against disease.

Vaccinate Before You Graduate (VBYG) Program - "To ensure all Rhode Island students have a chance to be fully immunized against vaccine-preventable diseases before high school graduation. VBYG was developed in 2001 as a catch-up program for 12th grade students who either missed or did not complete the Hepatitis B vaccination series. In 2010, the program expanded to include high school students, in both public and private schools statewide and offers all routinely-recommended ACIP adolescent immunizations." (Which includes HPV)

ACKNOWLEDGMENTS

The trouble with acknowledgments is someone invariably gets forgotten. Rather than taking that risk, I wish to thank everyone who played a role in Neil's saga – his family, medical advisors, dearest friends and advocates from all over the world. I also wish to express special thanks to:

My wife, Wendy, for her steadfast patience and encouragement,

Raffaele, for his uplifting empathy and guidance,

Eric Merola, for granting us permission to quote from his documentary,

Dr. Stanislaw Burzynski, for giving us full access to any and all documents we needed to help us address Neil's situation with the FDA,

And our publishers, Dawn and Steven Porter at Stillwater River Publications, along with their talented team of editors and artists.

SUGGESTED READING

Defeat Cancer: 15 Doctors of Integrative and Naturopathic Medicine Tell You How by Connie Strasheim

Intensive interviews with fifteen highly regarded doctors who specialize in cancer treatment, who share the core principles upon which they bast their approach to healing cancer, from anti-neoplastic remedies and immune system support to dietary and life-style choices.

Beating Cancer with Nutrition by Patrick Quillin, Ph.D., RD, CNS

Chemotherapy, radiation, and surgery can temporarily reduce tumor burden, however, these therapies fail to change the underlying cause of the disease. Comprehensive cancer treatment must include an aggressive nutrition component, which can increase life expectancy by 12 to 21 fold along with better chances for remission.

Anticancer: A New Way of Life by David Servan-Schreiber, M.D., Ph.D.

This personal memoir comes with a clear scientific explanation of what makes cancer cells thrive and what inhibits them. It is filled with easy-to-understand charts and diagrams and a sixteen-page color "Anticancer Action" insert that enables readers to make small but essential changes in lifestyle and diet. The body knows how to heal itself, and it is better able to fight, and prevent, cancer with nutrition, physical exercise, stress management, and the avoidance of environmental toxins.

The Metabolic Approach to Cancer: Integrating Deep Nutrition, the Ketogenic Diet, and Nontoxic Bio-Individualized Therapies by Dr. Nasha Winters, ND, L.Ac., FABNO and Jess Higgins Kelley, MNT

The authors identify ten key elements of a person's terrain – including the microbiome, the immune system, and blood sugar balance – as they relate to the cancer process. They prescribe a researched, tested, and nontoxic metabolic therapeutic approach that encompasses the ketogenic diet, fasting, specified phytonutrients, herbal treatments and more.

A Parent's Guide to Childhood Cancer: Supporting Your Child with Integrative Therapies Based on a Metabolic Approach by Dagmara Beine, PhD, PA-C

Based on Winter's work, this comprehensive, patient-centered, evidence-informed approach to treating pediatric cancer teaches parents how to effectively incorporate integrative therapies and nutrition alongside conventional oncology.

Cancer: Step Outside the Box by Ty Bollinger

"Discover the TRUTH about cancer that your doctor probably doesn't know and the drug companies hope you never find out. If you're concerned about the "C" word, then Cancer - Step Outside the Box is the book you've been waiting for. It reveals the most potent and well-proven strategies for preventing and treating cancer... without barbaric procedures like surgery, chemotherapy, or radiation."

The Burzynski Breakthrough by Thomas D. Elias

"An explosive true story of Burzynski's revolutionary discovery of antineoplastons – the century's most promising cancer treatment – and the government's relentless 14-year campaign to not only suppress this controversial medications but also to destroy Burzynski' s career."

The Gerson Therapy: The Proven Nutritional Program For Cancer and Other Illnesses by Charlotte Gerson and Morton Walker, D.P.M.

An alternative medicine therapist and medical journalist reveals the powerful effects of organic fruits and vegetables. She shares simple recipes, and she explains how juicing can reverse the effects of many degenerative illnesses to save lives.

ABOUT THE AUTHOR

Dean Fachon has a Bachelors Degree in English Literature from Colgate University, and a Masters Degree in Technical Communication from Rensselaer Polytechnic Institute. For several years, Dean wrote computer-related documents, first for International Business Machines and then for Digital Equipment Corporation. Dean later joined a small marketing-communications firm for two years before co-founding a website development group in the mid-1990s. After 9/11 – in which Dean's brother-in-law, Ed Straub, lost his life – Dean turned his attention towards government and world affairs. He became very involved in the early 'Tea Party' movement and authored an on-line petition called the 'Pledge of Renewal' (PoR) – a document intended to rekindle interest in the US Constitution. The PoR garnered nearly 12,000 signatures in a year. Dean's most recent published work, 'The Grand Illusion,' is a brief examination of fiat-currency and its debilitating effects on our government, economy and culture. This e-book is freely available at grandillusion.info.